Clinical Nutrition and Metabolic Research

European Society of
Parenteral and Enteral Nutrition

ESPEN
85

Proceedings of the 7th Congress of the
European Society of Parenteral and Enteral Nutrition (ESPEN),
Munich, September 9–11, 1985

Clinical Nutrition and Metabolic Research

Editors
G. Dietze, Munich; *A. Grünert,* Ulm; *G. Kleinberger,* Steyr;
G. Wolfram, Munich

126 figures and 72 tables, 1986

KARGER

Basel · München · Paris · London · New York · New Delhi · Singapore · Tokyo · Sydney

Drug Dosage

The authors and publisher have exerted every effort to ensure that drug selection and dosage set forth in this text are in accord with current recommendations and practice at the time of publication. However, in view of ongoing research, changes in government regulations, and the constant flow of information relating to drug therapy and drug reactions, the reader is urged to check the package insert for each drug for any change in indications and dosage and for added warnings and precautions. This is particularly important when the recommended agent is a new and/or infrequently employed drug.

Printed in Germany by Mühlberger GmbH, D-8900 Augsburg
ISBN 3-8055-4388-3

Contents

Preface . . . VII

Tissue Metabolism in Traumatized Patients

MacFie, J. (Leeds): Energy Substrate Utilisation in Trauma . . . 1

Johnson, D. J.; Wilmore, D. W. (Boston, Mass.): Substrate-Organ Interrelationships Following Trauma . . . 18

Guarnieri, G.; Toigo, G.; Situlin, R.; Del Bianco, A.; Capresi, L.; Zanettovich, A.; Romano, E.; Iscra, F.; Mocavero, G. (Trieste): Muscle-Biopsy Studies on Protein Metabolism in Traumatized Patients . . . 28

Tischler, M. E.; Leng, E.; Al-Kanhal, M.; Mnichowicz, J.; Reiser, J.; Norton, L. W. (Tucson, Ariz.): Metabolic Response of Muscle to Trauma: Altered Control of Protein Turnover . . . 40

Greig, P. D.; Grote, A. E.; Askanazi, J.; Michelsen, Ch. B.; Elwyn, D. H.; Kinney, J. M. (New York, N. Y.): Effect of Nutritional Substrates on Muscle Amino Acid and Protein Metabolism in Surgical Patients . . . 54

Wernermann, J.; Decken, A. von der; Vinnars, E. (Stockholm): Protein Synthesis after Trauma as Studied by Muscle Ribosome Profiles . . . 66

Intestinal Absorption of Nutrients During Enteral Nutrition in the Critically Ill

Spiller, R. C. (Rochester, Minn.): Intestinal Motility in the Critically Ill – Influences on Enteral Feeding . . . 86

Fölsch, U. R. (Göttingen): Exocrine Pancreatic Function in the Critically Ill: Effect of Enteral and Parenteral Feeding . . . 93

Stremmel, W. (Düsseldorf): Intestinal Absorption of Fat and Fat-Soluble Vitamins . . . 101

Adibi, S. A. (Pittsburgh, Pa.): Optimal Nitrogen Source for Enteral Nutrition: Dipeptides versus Free Amino Acids . . . 119

Jones, B. J. M. (London): Carbohydrate Absorption and Related Sodium and Water Absorption in the Critically Ill . . . 133

Shenkin, A.; Richardson, R.; Garden, O. J. (Glasgow): Intestinal Absorption of Water-Soluble Vitamins and Essential Trace Elements . . . 143

Stable Isotopes in Nutrition Research

Schmidt, H.-L.; Metges, C. (Munich): Variations of the Natural Isotope Abundance in Diet – Causes of Artifacts or the Base of New Possibilities in Stable Isotope Tracer Work? . . . 156
Coward, W. A.; Roberts, S. B.; Prentice, A. M.; Lucas, A. (Cambridge): The $^{2}H_{2}{}^{18}O$ Method for Energy Expenditure Measurements – Clinical Possibilities, Necessary Assumptions and Limitations . . . 169
Millward, D. J.; De Benoist, B. (London); *Halliday, D.* (Harrow): The Use of Stable Isotopes in the Measurement of Whole-Body Protein Turnover in the Human Neonate . . . 178
Ghoos, Y.; Rutgeerts, P.; Vantrappen, G. (Leuven): $^{13}CO_2$-Breath Tests in Nutritional Diagnosis: Present Applications and Future Possibilities . . . 192
Matthews, D. E. (St. Louis, Miss.): Amino Acid and Substrate Turnover in Man Using GCMS . . . 208
Hartig, W.; Matkowitz, R. (Leipzig): *Czarnetzki, H.-D.* (Rostock); *Metzner, Ch.; Ritter, R.; Jung, K.; Faust, H.; Junghans, P.* (Leipzig): Protein Turnover after Operation . . . 223
Bougnères, P. F. (Paris): Ketone Body Turnover Rates in the Human Neonate and Infant . . . 236
Jackson, M. J. (Liverpool): Stable Isotope Techniques in Studies of Trace Element Metabolism and Possible Clinical Applications . . . 242

Clinical Nutrition of the Traumatized Diabetic Patient

Owen, O. E.; Mozzoli, M. A.; Caprio, S.; Boden, G. (Philadelphia, Pa.): Resting and Postprandial Fuel Utilization in Normal and Diabetic Humans . . . 247
Wicklmayr, M.; Dietze, G.; Grunst, J.; Rett, K.; Sauter, B.; Mehnert, H. (Munich): Glucose versus Sugar Substitutes in Parenteral Nutrition of Diabetics . . . 260
Bergman, M.; RaviKumar, S.; Auerhahn, C.; Del Savio, N.; Savino, J. (New York, N. Y.); *Hendler, R.; Jacob, R.; Felig, P.* (New Haven, Conn.): Use of Insulin Infusion Pumps during Hyperalimentation of the Stressed Diabetic Patient . . . 269
Gunnarsson, R. (Stockholm): Perioperative Management of Diabetes Mellitus . . . 280
Kleinberger, G. (Steyr): All-in-One Solutions for TPN of Diabetic Patients . . . 291
Allison, S. P. (Nottingham): Parenteral versus Tube Feeding in the Diabetic Patient . . . 300

Animal Models in Nutrition Research

Giesecke, D. (Munich): Species Differences Relevant to Nutrition and Metabolism Research . . . 311
Hackbarth, H.; Gärtner, K. (Hannover): Requirements of Energy and Essential Nutrients with Regard to Body Mass . . . 329
Soeters, P.; de Boer, J. E. G. (Maastricht): Specificity of Animal Models in Liver Research . . . 333
Holm, E.; Behne, F.; Leweling, H.; Staedt, U.; Striebel, J.-P.; Tschepe, A. (Heidelberg): Animal Models of Hepatic Failure. Metabolic Characteristics and Effects of TPN 343
Jeppsson, B.; Hansson, L. (Lund): Animal Models of Sepsis in Relation to Metabolism and Nutrition . . . 375
Torosian, M. H.; Daly, J. M. (New York, N. Y.): Tumor-Bearing Animal Models of Nutrition Research . . . 385

Preface

This volume contains all invited papers presented by experts from all over the world during two symposia and three workshops held at the 7th Annual Meeting of the European Society of Parenteral and Enteral Nutrition (ESPEN) in Munich, September 9–11, 1985.

The two symposia were devoted to therapeutically related problems:

The first one dealt with 'Intestinal Absorption of Nutrients during Enteral Nutrition in the Critically Ill', covering contributions on intestinal motility, absorption of fat, of protein, amino acids and peptides, of carbohydrates, water and electrolytes, of water-soluble vitamins, trace elements and hemotinics.

The second was concerned with 'Clinical Nutrition of the Traumatized Diabetic Patient' comprising presentations on postprandial fuel utilization, glucose versus sugar substitutes, use of insulin infusion pumps, perioperative management, all-in-one solutions, parenteral versus tube feeding.

The workshops were addressed to technical problems in clinical and basic research:

Under the heading of 'Tissue Metabolism in Traumatized Patients' the first workshop included papers on changes in energy substrate utilization, substrate-organ interrelationships, muscle energy rich compound, DNA, RNA, alkali-soluble protein content and protease activity, metabolic response of muscle, effect of nutrition on substrates in muscle amino acid and protein metabolism and protein synthesis as studied by muscle ribosome profile.

During the second workshop on 'Stable Isotopes in Nutrition Research', the experts in this field drew the participant's attention to variations of the natural isotope abundance in diet, to clinical possibilities and limitations of the $D_2{}^{18}O$-method for energy expenditure, to the use of stable isotopes in nutritional research in neonates, to the present application and possibilities of the $^{13}CO_2$-breath test, to the use of GC-MS in measuring amino acid and substrate turnover to protein turnover after operations, to ketone body turnover measurements, to the clinical application of stable isotopes in studies of trace element metabolism.

The third workshop was committed to give an overview of the actual 'Animal Models in Nutrition Research'. The lectures were concerned with species differences with relevance for nutrition and metabolic research, with requirements of energy and essential nutrients with regard to body mass, with specificity of animals in liver research, with metabolic characteristics and effects of total parenteral nutrition in animal models of the hepatic failure, with animal models of sepsis and with tumor-bearing animal models.

After all, we would like to express our gratitude to the participants of the symposia and workshops: to the chairmen, the speakers and to the audience who offered their experience and support and gave their personal enthusiasm providing the creative atmosphere of the Munich Annual Meeting 1985.

We are extremely thankful to Mrs. *Gisela Schnell* who with her energy and kindness was essential for the successful work of the Organizing Committee.

Finally, the editors wish to acknowledge the excellent cooperation with the staff of Karger, Munich – particularly with *Walter Kunz* and *Siegfried H. Bezold*.

Munich, June 1986

Günther J. Dietze
Gunter Kleinberger
Ad Grünert
Günther Wolfram

Dietze, Grünert, Kleinberger, Wolfram (eds.), Clinical Nutrition and Metabolic Research. Proc. 7th Congr. ESPEN, Munich 1985, pp. 1–17 (Karger, Basel 1986)

Energy Substrate Utilisation in Trauma

J. MacFie

St. James's University Hospital, Leeds, UK

One feature that is common to all types of injury is weight loss, the rate and magnitude of which is roughly proportional to the severity of the injury [1]. This loss is primarily caused by the breakdown of body protein and fat which together constitute the major part of the body stores of energy. Consequently, weight loss reflects an increased demand for tissue fuel which is needed to meet the additional energy requirements that are characteristic of the catabolic state.

Over twenty years ago, it was recognised that breakdown of the body energy stores could be minimised and sometimes reversed by the administration of exogenous calories and nitrogen [2]. Today the value of nutritional support in the management of these patients is beyond doubt [3], but controversy persists as to the best way in which this should be given.

This paper will briefly review recent developments in energy substrate metabolism in the traumatised and septic patient and then discuss the relevance of these to the provision of total parenteral nutrition (TPN).

Carbohydrate Metabolism

In 1877, Claude Bernard documented an increase in the blood sugar as a feature of the response to injury [4]. It is now known that this increase is roughly proportional to the severity of the injury and occurs in the presence of inappropriately high levels of plasma insulin. The term 'diabetes of injury' is now frequently used to describe this phenomenon of insulin resistance which always occurs in conjunction with glucose intolerance. Evans and Butterfield used the term pseudodiabetes to emphasize that the hyperglycaemia occurred in the absence of ketosis which reflects the increased and uncontrolled lipolysis of classical diabetes mellitus [5].

Carbohydrate metabolism in trauma is, then, characterised by abnormal glucose tolerance, insulin resistance and hyperglycaemia. To this should be added the invariable phenomenon of a massive increase in gluconeogenesis which cannot be easily reversed by infusions of glucose which is in marked contra-distinction to the gluconeogenesis that occurs in starvation states [6]. Gluconeogenesis is the synthesis of glucose from non-carbohydrate precursors such as amino acids, lactate and pyruvate. The explanation for the increased gluconeogenesis of trauma remains unclear. Until recently, it was considered an adaptive response by which increased energy requirements were met. In particular, it was felt that increased protein breakdown occurred following trauma to provide amino acid as the main substrate for gluconeogenesis. This view is no longer accepted as a complete explanation for a number of reasons; firstly, with the exception of major trauma or severe burns, only moderate increases in energy expenditure occur following injury and these could easily be met by endogenous energy sources other than protein [7–9]. Secondly, studies of the tissue composition of weight loss after injury show that protein losses do not occur simply to meet an increased energy demand [10] and finally, but most importantly, measurement of body composition and of indirect calorimetry show quite clearly that fat oxidation remains the most important energy source in injury with protein oxidation accounting for no more than 20–30% of total energy requirements [10, 11]. One possible explanation is that amino acid oxidation occurs to ensure that there is more than adequate glucose available for reparative tissue metabolism which is completely dependent on glucose as its energy source [12]. After all, in starvation states virtually all tissues adapt to the use of fat as a fuel source and it is not, therefore, surprising that the distinctive differences in carbohydrate metabolism between starvation and injury are related to the presence of glucose-dependent reparative tissue. The relative inability of exogenous glucose to inhibit this protein-derived gluconeogenesis may be partly explained by the fact that in the injured patient the rates of uptake of glucose are already significantly increased and the glucose intolerance of these patients is not related to reduced peripheral utilisation [13, 14].

The increases in circulating lactate and pyruvate are generally considered to occur as a result of an increase in anaerobic glycolysis consequent upon a reduced perfusion of muscle [15]. Lactate accumulation may be potentiated by a relative functional failure of the liver and other tissues that remove it under normal conditions. If this is so then it is possible that increased gluconeogenesis (from lactate) may itself be an adaptive response to ensure that these metabolites do not accumulate to toxic levels rather than a further homeostatic mechanism to meet increased energy demands [16]. On any account, both lactate and pyruvate are inefficient energetically as gluconeogenic precursors and are therefore unlikely to be produced solely to meet energy requirements [17]. One further point regarding lactate production in the injured patient is worth making. Although it is generally regarded as being a potentially harmful byproduct of anaerobic glycolysis, it may be that lactate production itself occurs to aid metabolic recovery in damaged tissue. The reason for suggesting this is that there are many properties of lactate which are beneficial to tissue metabolism. These include its vasodilator effect, its bactericidal properties and the fact that it aids hydroxylation of proline to form collagen which may speed the process of repair.

The nature of the metabolic regulators to glucose metabolism in trauma remains unclear. Insulin levels are inappropriately high throughout the flow-phase of injury and glucagon levels show little change [18, 19]. Although diabetogenic hormones such as the catecholamines are high in association with any stress and clearly play a part in the insulin resistance of trauma, it is unlikely that they are the primary regulators. It is interesting to speculate that availability of high energy phosphate compounds such as ATP are themselves regulatory. The evidence for this is admittedly somewhat tenuous. For instance, it is well known that glucose turnover in injury correlates well with oxygen consumption which is, after all, a measure of total body oxidative metabolism [20]. Following trauma, oxygen consumption is increased, although measurements of respiratory quotient remain low pointing to continued fat oxidation [21]. The increased flow of glucose is always associated with an increasing flow of 3 carbon intermediates (lactate, pyruvate and alanine) as gluconeogenic precursors. This cycling of glucose has a marked effect on the availability of ATP and ADP and it is the concentration of these that may control the rate and nature of fuel oxidation. This altered glucose cycling, namely glycolysis and gluconeogenesis, is an invariable accompaniment to the metabolic response to trauma. Endogenous glucose cycling is now thought to be crucially important in the control of thermogenesis [22] and it is possible that altered cycling rates in trauma reflect changing demands for ATP and ADP. In this regard, it is interesting to look at the evidence for alterations in glucose cycling in the presence of trauma. Studies using labelled isotopes all find that endogenous glucose cycling is increased and cannot be easily suppressed by exogenous glucose [23, 24]. However, these studies do not throw any light on the metabolic regulation of such cycling. Recently Newsholme and Crabtree from Oxford have described certain metabolic substrate cycles, formally referred to as futile cycles, in glycolysis which are controlled by the concentration of certain key or regulatory enzymes (fig. 1) [25]. These enzymes are distinct from most

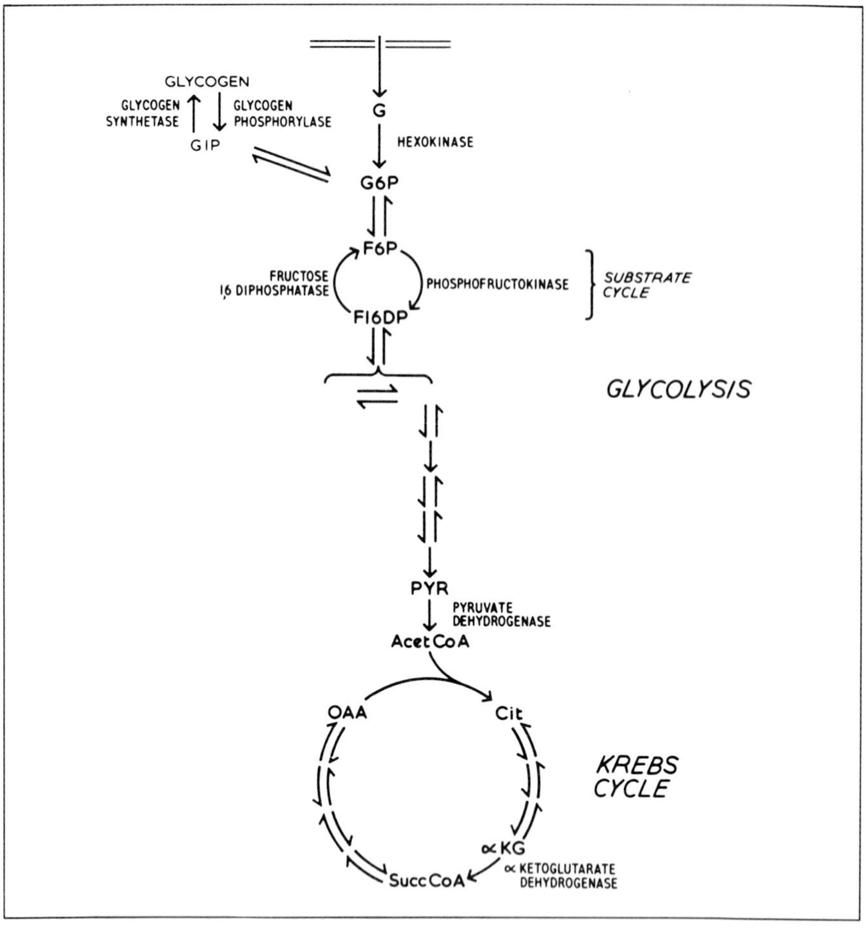

Fig. 1. Key enzymes of muscle glucose oxidation.

other near equilibrium enzymes in as much as their acitivities are not controlled by the concentration of substrates or products of any particular reaction but rather by allosteric mediators such as ADP, citrate, and acetyl CoA [26]. The maximum activity of these enzymes has been shown to closely correlate with in-vivo rates of flux of subtrates, and alterations in their values have been described in patients with peripheral vascular disease, following physical training and in obesity, suggesting that they may have an important role in metabolic regulation [27, 28]. We have recently measured the maximum activities of hexokinase, which controls phosphorylation of glucose on entry into the cell, phosphofructokinase and fructose-bisphosphatase which together constitute a substrate cycle and are regulatory in glycolysis and, lastly, alpha-ketoglutarate-dehydrogenase which is considered by some authorities to be regulatory in Krebs cycling activity. All these enzymes were measured in muscle obtained from critically ill surgical patients following major abdominal surgery [29]. The results of this study showed that phosphofructokinase and fructose-bisphosphatase were both significantly reduced suggesting that the maximum capacity for anaerobic glycolysis and thereby glucose utilisation would also be significantly reduced in these patients compared to controls. The decrease in these enzymes could occur as a result of inhibition secondary to decreased levels of ATP or the accumulation of acetyl CoA or citrate which might result as a consequence of increased free fatty acid oxidation. Fat may be the preferred energy source in injury (see later) and if so, the increased utilisation of free fatty acids may be responsible for decreasing glucose oxidation, possibly mediated via effects on these regulatory enzymes. This hypothesis coincides with the glucose/fatty acid cycle as described by Randle et al. [30].

Fat Metabolism

In 1969, Kinney and colleagues demonstrated that proteolysis accounts for no more than 20–30% of energy requirements and that fat oxidation was responsible for the remaining 70–80% [11]. These conclusions were based on repeated measurements of gas exchange performed in trauma patients. Indeed, it was found that their values of RQ remained persistently low indicating continued fat oxidation. The importance of fat as a fuel source in trauma and sepsis has since been confirmed by many others [31–37]. For instance, Moore emphasised the significance of the large loss of adipose tissue that can occur after injury [31] and more recent body composition studies such as that illustrated in figure 2 confirm this. Shoemaker et al. examined the changes in circulating lipids during successive stages of hypovolaemic shock [32]. In the early stage, there was a net increase in the release of triglycerides and an increased uptake of free fatty acids suggesting that these fat fuels were important to survival. The appearance of fat macroglobules following injury or sepsis has been commented upon by other authors who emphasise that this reflects a homeostatic response to injury in which rapid mobilisation of fat stores occurs to meet the increased demand for energy [33–35]. Indeed, based on meas-

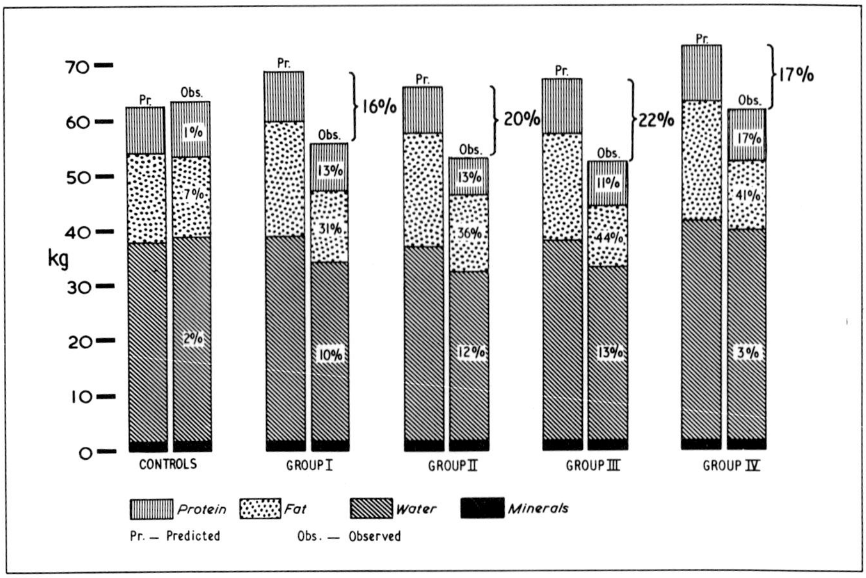

Fig. 2. For each of the 5 groups the histogram on the left was calculated from a predicted value of weight, protein, fat and water. These predicted values were derived from a series of regression equations obtained from a study of healthy volunteers in whom body protein was measured by in vivo neutron activation analysis, body fat by anthropometric measurements and body water by tritium dilution. The histogram on the right was calculated from the summation of the observed (i.e. measured) values in the same patients. Thus each histogram represents the mean value of body weight with the relative amounts of protein, fat and water indicated for predicted on the left and observed on the right in each of the 5 groups. The figures show the difference between the predicted and the observed values for weight, indicated by the parentheses, and for protein, fat and water expressed as a percentage of the predicted value. They represent an estimate of the loss of weight, protein, fat and water that occurs in each of these groups prior to the commencement of IVN [59].

urements of free fatty acid concentration, Carlson and Liljedahl suggested that injury was associated with an excessive free fatty acid mobilisation, i.e. mobilisation above calorie needs [36]. More recently, Shaw and Wolfe, in an elegant kinetic analysis performed in a septic dog model, found that the ability to oxidise fat was enhanced in sepsis and that in contrast the potential for glucose oxidation was reduced [38].

Despite these studies, which emphasise the importance of fat as a fuel source in trauma and sepsis, controversy still persists. For instance, Daniel and colleagues in 1978 reported the results of a well-designed study in dogs subjected to hypovolaemic or endotoxic shock [39]. They found, in marked contrast to the studies described above, that shock resulted in a decreased oxidation of circulating free fatty acids and, at the same time, increased urea production indicating accelerated protein breakdown and amino acid oxidation. They postulated that shock results in an increased reliance on endogenous fuels which form lactate and pyruvate as intermediary metabolites, i.e. carbohydrates and amino acids. A few other studies have also suggested that fat oxidation may be impaired in trauma or sepsis [40, 41]. Furthermore, it is generally accepted that in shock decreased mobilisation of free fatty acids from adipose tissue may occur due to poor perfusion or as a result of the inhibitory effect of lactate on lipolysis. Abnormally low values of ATP may impair the ability of catecholamines to stimulate lipolysis and this may be important in certain states of shock.

The explanation for these apparently contradictory results is unclear. It is possible that differences have occurred because of variations in the degree of severity of the shock states examined. Thus, for instance, in the study reported by Daniel et al., it is possible that the decrease in free fatty acid oxidation resulted simply from a decrease in availability which occurred as a consequence of severe hypoperfusion in their shock model. No information is given in their paper, for instance, as to the mortality of the dogs studied.

In summary, injury or sepsis results in an increased energy expenditure. This increase in metabolism results in mobilisation of all available energy stores. Gluconeogenesis is essential as glucose is required by damaged tissue. Lactate, pyruvate and amino acid oxidation provide gluconeogenic precursors but the controlling interrelationships of these substrates remain unclear. It is possible that cycling rates are determined by ATP availability. Whatever the mechanism of regulation, energy production from amino acid oxidation and anaerobic glycolysis of lactate does not account for the bulk of energy supply. This is achieved by continued fat oxidation which persists in both the injured and the septic state.

Nutritional Considerations

It is axiomatic that if protein losses in the injured patient are not reversed or at least diminished, either by improvement in the clinical condition of the patient or by artificial nutrition, then increased morbidity and mortality will result. Depletion of lean body mass is inexorably associated with impaired immunocompetence, reduced synthesis of visceral protein, poor wound healing and ultimately organ failure. This is the justification for nutritional support in the injured patient and many studies have amply demonstrated its clinical value [2, 42].

Despite this fact that TPN is of proven value, there is still considerable controversy as to what constitutes optimal nutritional support. The following paragraphs briefly outline our approach in St. James's University Hospital, Leeds, to TPN in the injured and septic patient and summarise those studies which have, in particular, influenced our own clinical practice.

Protein Requirements

About 10% of the body mass is protein. As there are no dispensible protein stores (in contrast to fat), loss of body protein leads to functional impairment. The protein requirement then for any individual patient is the amount needed to maintain normal body stores as well as that needed to return stores to normal.

A nitrogen intake of the order of 150 mg/kg/day is required to maintain nitrogen equilibrium in normal persons [43]. In the 'ebb-phase' immediately following major surgery, nitrogen losses range between 300 mg/kg/day and 600 mg/kg/day and after severe burns may approach 1.5 g/kg/day. One gram of nitrogen is equivalent to 6.25 g of protein, or 25 g of muscle tissue. A 70 kg man losing 1.5 g/kg/day would lose the equivalent of 2.6 kg of muscle each day! Clearly this loss could not be sustained for anything more than very short periods. Fortunately, however, such losses are very rarely prolonged and, for this reason, it is not usually necessary to provide nitrogen intakes that are equivalent to the nitrogen losses that can occur in the early ebb-phase following trauma. Nitrogen intakes of 300 mg/kg/day are usually sufficient following major surgery and amounts greater than this are only needed in patients with severe trauma.

Two additional points regarding protein requirements in trauma are worth making: firstly, it was considered for a long time that a negative nitrogen balance following trauma was inevitable. Recent evidence would suggest that this is not necessarily the case [18]. Secondly, it is now well established that infused amino acids are ineffective in reversing protein losses unless sufficient energy is given concomitantly to ensure a positive energy balance [44].

Energy Requirements

Although there is no doubt that energy expenditure is increased in trauma or sepsis, there is no evidence whatever to justify calorie intakes of 5–6000 kcal/day as was frequently recommended in the past. The energy requirements of surgical patients who have sustained major operative trauma or who are hypermetabolic from some septic complication will rarely exceed 2500 kcal/day [7–9]. Many of these patients have already sustained significant weight loss prior to surgery and this effectively decreases their value of resting energy expenditure. Increments in energy expenditure of about 10% occur with elective surgery and up to 25% with sepsis. However, increases of this magnitude do not result in large increases in absolute calorie requirements because base-line values of resting energy expenditure in these patients may only be 1500 kcal/day [9]. Even in patients with severe burns, or those with multiple trauma, total energy requirements will rarely exceed 3500 kcal/day.

The prescription of calories during TPN should aim to ensure a positive energy balance. The administration of calories greatly in excess of requirements is to be deprecated, not only because it is extremely wasteful but also because it significantly increases TPN-related morbidity.

Energy Source

The nature of the energy source that should be used in TPN in trauma patients has caused considerable debate. Glucose alone is still recommended by many authorities as it is cheap, easily monitored and its nitrogen-sparing effects are well known [45]. Also, it must be said that hypertonic glucose solutions represent conventional, almost traditional, TPN. The original studies of Long et al. were all, by necessity, performed using glucose as the only energy source [46]. As TPN became more widely practised, it was only natural that glucose would be used in all patients who required nutritional support. This conventional TPN using glucose was encouraged by the fact that early lipid emulsions were associated with a high incidence of toxic side effects and adverse reactions. The development of a safe fat emulsion by Schuberth and Wretlind in 1961 [47] occurred at a time when so-called conventional glucose-based TPN was being widely practised in both the United States and the United Kingdom. As such, clinicians were understandably reticent to suddenly change their TPN regimes for a relatively new and untried energy source. During the 1970s however, numerous studies were published, all of which attested not only to the safety of this fat emulsion but also to the fact that it was effective in terms of nitrogen sparing [48–51].

The situation is now, however, very different. As already described, the metabolic response to trauma and infection is characterised by insulin resistance and glucose intolerance and, partly as a result of this, many authorities are now questioning the validity of using glucose as the only energy source in this type of patient. There are two further reasons for this change in attitude: firstly, the work of Kinney and colleagues in 1969 showed that endogenous fat is the main fuel source in traumatised and septic patients [11]. Secondly, many recent studies have found that there is a physiological maximum to the amount of exogenous glucose that may be oxidised by man [23, 52, 53]. The absolute value of this maximum is difficult to define but it would appear to be in the order of 4 mg/kg/min in normal subjects, slightly less in depleted subjects and marginally higher in burned patients. Clearly, if sufficient calories are to be provided such that a positive energy balance is ensured, then glucose infusion rates in excess of these postulated maximums would be required. This is illogical practice as a significant proportion of the infused glucose will simply not be oxidised and is therefore not immediately available for ATP production. The fate of any non-oxidised glucose must be that it is either converted into fat or deposited as glycogen (assuming no urinary losses and no increase in endogenous cycling rates). Lipogenesis, manifested by respiratory quotients of greater than one, frequently occurs during glucose-based TPN, particularly in depleted patients [54]. Unless the aim of TPN is to replete fat stores, there is nothing to be gained by this. Indeed lipogenesis is itself energy consumptive and, consequently, its occurrence indicates an increased energy requirement by the patient. Furthermore, the increased carbon dioxide production in these patients may be detrimental to their respiratory function. In contrast to the depleted patient, non-oxidised glucose in the traumatised or septic patient is not invariably associated with lipogenesis but is probably deposited as glycogen [24]. This may account for the increased noradrenaline excretion that occurs in these patients with large glucose infusions and this is said to reflect an additional physiological stress to these patients [24].

For all these reasons, the use of glucose as the only energy source during TPN in the injured patient probably does not represent optimal nutritional support. What, then, about fat emulsions?

As already pointed out, there are discrepancies in the results of studies that have investigated fat metabolism in patients with trauma and sepsis. These may be accounted for by differences in the extent or severity of shock or sepsis present, the prior nutritional status of the host as well as by differences between species. Further studies may clarify the situation further but at present the consensus view is as follows: The work of Robin et al. in Kinney's Department in N.Y. has demonstrated that fractional removal rates (first order kinetics) and maximal clearance rates (zero order kinetics) of labelled Intralipid are both increased in trauma and sepsis [55]. However, these parameters did not correlate with rates of oxidation of exogenous fat indicating that plasma removal of fat does not necessarily indicate its oxidation. Rates of oxidation of Intralipid were, though, increased in traumatised and septic patients supporting the use of this emulsion as an energy source in this type of patient [54]. Both clearance and removal rates were significantly increased compared to normal when measured in patients receiving TPN with glucose. Despite this, oxidation of fat in these patients was reduced suggesting that exogenous fat was simply being stored in adipose tissue. The increased plasma removal may reflect the increased lipoprotein lipase activity consequent upon increased values of plasma insulin. It is interesting to note that even in patients with elevated plasma insulins that although decreased, some fat oxidation persisted, again emphasising the importance of fat as a fuel source in this type of patient. Indeed, this persistent fat oxidation at high levels of carbohydrate intake has been shown to be characteristic of injury and sepsis, and is possibly related to the high levels of counter-regulatory hormones. These ensure a continued lipolytic milieu. The foregoing observations are supported by work reported by Stoner et al. in Manchester [56] who emphasised the importance of insulin resistance and cortisol concentrations in the presence of sepsis and also by Shaw and Wolfe who, using a septic dog model, concluded that the practice of giving patients with sepsis exogenous glucose at rates sufficient to meet their total calorie requirements was probably not justified [38].

Consideration should also be given to interaction between exogenous glucose and fat during TPN. Oxidation rates of free fatty acids are negatively correlated with carbohydrate intakes and also insulin [37]. However, as already stated, clearance and fractional removal rates are increased. The fate of the non-oxidised free fatty acid is probably as re-esterification through increased formation of α-glycerophosphate [37]. There is continuous hydrolysis of triglyceride and, as such, a futile substrate cycle is established. The provision of large amounts of glucose will theoretically increase the rates of this futile cycle which conforms to the glucose-fatty acid cycle as postulated by Randle et al. [30]. This regulatory mechanism in the control of free fatty acid oxidation in relation to glucose availability is supported by the work of Nanni et al. [57] who, using indirect calorimetry, found that the concomitant administration of fat with glucose actually enhanced glucose oxidation rates. This potential for glucose-lipid interaction during TPN and the possible detrimental effects of giving large volumes of glucose in conjunction with fat emulsions were the stimulus for a clinical study in which the effects of a continuous fat infusion were compared with administering fat on an intermittent basis alternating the emulsion with glucose [58]. Patients were randomly allocated to receive one of 2 alternative nutritional regimens. These regimens were equicaloric and equinitrogenous. During Regimen A (continuous fat), a crystalline amino acid solution was given concurrently with a fat emulsion together with 25% dextrose for the first 3 days of the study. After this, patients were 'crossed over' to receive the alternative regimen, Regimen B (intermittent fat), which consisted of crystalline amino acid given for 12 h with 25% dextrose and in the next 12 h given with a 10% fat emulsion. The results are illustrated in figure 3. The hyperinsulinaemia that occurs during the intermittent infusion of fat will almost certainly impair the oxidation of plasma free fatty acids. Furthermore, it can be seen that the substrate hormonal profiles were more stable during the continuous infusion of fat and were similar to those one would expect in normal post-absorptive man (figs. 4, 5). On the basis of this study, we advocate that fat emulsions should always be given on a continuous basis together with an

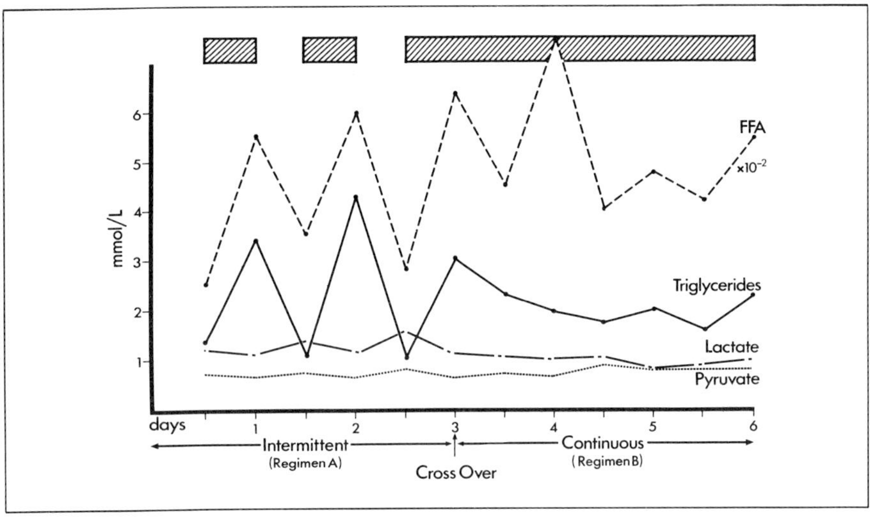

Fig. 3. Changes in plasma insulin and glucose in those patients who received the intermittent fat regimen for the first 3 days, followed by the continuous fat regimen. The shaded areas denote those time periods during which some fat was being infused. The results are expressed as means ± 1 standard deviation of the mean.

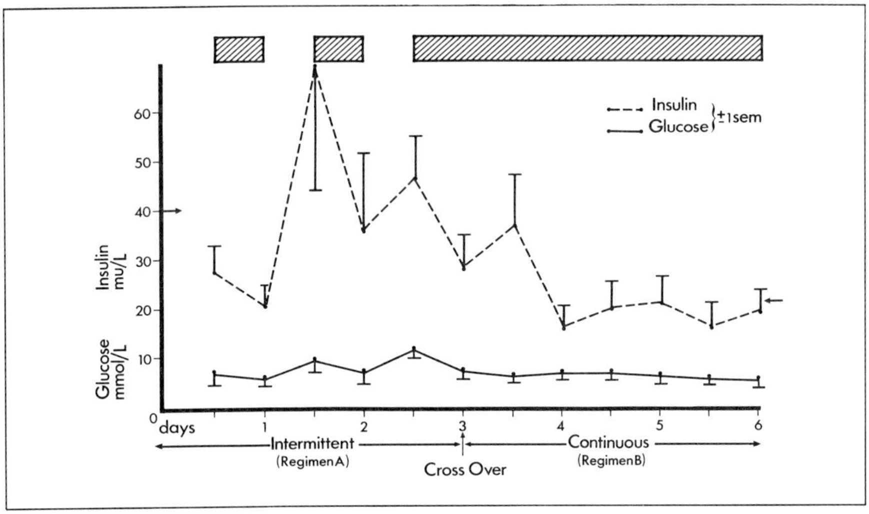

Fig. 4. The values of plasma free fatty acids, triglycerides, lactate and pyruvate are shown for those patients who received the intermittent fat regimen followed by the continuous fat regimen.

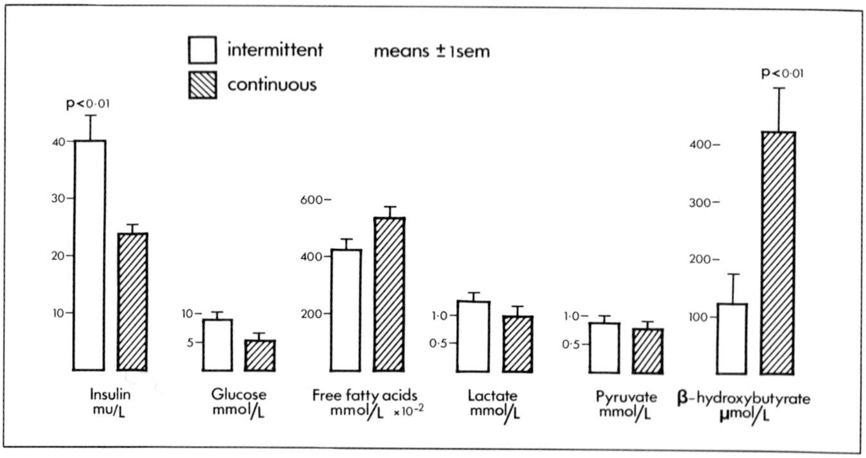

Fig. 5. Means ± 1 sem for plasma insulin and these substrates by combining all results for regimen A and all results for regimen B irrespective of whether it was given in the first or second 3-day period.

amino acid and glucose. Indeed, this provides a metabolic justification for the 3-l bag system.

In summary, there are distinct differences in the metabolic response to starvation and to injury. There is no doubt that TPN is of value in both groups of patients although their requirements may differ. In trauma patients, energy and protein requirements are higher and, in addition, protein anabolism is more difficult to achieve. Fat is the preferred fuel source and should be given as a continuous infusion with glucose. Large volumes of glucose should be avoided to ensure its complete oxidation and also to minimise the risks of TPN-related morbidity.

References

1 Kinney, J. M.; Long, C. L.; Duke, J. H.: Energy demands in the surgical patient; in Fox, Nahas, Body fluid replacement in the surgical patient, pp. 296–300 (Grune and Stratton, New York 1970).
2 Dudrick, S. J.; Wilmore, D. W.; Vars, H. M.; Rhoads, J. E.: Long-term total parenteral nutrition with growth, development and positive nitrogen balance. Surgery *64:* 134–142 (1968).
3 Abbott, W. M.: Indications for parenteral nutrition; in Fischer, Total parenteral nutrition, pp. 3–14 (Little, Brown and Co., Boston 1976).

4 Bernard, C.: Leçons sur le Diabète, p. 408 (Librairie J. B. Baillere, Paris 1877).
5 Evans, E. I.; Butterfield, W. J. H.: The stress response in the severely burned. Ann. Surg. *134:* 588–613 (1951).
6 Long, C. L.; Kinney, J. M.; Geiger, J. W.: Non-suppressability of gluconeogenesis by glucose in septic patients. Metabolism *25:* 193–200 (1976).
7 Kinney, J. M.; Duke, J. H., Jr.; Long, C. L.; Gump, F. E.: Tissue fuel and weight loss after injury. Proceedings from Symposium on the Pathology of Trauma. J. clin. Path. *4:* 65–72 (1970).
8 Gump, F. E.; Kinney, J. M.: Calorie and fluid losses through the burn wound. Surg. Clins. N. Am. *50:* 1235–1248 (1970).
9 MacFie, J.: Energy requirements of surgical patients during intravenous nutrition. Ann. R. Coll. Surg. *66:* 39–42 (1984).
10 Duke, J. H.; Jorgensen, S. B.; Broell, J. R. et al.: Contribution of protein to calorie expenditure following injury. Surgery *68:* 168–174 (1970).
11 Kinney, J. M.: Surgical diagnosis, patterns of energy, weight and tissue change; in Wilkinson, Cuthbertson, Metabolism and the response to injury, p. 121 (Pitman Medical, Kent 1976).
12 Aoki, T. T.; Brennan, M. F.; Muller, W. A.; Cahill, G. F., Jr.: Nitrogen balance, insulin and amino acid metabolism; in Brown, Protein nutrition, p. 180 (Charles C. Thomas, Springfield 1974).
13 Hayes, M. A.; Brandt, R. L.: Carbohydrate metabolism in the immediate postoperative period. Surgery *32:* 819–827 (1952).
14 Giddings, A. E. B.; Rowlands, B. J.; Mangnall, D.; Clark, R. G.: Plasma insulin and surgery II. Later changes and the effect of intravenous carbohydrates. Ann. Surg. *186:* 687–693 (1977).
15 Broder, G.; Weil, M. H.: Excess lactate: An index of reversibility of shock in human patients. Science *143:* 1457–1459 (1964).
16 Clowes, G. H. A., Jr.; O'Donnell, T. F.; Ryan, N. T.; Blackburn, G. L.: Energy metabolism in sepsis: Treatment based on different patterns in shock and high output state. Ann. Surg. *180:* 684 (1974).
17 Gold, J.: Cancer cachexia and gluconeogenesis. Ann. N.Y. Acad. Sci. *230:* 103–110 (1974).
18 Kinney, J. M.; Felig, P.: The Metabolic Response to Injury and Infection; in DeGroot, Endocrinology, pp. 1963–1985 (Grune and Stratton, New York 1979).
19 Clowes, G. H. A., Jr.; O'Donnell, T. F.; Blackburn, G. L.; Maki, T. N.: Energy metabolism and proteolysis in traumatized and septic man. Surg. Clins. N. Am. *56:* 1169–1184 (1976).
20 Wilmore, D. W.; Mason, A. D., Jr.; Pruitt, B. A., Jr.: Insulin response to glucose in hypermetabolic burn patients. Ann. Surg. *183:* 314–320 (1976).
21 Giovannini, I.; Boldrini, G.; Castagneto, M. et al.: Respiratory quotient and patterns of substrate utilisation in human sepsis and trauma. J. parent. ent. Nutr. *7:* 226–230 (1983).
22 Newsholme, E. A.; Crabtree, B.: Substrate cycles in metabolic regulation and in heat generation. Biochem. Soc. Symp. *41:* 61–110 (1976).
23 Wolfe, R. R.; Allsop, J. R.; Burke, J. F.: Glucose metabolism in man: Responses to intravenous glucose infusion. Metabolism *28:* 210–220 (1979).

24 Elwyn, D. H.; Kinney, J. M.; Jeevanordan, M. et al.: Influence of increasing carbohydrate intake on glucose kinetics in injured patients. Ann. Surg. *190:* 117–127 (1979).
25 Newsholme, E. A.; Crabtree, B.: The role of fructose 1-6 disphosphatase in the regulation of glycolysis in skeletal muscle. FEBS Lett. *7:* 195–198 (1970).
26 Crabtree, B.; Newsholme, E. A.: The activity of phosphorylase, hexokinase, phosphofructokinase, lactate dehydrogenase and the glycerol 3-phosphate dehydrogenases in muscles from vertebrates and invertebrates. Biochem. J. *126:* 49–68 (1971).
27 Bylund, A. C.; Holm, J.; Lundholm, K.; Schersten, T.: Incorporation rate of glucose carbon, palmitate carbon and leucine carbon into metabolites in relation to enzyme activities and RNA levels in human skeletal muscles. Enzyme *21:* 39–52 (1976).
28 Holm, J.; Dahllof, A. G.; Schersten, T.: Metabolic activity of skeletal muscle in patients with peripheral arterial insufficiency. Effect of arterial reconstructive surgery. Scand. J. clin. Lab. Invest. *35:* 81–86 (1975).
29 King. R. F. G. J.; MacFie, J.; Hill, G.: Activities of hexokinase, phosphofructokinase, fructose bisphosphatase and 2-oxoglutarate dehydrogenase in muscle of normal subjects and very ill surgical patients. Clin. Sci. mol. Med. *60:* 451–456 (1981).
30 Randle, P. J.; Garland, P. B.; Hales, C. N.; Newsholme, E. A.: The glucose fatty-acid cycle, its role in insulin sensitivity and the metabolic disturbances of diabetes mellitus. Lancet *ii:* 785–789 (1963).
31 Moore, F. D.: Metabolic care of the surgical patient, p. 15 (Saunders, Philadelphia 1959).
32 Shoemaker, W. C.; Stahr, L. J.; Kim, S. I.; Elwyn, D. H.: Sequential circulatory and metabolic changes in the liver and whole body during haemorrhagic shock; in Kovach, Stoner, Spitzer, Neurohumeral and metabolic aspects of injury, p. 243 (Plenum Press, New York 1973).
33 Lepisto, P. V.: Post-traumatic blood lipid changes and fat embolism. J. Trauma *16:* 52–57 (1976).
34 Carlson, L. A.: Mobilisation and utilisation of lipids after trauma: Relation to calorie homeostasis; in Porter, Knight, Energy metabolism in trauma. Ciba Foundation Symposium (Churchill, London 1970).
35 Carlson, L. A.; Liljedahl, S. O.; Wirsen, C.: Blood and tissue changes in the dog during and after excessive free fatty acid mobilisation: A biochemical and morphological study. Acta med. scand. *178:* 81–102 (1965).
36 Carlson, L. A.; Liljedahl, S. O.: Lipid metabolism and trauma. Acta chir. scand. *137:* 123–129 (1971).
37 Nordenstrom, J.; Carpentier, Y. A.; Askanazi, J. et al.: Free fatty acid mobilisation and oxidation during total parenteral nutrition in trauma and infection. Ann. Surg. *6:* 725–735 (1983).
38 Shaw, J. H. F.; Wolfe, R. R.: Response to glucose and lipid infusions in sepsis: A kinetic analysis. Metabolism *34:* 442–449 (1985).
39 Daniel, A. M.; Pierce, G. H.; Shizgal, H. M.; Machean, L. D.: Protein and fat utilisation in shock. Surgery *84:* 588–594 (1978).
40 Daniel, A. M.; Pierce, G. H.; Machean, L. D.; Shizgal, H. M.: Lactate metabolism during canine shock from haemorrhage, cardiac tamponade or endotoxin. Surgery Gyn. Obstet. *143:* 581–583 (1976).
41 Long, J. M.; Wilmore, D. W.; Masson, A. D., Jr.; Pruitt, A. D., Jr.: Fat-carbohydrate

interaction: Nitrogen sparing effect of varying caloric sources for total intravenous feeding. Surg. Forum *25:* 61–63 (1974).
42 Woolfson, A. M. J.: Artificial nutrition in hospital. Br. Med. J. *287:* 1004–1006 (1983).
43 Hill, G. L.; Church, J.: Energy and protein requirements of general surgical patients requiring intravenous nutrition. Br. J. Surg. *71:* 1–9 (1984).
44 O'Connell, R. C.; Morgan, H. P.; Aoki, T. T. et al.: Nitrogen conservation in starvation: Graded responses to intravenous glucose. J. clin. Endocr. Metab. *39:* 555–563 (1974).
45 Gamble, J. L.: Physiological information gained from studies on the life raft ration. Harvey Lect. *42:* 247 (1947).
46 Long, J. M.; Dudrick, S. J.; Duke, J. R.: A rationale for glucose as the primary energy source; in Richards, Kinney, Nutritional aspects of care in the critically ill, pp. 331–344 (Churchill Livingstone, London, New York 1977).
47 Schuberth, O.; Wretlind, A.: Intravenous infusion of fat emulsions, phosphatides and emulsifying agents. Clinical and experimental studies. Acta chir. scand., suppl. 278 (1961).
48 Jeejeebhoy, K. N.; Anderson, G. H.; Nakoda, A. F. et al.: Metabolic studies in total parenteral nutrition in man. J. clin. Invest. *57:* 125–136 (1976).
49 MacFie, J.; Smith, R. C.; Hill, G. L.: Glucose or fat as non-protein energy source? A controlled clinical trial in gastroenterological patients requiring intravenous nutrition. Gastroenterology *80:* 102–107 (1981).
50 Kirkpatrick, J. R.; Dahn, M.; Lewis, L.: Selective versus standard hyperalimentation. Am. J. Surg. *141:* 116–121 (1980).
51 Bark, S.; Holm, E.; Hakansson, I.; Wretlind, A.: Nitrogen-sparing effect of fat emulsion compared with glucose in the post-operative period. Acta chir. scand. *142:* 423–427 (1976).
52 Burke, J. F.; Wolfe, R. R.; Mullaney, C. J.: Glucose requirements following burn injury. Ann. Surg. *190:* 274–285 (1979).
53 Wolfe, R. R.; Burke, J. F.: Isotopic studies of glucose metabolism in humans. J. clin. Surg. *1:* 180–193 (1982).
54 Askanazi, J.; Carpentier, Y. A.; Elwyn, D. H. et al.: Influence of total parenteral nutrition on fuel utilisation in injury and sepsis. Ann. Surg. *1:* 40–46 (1980).
55 Robin, A. P.; Nordenstrom, J.; Askenazis, J. et al.: Plasma clearance of fat emulsion in trauma and sepsis: Use of a 3-stage lipid clearance test. J. parent. ent. Nutr. *4:* 505–510 (1980).
56 Stoner, H. B.; Little, R. A.; Frayn, K. N. et al.: The effect of sepsis on the oxidation of carbohydrate and fat. Br. J. Surg. *70:* 31–35 (1983).
57 Nanni, G.; Siegel, J. H.; Coleman, B. et al.: Increased lipid fuel dependence in critically ill septic patients. J. Trauma *24:* 14–30 (1984).
58 MacFie, J.; Courtney, D. F.; Brennan, T. G.: Continuous versus intermittent infusion of fat emulsion during T.P.N.? A prospective clinical trial. Br. J. Surg. (in press).

John MacFie, MD, FRCS, St. James's University Hospital, 88, Ash Hill Drive, Shadwell, GB-Leeds, LS17 8JR (UK)

Dietze, Grünert, Kleinberger, Wolfram (eds.), Clinical Nutrition and Metabolic Research. Proc. 7th Congr. ESPEN, Munich 1985, pp. 18–27 (Karger, Basel 1986)

Substrate-Organ Interrelationships Following Trauma

D. J. Johnson, D. W. Wilmore

Department of Surgery, Harvard Medical School, Brigham and Women's Hospital, Boston, Mass., USA

Introduction

Following injury, a series of neural-hormonal responses initiate complex biochemical activity which results in the movement of substrate between organs. The catabolic hormones (catecholamines, glucagon, and cortisol) increase glucose production in the visceral organs and confer insulin resistance to peripheral tissue, particularly skeletal muscle [5]. These hormones, especially cortisol, are responsible in part for skeletal muscle proteolysis and increased release of amino acids [17]. Visceral organs (i.e., liver and gastrointestinal tract) process the mobilized amino acids for conversion to glucose and necessary proteins for wound repair, immunocompetence, and recovery. Triglyceride is also mobilized and utilized as a primary fuel source in non-glucose dependent tissue.

Multiple investigators in our laboratory have studied these post-traumatic substrate-organ interactions. Patients, normal human volunteers, and animal models have been utilized; substrate flux has been measured by isolating the blood supply to certain organs or regions, and measuring arteriovenous substrate concentration difference and blood flow across the regional bed under study. In this way, dynamic exchange rates can be estimated for various substrates across multiple organs. Movement of glucose and its 3-carbon precursors, amino acids, as well as fat and ketones has been examined using these techniques for skeletal muscle, liver, gastrointestinal tract, and kidney.

This paper will review these findings and construct a post-injury interorgan substrate flux model. In addition, certain attempts to modify these interactions using nutritional and hormonal means will be discussed.

Methodology

Various studies of post-injury metabolism have been conducted in humans following accidental injury, in burn patients, and in canines following operation. Skeletal muscle exchange has been measured by forearm flux studies in trauma patients and normal volunteers [8]. Leg and splanchnic arteriovenous substrate exchange were measured in burn patients [3]. And, finally, hindquarter skeletal muscle and more detailed splanchnic (liver, intestinal, and kidney) flux determinations were performed in awake animals following laparotomy and retroperitoneal dissection [15, 22].

Forearm flux studies in humans utilized a catheter positioned in the deep antecubital vein of one arm for deep venous sampling. Arterialized blood was obtained from the contralateral 'hot hand' [16]. Blood flow was measured by plethysmography with the hand excluded. Leg exchange was measured by placement of arterial and femoral vein catheters, and blood flow was measured by plethysmography. Splanchnic exchange in humans was determined after fluoroscopically guided placement of a sampling catheter in the hepatic or renal vein; appropriate dye extraction studies were performed to calculate blood flow [2, 25]. Canine hindquarter studies were performed after placement of a proximal aortic sampling catheter and a distal aortic dye infusion catheter. A third catheter was placed in the distal vena cava for venous sampling [15]. In this way, the blood supply to the hindquarter, which is approximately 50% skeletal muscle, was isolated. The canine catheters were implanted subcutaneously for repeated use in multiple postoperative studies. Finally, canine visceral flux was measured after implantation of arterial, portal vein, and renal or hepatic vein sampling catheters. A mesenteric vein catheter was placed for dye infusion and blood flow was determined using a dye dilution technique [22].

Flux for individual substrates is calculated as the product of arteriovenous concentration difference and blood flow. Therefore, net flux values preceded by a positive sign (+) represent organ uptake, and those preceded by a negative sign (−) represent organ release.

Other special studies performed included euglycemic insulin clamps (human studies) [9] and hindlimb skeletal muscle biopsies for the quantitation of intracellular amino acid levels [4]. These methods are described in detail elsewhere.

Experimental Data

The following data were collected from various human and animal studies and will be consolidated to form a logical interorgan flux model for each of the substrates discussed.

Glucose

In splanchnic organs, liver is the major glucose producer following injury [25]. However, small intestine may play a role in overall production as demonstrated by Souba and Wilmore [23] in canines subjected to

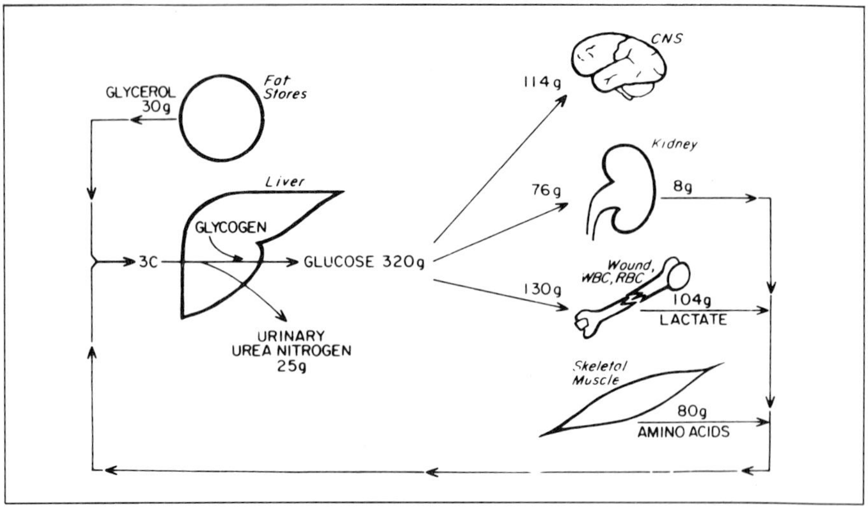

Fig. 1. 24-h flux of glucose and gluconeogenic precursors post-injury.

chronic administration of corticosteroids. The kidney is capable of gluconeogenesis and produces glucose primarily as its own energy source; however, Wilmore et al. have demonstrated increased renal uptake of glucose in burn patients [25]. The increase in visceral glucose production following trauma is primarily under control of certain catabolic and gluconeogenic hormones (catecholamines, cortisol, glucagon), as this combination produces hyperglycemia in human volunteers [19] and circulating levels of all three are increased post-injury [5].

Substrates for glucose production are derived from a wide variety of sources (fig. 1). Lactate and pyruvate are produced in the periphery by the wound [24]. Gluconeogenic amino acids are released by skeletal muscle. Alanine and glutamine are principal gluconeogenic precursors and, in addition to peripheral release of these amino acids, alanine can be produced in the small intestine by conversion from glutamine following deamination to glutamate and a transamination reaction [26]. Other glucose precursors include glycerol which is released through lipolysis of peripheral adipose stores.

Glucose is directed toward tissues which are obligated to use this substrate as their only fuel source. These tissues are the central and peripheral nervous system, red and white cells, renal medulla and inflammatory tissue. Other tissues such as skeletal muscle and adipose tissue will consume glucose in the presence of increases in insulin concentration. However, after trauma glucose uptake by the forearm is blunted [7, 8], and this response can be mimicked in normal volunteers by infusing the 'stress' hormones glucagon, cortisol, and epinephrine [5]. In addition, intra-arterial infusion of insulin in dogs that have undergone major laparotomy and bilateral groin dissection increases hindlimb glucose uptake only slightly over basal (0.48 ± 0.22 to 0.73 ± 0.26 mg/min/kg; NS) compared to the opposite non-infused limb (0.27 ± 0.08 to 0.41 ± 0.15 mg/min/kg; NS) [14]. This dose of insulin (180 μU/min/kg) raises insulin concentration five-fold in the experimental limb, while systemic levels remain constant.

Amino Acids

Net skeletal muscle proteolysis occurs following injury. The stimulus for this event is complex and may be related to hormones, inflammatory mediators such as interleukin-1 [10], acidosis, altered perfusion, prostaglandin generation, or other factors. Increased peripheral release of many amino acids from the skeletal muscle bed has been demonstrated in burn patients [3], multiple trauma victims [8], and in postoperative dogs [15]. Glutamine and alanine comprise a large percentage of the amino acid nitrogen released under these circumstances (fig. 2).

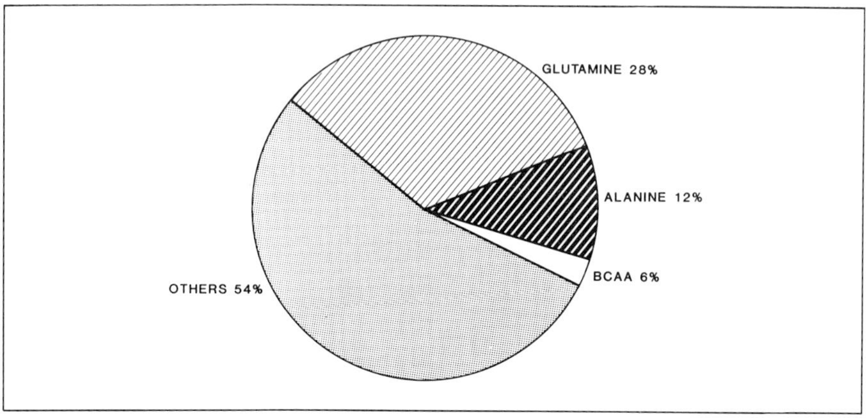

Fig. 2. Components of skeletal muscle amino acid nitrogen release 6 h after laparotomy and retroperitoneal dissection in a canine model.

Table I. Glutamine consumption by visceral organs during stress (μmol/min – kg, mean ± SEM) [22, 23]

	Control	Postoperative day #2	Dexamethasone day #2
Intestinal	0.96 ± 0.14	1.47 ± 0.19*	2.23 ± 0.24**
Kidney	0.64 ± 0.10	1.13 ± 0.24	2.11 ± 0.23**

* diff. from control $p < 0.05$
** diff. from control $p < 0.001$

The liberated amino acids appear to be taken up by the liver and gastrointestinal tract. Amino acids serve as precursors for gluconeogenesis and protein synthesis in these organs. Following burn injury, the splanchnic uptake of these substrates is increased 2–4 times greater than the uptake in normal individuals [25]. More specifically, glutamine is consumed in increased amounts by the small intestine and kidney, which has been demonstrated by Souba in postoperative and dexamethasone-treated canines [22, 23] (table I). In the small intestine, glutamine serves as fuel, nitrogen donor for ammonia production, and gluconeogenic precursor [26]. Glutamine infusion has been shown to increase intestinal consumption while the infusions of other intestinal substrates, glucose and ketones, are unable to alter what appears to be obligatory uptake of glutamine [21].

Attempts have been made to alter skeletal muscle release and inter-organ movement of amino acids using nutritional and hormonal manipulations. The postoperative canine model was studied to evaluate the effects of various therapies. We compared saline with two isonitrogenous amino acid infusions, one with glutamine and the other without. Both formulas maintained skeletal muscle intracellular nitrogen and reduced amino acid release from the hindquarter equally well [15] (fig. 3). On the other hand, when branched chain amino acids (BCAA) were provided in

Fig. 3. Comparable reduction of postoperative skeletal muscle amino acid nitrogen release using intravenous isonitrogenous amino acid solutions, one containing glutamine and the other, standard amino acids.

Fig. 4. Skeletal muscle nitrogen release is reduced 6 h postoperatively as the rate of total BCAA uptake increases.

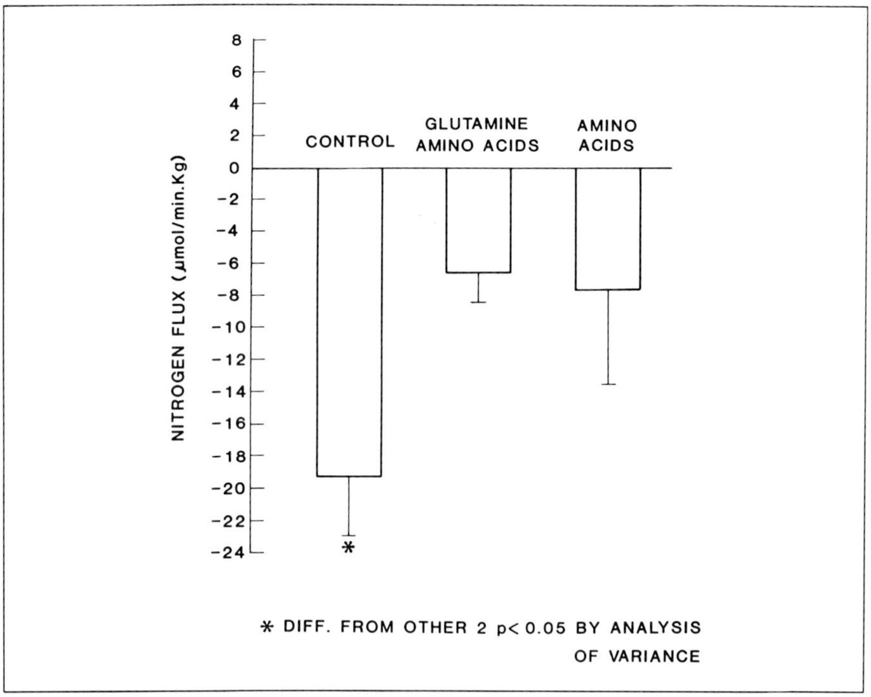
NITROGEN FLUX (μmol/min.Kg)
8
6
4
2
0
-2
-4
-6
-8
-10
-12
-14
-16
-18
-20
-22
-24
CONTROL
GLUTAMINE AMINO ACIDS
AMINO ACIDS
*
* DIFF. FROM OTHER 2 p< 0.05 BY ANALYSIS OF VARIANCE

3

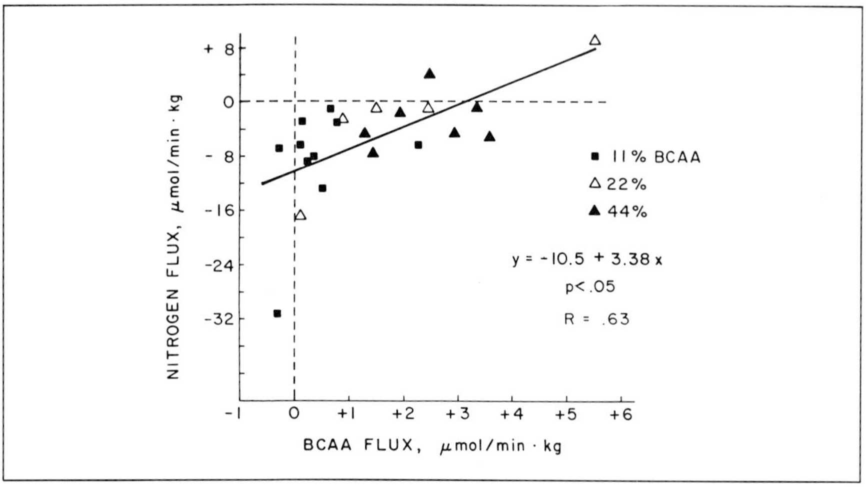
NITROGEN FLUX, μmol/min · kg
+ 8
0
- 8
-16
-24
-32
-1
0
+1
+2
+3
+4
+5
+6
BCAA FLUX, μmol/min · kg
■ 11% BCAA
△ 22%
▲ 44%
y = -10.5 + 3.38 x
p<.05
R = .63

4

Table II. Modification of postoperative skeletal muscle amino acid release (μmol/min – kg)

	Control	Infused
Insulin	– 3.45 ± 1.68	– 1.66 ± 0.58
Insulin and ketones	– 3.08 ± 0.34	– 0.87 ± 0.52*

* $p < 0.05$ diff. from control

three different doses, hindquarter nitrogen release was not related to the rate of BCAA administration but was reduced as total BCAA uptake increased [13] (fig. 4). This finding suggests a skeletal muscle-sparing effect of BCAA which is not related to the rate of administration.

Insulin elaboration may be an important variable in the skeletal muscle-amino acid relationship following injury. Brooks et al. [8] have shown diminished forearm amino acid release as well as BCAA uptake during an euglycemic insulin clamp conducted on multiple-trauma patients. During a similar control period, these patients demonstrated a high rate of efflux of many amino acids including the BCAA. Further studies in postoperative canines have demonstrated reduced amino acid nitrogen release from the hindlimb with intra-arterial insulin infusion [14]. This reduction became significantly less than control when infusion of ketones was added to the insulin (table II). The effects of BCAA on skeletal muscle may be mediated through this substrate-hormone interaction. Other hormonal manipulations using either epidural anesthesia or combined catecholamine receptor blockade with phentolamine and propranolol have both effectively reduced hindquarter amino acid nitrogen release in postoperative dogs [12].

Fats and Ketones

Peripheral adipose stores, which can be mobilized following injury, serve as an efficient energy source. The catecholamines serve as mediators of lipolysis in critically ill patients, releasing glycerol and free fatty acids which are taken up by the liver and used in the tricarboxylic acid cycle for energy and gluconeogenesis. The degree to which fat mobilization occurs depends on the insulin response following injury, as insulin exerts a lipogenic effect on fat stores. Free fatty acid levels are often depressed in injured and septic patients, but labeled lipid infusions have shown that oxidation of these substrates is increased following injury [18].

In addition to depressed free fatty acid levels, a blunted ketonemic response to starvation has been observed in multiple trauma patients [6]. Hypoketonemia of injury may again be related to the insulin response [11], but may also be a variable finding. It appears that patients with a greater ketosis may in fact conserve more body nitrogen [20]. This relationship becomes important with regard to the recent discussion about the protein-sparing effects of BCAA. Leucine, in particular, is ketogenic, and leucine infusion in normal humans produces a mild ketonemia [1]. The effects of insulin-ketone combinations have been examined in postoperative dogs and are particularly effective as described above.

Discussion

Interorgan movement of glucose, amino acids, free fatty acids, and other substrates occurs at accelerated rates following traumatic injury or major operation. Carbon skeletons from these substrates are used for energy and gluconeogenesis, while amino acids are also used to reform proteins necessary for wound repair and recovery. Exchange of these substrates has been described in detail, but the factors that initiate these responses are not completely understood. However, hormonal infusion into normals initiates many of these responses; thus, the hormonal environment must be one factor which determines complex substrate movements.

In summary, increased energy demands in the injured host necessitate the synthesis of glucose and other substrates by visceral organs for distribution throughout the body. The periphery appears to support this increased production by providing amino acids through skeletal muscle proteolysis, glycerol and free fatty acids through lipolysis, and lactate and pyruvate by anaerobic glycolysis. Provision of substrates by parenteral or enteral means may offset some of the obligatory peripheral tissue destruction that occurs to provide energy and substrate to repair wounds and fight infection. Hormonal manipulation may effectively offset peripheral amino acid release, but splanchnic uptake and ureagenesis continue unchecked.

Progress has been made toward defining the mechanisms of substrate-organ exchange following trauma. However, the complexity of these processes as well as the relative independence of organ responses within the host make whole-animal study of these relationships difficult. Therefore,. substrate provision through accepted means of nutritional support in addition to fundamental surgical and medical management continue to be sound methods for satisfying organ and tissue needs following trauma.

References

1 Abumrad, N. N.; Robinson, R. P.; Gooch, B. R. et al.: The effect of leucine infusion on substrate flux across human forearm. J. surg. Res. *32:* 453 (1982).

2 Aulick, L. H.; Goodwin, C. W.; Becker, R. A. et al.: Visceral blood flow following thermal injury. Ann. Surg. *193:* 112 (1981).

3 Aulick, L. H.; Wilmore, D. W.: Increased peripheral amino acid release following burn injury. Surgery *85:* 560 (1979).

4 Bergstrom, J.; Furst, P.; Noree, L.-O. et al.: Intracellular free amino acid concentration in human muscle tissue. J. appl. Physiol. *36:* 693 (1974).

5 Bessey, P. Q.; Watters, J. M.; Aokin, T. I. et al.: Combined hormonal infusion simulates the metabolic response to injury. Ann. Surg. *200:* 264 (1984).

6 Birkhahn, R. H.; Long, C. L.; Fitkin, D. L. et al.: A comparison of the effects of skeletal trauma in surgery on the ketosis of starvation in man. J. Trauma *21:* 513 (1981).

7 Black, P. R.; Brooks, D. C.; Bessey, P. Q. et al.: Mechanism of insulin resistance following injury. Ann. Surg. *196:* 420 (1982).

8 Brooks, D. C.; Bessey, P. Q.; Black, P. R. et al.: Insulin stimulates branched chain amino acid uptake and diminishes nitrogen flux from skeletal muscle of injured patients. J. surg. Res. (in press).

9 De Fronzo, R. A.; Jacot, E.; Jequier, E. et al.: The effect of insulin on the disposal of intravenous glucose: Results from indirect calorimetry and hepatic and femoral venous catheterization. Diabetes *30:* 1000 (1981).

10 Goldberg, A. L.; Baracos, V.; Rodemann, P. et al.: Control of protein degradation in muscle by prostaglandins, Ca^{++} and leukocytic pyrogen (interleukin-1). Fed. Proc. *43:* 1301 (1984).

11 Grecos, G. P.; Abbott, W. C.; Schiller, W. R. et al.: The effect of major thermal injury and carbohydrate-free intake on serum triglycerides, insulin and 3-methylhistidine excretion. Ann. Surg. *200:* 632 (1984).

12 Hulton, N. R.; Johnson, D. J.; Wilmore, D. W.: Hormonal blockade modifies post-traumatic protein catabolism. J. surg. Res. (in press).

13 Johnson, D. J.; Kapadia, C. R.; Liang, Z. M. et al.: Branched chain amino acid supplementation fails to reduce post-traumatic protein catabolism. Surg. Forum *35:* 102 (1984).

14 Johnson, D. J.; Pressler, V. M.; Colpoys, M. F. et al.: Insulin-ketone interaction: A possible mechanism for post-injury branched chain amino acid anticatabolic properties. Surg. Forum (in press).

15 Kapadia, C. R.; Liang, Z. M.; Colpoys, M. F. et al.: Maintenance of skeletal muscle intracellular glutamine during standard surgical trauma. J. parent. ent. Nutr. (in press).
16 McGuire, E. A. H.; Helderman, J. H.; Tobin, J. D. et al.: Effects of arterial versus venous sampling on analysis of glucose kinetics in man. J. appl. Physiol. *41:* 5651 (1976).
17 Muhlbacher, F.; Kapadia, C. R.; Colpoys, M. F. et al.: Effects of glucocorticoids on glutamine metabolism in skeletal muscle. Am. J. Physiol. *247:* E 75 (1984).
18 Nordenstrom, J.; Carpentier, Y. A.; Askanazi, J. et al.: Metabolic utilization of intravenous fat emulsion during total parenteral nutrition. Ann. Surg. *196:* 221 (1982).
19 Sharmoon, H. M.; Hendler, R.; Sherwin, R. S.: Synergistic interactions among anti-insulin hormones in the pathogenesis of stress hyperglycemia in humans. J. clin. Endocr. Metab. *52:* 1235 (1981).
20 Smith, R.; Fuller, B. J.; Wedge, J. H. et al.: Initial effect of injury on ketone bodies and other blood metabolites. Lancet *i:* 1 (1975).
21 Souba, W. W.; Scott, T. E.; Wilmore, D. W.: Intestinal consumption of intravenously administered fuels. J. parent. ent. Nutr. *9:* 18 (1985).
22 Souba, W. W.; Wilmore, D. W.: Postoperative alteration in arteriovenous exchange of amino acids across the gastrointestinal tract. Surgery *94:* 342 (1983).
23 Souba, W. W.; Wilmore, D. W.: Gut-liver interaction during accelerated gluconeogenesis. Archs. Surg. *120:* 66 (1985).
24 Wilmore, D. W.; Aulick, L. H.; Mason, A. D. et al.: The influence of the burn wound on local and systemic response to injury. Ann. Surg. *186:* 444 (1977).
25 Wilmore, D. W.; Goodwin, C. W.; Aulick, L. H. et al.: Effect of injury and infection on visceral metabolism and circulation. Am. Surg. *192:* 491 (1980).
26 Windmueller, H. G.; Spaeth, A. E.: Uptake and metabolism of plasma glutamine by the small intestine. J. biol. Chem. *249:* 5070 (1974).

Daniel J. Johnson, MD, Department of Surgery, University of Cincinnati Medical Center, 231 Bethesda Avenue, Cincinnati, OH 452 67-0558 (USA)

Dietze, Grünert, Kleinberger, Wolfram (eds.), Clinical Nutrition and Metabolic Research. Proc. 7th Congr. ESPEN, Munich 1985, pp. 28–39 (Karger, Basel 1986)

Muscle-Biopsy Studies on Protein Metabolism in Traumatized Patients[1]

G. Guarnieri[a], G. Toigo[a], R. Situlin[a], A. Del Bianco[a], L. Crapesi[a], A. Zanettovich[a], E. Romano[b], F. Iscra[b], G. Mocavero[b]

[a] Institute of Medical Pathology, University of Trieste
[b] Institute of Anesthesiology and Intensive Care, University of Trieste, Italy

Skeletal muscle is an important compartment for the study of protein metabolism in traumatized patients. According to Heymsfield et al., in a diseased state skeletal muscle remains very responsive to negative protein and energy balance, whereas the protein pools of many other tissues and organs become metabolically unavailable [1]. The same authors point out a size-composition dissociation in malnutrition: measurements of muscle mass or size do not necessarily reflect underlying muscle composition [1]. Moreover, about 40% of total body proteins is localized in skeletal muscles in humans (table I) and the other main constituents of this tissue are

Table I. The normal human skeletal muscle

- ≃40% of body weight
- Minerals: 1% of wet weight
- Water: 77–79% of wet weight (82% as intracellular water)
- Solids: 21–23% of wet weight
- Proteins (structural and non structural): ≃20% of wet weight (≃40% of total body protein)
- Collagen: ≃5% of muscle protein
- Energy content: 20,000–30,000 kcal (70–80% metabolizable, i.e. ≃1 kcal/kg of muscle)
- Other major constituents: RNA, DNA, glycogen, lipids, potassium (60–70% of TBK)
- 17–20 kg of muscle = 1 g of urinary creatinine

[1] This work was partly supported by a grant from CNR.

water, DNA, RNA, lipids, and glycogen. In man, skeletal muscle protein is the largest store of nitrogen and non-fat energy, and losses in response to undernutrition can be very extensive [2–5].

For these reasons we started a study of muscle protein metabolism in traumatized patients by direct chemical analysis of biopsy specimens obtained by Bergström's needle. We determined the muscle content of DNA, RNA, ASP (non collagen, alkali-soluble proteins), and the activity of phosphofructokinase and cathepsin B and D by methods previously reported [6–8] (fig. 1).

Muscle DNA content in adults is considered a satisfactory reference standard [9] and in protein-energy malnutrition the total number of nuclei in muscle is slightly affected [10]. The ASP : DNA ratio is an index of a hypothetical muscle cell size, i. e. the imaginary volume of cytoplasm managed by a single nucleus [2–5]. Total muscle RNA content, which is about 80% ribosomal RNA, and the RNA : DNA and RNA : ASP ratios are a measure of the capacity of the cell to synthesize proteins [2–5]. Starvation and refeeding are accompanied by progressive changes in muscle RNA content and in muscle protein synthesis and content [2–5]. Cathepsin B

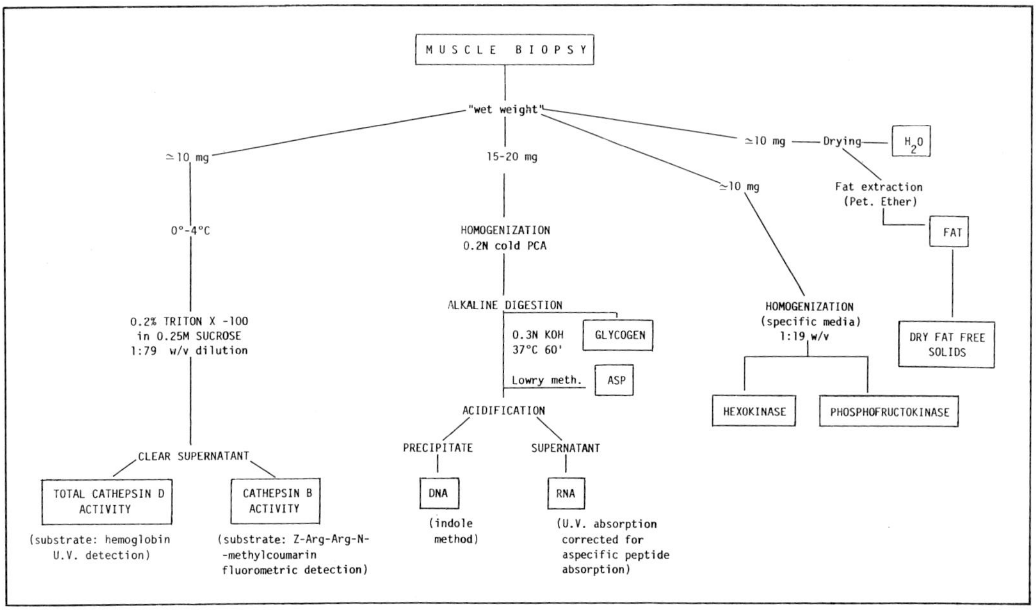

Fig. 1. A schematic illustration of methods used.

Table II. Degradability of myofibrillar proteins by muscle cathepsins B and D (modified from [11])

	Cathepsin B		Cathepsin D	
	SP	MP	SP	MP
Thick filament				
Myosin				
– heavy chain	+		+	+
– light chain LC_1	(+)		+	
LC_2	(+)		+	
LC_3				
C-protein				
Thin filament				
Actin	+		+	
Tropomyosin	+			
Troponin TN-C	–			
TN-I	+			
TN-T	+			
M-line				
M-protein		+		
Z-line				
4a-actinin	–			

SP = single protein; MP = myofibrillar-bound protein; + = degraded

(E. C. 3.4.22.1, molecular weight about 25,000 daltons) is an acid lysosomal cysteine proteinase and cathepsin D (E. C. 3.4.23.5, molecular weight about 42,000 daltons) is an acid lysosomal aspartic-proteinase [11]. They are present in all mammals and are capable of degrading myofibrillar proteins [11] (table II).

Protein Catabolism and Proteinase Activity in Skeletal Muscle

The mechanisms of protein degradation in skeletal muscle are not well understood. It has been reported that the rate of proteolysis in muscle is coupled with the activity of cathepsin B and D and other myofibrillar proteinases [8, 12–18]. According to these and other studies, cathepsins B and D participate in lysosomal proteolysis, but a great deal remains to be learnt about their role in physiological and pathological conditions. The requirement of cathepsin B and D for acidic conditions suggests that they are likely to function in vivo only within cells, or possibly also in very restricted extracellular location [19, 20]. Lysosomal acid proteinases probably cooperate with sarcoplasmic neutral and calcium-activated neutral proteinases for muscle protein degradation [21, 22]. However, it is not clear whether muscle proteinases do have a regulatory role on muscle protein degradation or the changes of their activity with changing protein catabolism are merely an epiphenomenon. It has even been suggested that an increased cathepsin D activity might be related to repair processes, rather than degradative activity [18].

A soluble, non lysosomal proteolytic system probably plays a minor role in muscle protein degradation [23]. Both the lysosomal and the cell-free systems have an absolute requirement for cellular energy, although proteolysis per se is an exergonic process [23]. This points out the important interrelationships between energy and protein metabolism.

Protein degradation in skeletal muscle is also linked to cellular redox state [24] and is under hormonal regulation both in physiological and pathological conditions [25]. Fever, sepsis, interleukin-1, and a peptide present in trauma and sepsis appear to increase muscle proteolysis by activating PGE_2 and subsequently cathepsin B [26–29].

Changes of muscle cathepsins B and D activities were reported in different conditions [8, 12, 13, 15, 17, 18, 20, 30–37] (table III). Moreover, inhibitors of cathepsins B and D reduce muscle proteolysis in experimental myopathies [15] and sepsis [26–29], and cathepsin B inactivates muscle aldolase, by this means possibly acting as a regulator of the glycolytic pathway [38]. This once more points out the links between protein and energy metabolism.

Table III. Muscle cathepsin D activity in different conditions

Increased activity	
	T_4, muscle dystrophy, denervation, prolonged running, ageing, dexamethasone (free), cancer
Decreased activity	
	trenbolone acetate (free), zeranol (free), insulin (free), wasted hemodialysis patients, patients with chronic pancreatitis
Unchanged activity	
	experimental acute renal failure

The recent discovery of the presence of endogenous inhibitors of cysteine proteinases and the existence of cathepsin D in the form of a precursor obviously add a great potential in the regulation of proteolysis [39].

Muscle Protein Metabolism in Trauma

Conflict exists over the mechanisms which give rise to the negative nitrogen balance in the stressed individual [40]. Both whole body protein synthesis and catabolism are probably affected by trauma. According to Clague et al. [41], injury may cause a rise in whole body protein turnover: both whole body synthesis and breakdown rise along with the degree of trauma, breakdown rising more rapidly than synthesis, thus accounting for the increased negative nitrogen balance with increasing severity of injury. Breakdown appears to be largely related to the severity of injury, whereas synthesis responds to substrate availability [41].

However, there is inconsistent information on the relative contributions of muscle and other tissues to these changes of whole body protein metabolism. In injury muscle protein synthesis is generally reduced, but there is no agreement on muscle protein breakdown changes. The discrepancies in the literature may reflect the differences in the severity of the injuries studied, the energy and nitrogen intake, the methods used to assess protein degradation, and the time following injury at which measurements were made. According to previous studies, muscle protein breakdown was considered to be increased after trauma [42]. However, this and other studies were based on urinary 3-methylhistidine determinations to assess muscle protein degradation, and this technique has been subsequently criticized [43]. By directly measuring the efflux of 3-methylhistidine from the leg, Rennie et al. recently concluded that the negative nitrogen balance across muscle tissue commonly observed in disease and injury is not associated with an increase in muscle protein breakdown [44, 45].

Experimental Results

To better define the role of muscle synthesis and breakdown, in this preliminary study we examined 9 traumatized patients from the intensive care unit of our hospital. All patients were previously healthy and were admitted for severe accidental injuries (category 1, according to the classification of the American College of Surgeons [46]). A muscle needle biopsy was taken from quadriceps femoris by Bergström's needle on the 3rd–4th day after trauma and then the patients were treated with TPN. Energy intake was about 25% above measured [47] energy expenditure, 50% as lipids (Intralipid®), and 50% as glucose. Nitrogen intake was 250–300 mg/kg ideal B.W./day as cristallin amino acids. Patients often received corticosteroids for head injury. In some patients a second muscle biopsy was taken after 2–3 weeks of parenteral nutrition.

Muscle phosphofructokinase activity increased after TPN in 4 out of 7 patients (fig. 2). Phosphofructokinase is the key enzyme of glycolysis and its activity has been found decreased in chronically uremic [6] and in malnourished cancer [48] and surgical patients [49]; enzyme activity

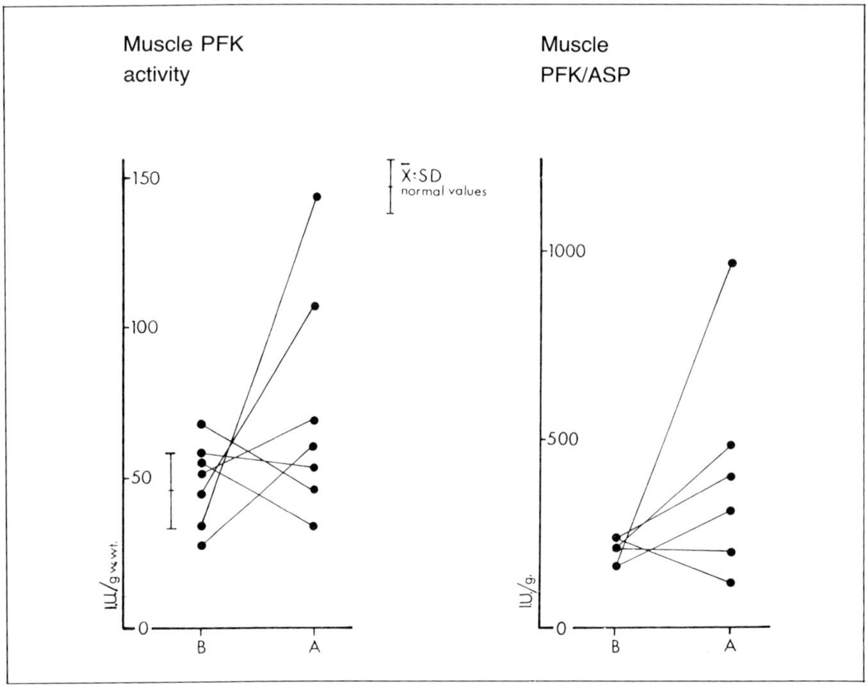

Fig. 2. Muscle phosphofructokinase activity before (B) and after (A) 2–3 weeks of TPN.

tended to increase after nutrition therapy [48, 49]. Elevated levels of muscle phosphofructokinase activity were observed after experimental thermal injury and this provided evidence that the capacity for glucose utilization increased after injury [50], as possibly in some of our patients after TPN.

Muscle DNA content was increased in 3 patients on the first assessment and definitely high, compared to controls, at the end of TPN, suggesting muscle hypotrophy and, possibly, dehydration (fig. 3). The RNA : DNA and ASP : DNA ratios were low in 2 patients before nutritional treatment and very low in the 7 patients re-examined after TPN. These results suggest that changes in muscle nucleic acid and protein concentration are already detectable in some patients a few days after trauma and are very evident at the end of treatment when both protein synthesis and content are decreased. However, in four patients the

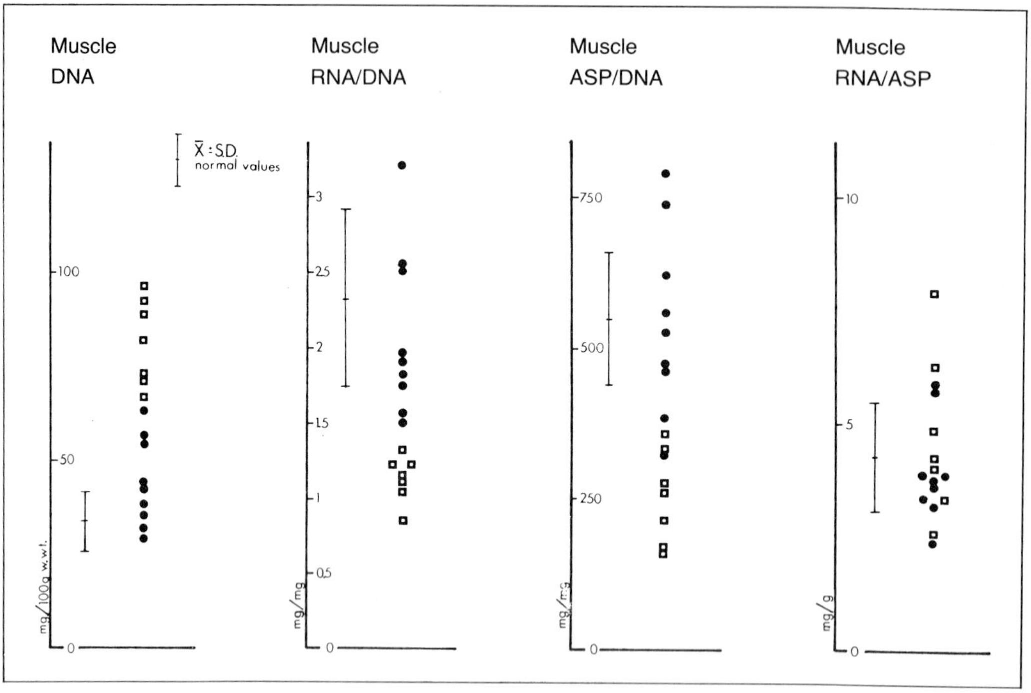

Fig. 3. Muscle DNA content and RNA : DNA, ASP : DNA and RNA : ASP ratios before (B) and after (A) 2–3 weeks of TPN.

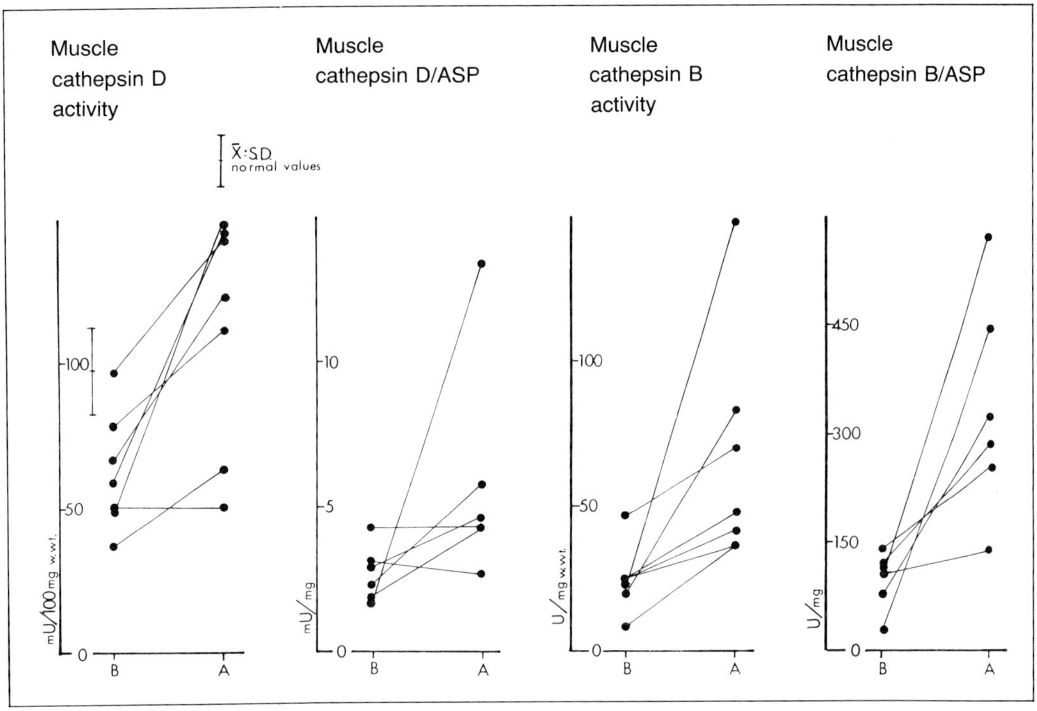

Fig. 4. Muscle cathepsin B and D activity before (B) and after (A) 2–3 weeks of TPN.

RNA : ASP ratio increased after TPN, suggesting an increasing ribosomal capacity for protein synthesis [2, 3] during recovery.

Total cathepsin D activity was generally low before TPN and increased at the end of treatment (fig. 4). Similar changes were observed for cathepsin B activity (fig. 4). As discussed above, a cause-effect relationship between muscle proteinase activity and protein degradation is not clear: changes over time of cathepsin B and D activities might have a regulatory role on protein degradation in vivo, in response to nutritional and hormonal signals, or might only be pathological responses in deteriorating tissues. Proteinase activities measured in vitro have been shown to follow rates of degradation in vivo or in vitro [12, 51]. Anyway, cathepsin B and D activities are presumably an index of muscle protein degradation rate.

Discussion and Conclusions

Shock, endogenous and exogenous hormone levels, and nutrient intake could all affect muscle metabolism in our patients. During the first days after injury they were resuscitated, treated for shock, fractures etc., and artificially ventilated. Their energy intake was actually very low and no nitrogen was supplied. According to Millward et al., muscle protein degradation falls in protein deficiency and in fasting adults and, interestingly, the changes in degradation occur in concert with changes in lysosomal proteinases [51]. Also ischemia, anoxia, and acidosis are known to inhibit proteolysis [52]. Opposite changes of muscle breakdown have been reported by Waterlow et al. [3] during experimental starvation: an adaptive decrease in breakdown was followed by an increase after many days of insufficient nutrient intake, when muscle proteins were probably drawn upon to provide substrates for energy generation. A two stage response is also apparent from our results: in muscle early changes after injury were often opposite to late changes, after TPN and corticosteroid administration, when muscle RNA : DNA and ASP : DNA ratios (namely muscle protein synthesis and content) were low and muscle cathepsin B and D activities (possibly an index of muscle protein degradation) were increased. Although being temptative to speculate that these changes of proteinase activity are an effort to spare some muscle protein in early stages and to provide substrates later on, other possible explanations exist. For the early changes, we should mention loss of enzyme from the sarcoplasm, enzyme inhibition, decreased enzyme synthesis or increased enzyme degradation. Besides, it is not clear from these preliminary results whether changes present at the end of treatment were related to an inadequate nutrient intake, to the metabolic abnormalities of trauma, not reversed by the medical and nutritional treatment, or to corticosteroid administration. As reported above, also changes after trauma and shock of tissue NADH : NAD^{1+} ratio and epinephrine levels and inactivity could affect muscle protein degradation in our patients.

References

1 Heymsfield, S. B.; McManus, C.; Stevens, V.; Smith, J.: Muscle mass: reliable indicator of protein-energy malnutrition severity and outcome. Am. J. clin. Nutr. *35:* 1192–1199 (1982).

2 Millward, D. J.; Waterlow, J. C.: Effect of nutrition on protein turnover in skeletal muscle. Fed. Proc. *37:* 2283–2290 (1978).

3 Waterlow, J. C.; Garlick, P. J.; Millward, D. J.: Protein turnover in mammalian tissues and in the whole body, pp. 625–695 (Elsevier/North-Holland Biomedical Press, Amsterdam 1978).

4 Li, J. B.; Goldberg, A. L.: Effect of food deprivation on protein synthesis and degradation in rat skeletal muscles. Am. J. Physiol. *231:* 441–448 (1976).

5 Cheek, D. B.; Graystone, J. E.: Insulin and growth hormone: regulators of growth with particular reference to muscle. Kidney int. *14:* 317–322 (1978).

6 Guarnieri, G. F.; Toigo, G.; De Marchi, S.; Situlin, R.; Campanacci, L.: Muscle hexokinase and phosphofructokinase activity in chronically uremic patients; in Giordano, Friedman, Uremia-pathobiology of patients treated for 10 years or more, pp. 278–282 (Wichtig, Milano 1981).

7 Guarnieri, G. F.; Toigo, G.; Situlin, R.; Faccini, L.; Coli, U.; Landini, S.; Bazzato, G.; Dardi, F.; Campanacci, L.: Muscle biopsy studies in chronically uremic patients: evidence for malnutrition. Kidney int. *16:* 187–193 (1983).

8 Guarnieri, G. F.; Toigo, G.; Situlin, R.; Faccini, L.; Rustia, R.; Dardi, F.: Muscle cathepsin D activity, and RNA, DNA and protein content in maintenance hemodialysis patients; in Hörl, Heidland, Proteases: potential role in health and disease, pp. 533–543 (Plenum Press, New York 1984).

9 Gordon, E. E.; Kowlasky, K.; Fritts, M.: Muscle proteins and DNA in rat quadriceps during growth. Am. J. Physiol. *210:* 1033–1040 (1966).

10 Alleyne, G. A. O.; Hay, R. W.; Picou, D. I.; Stanfield, J. P.; Whithehead, R.C.: Protein-energy malnutrition (Edward Arnold Publisher, Maidenhead 1977).

11 Dahlmann, B.; Kuehn, L.; Reinauer, H.: Proteolytic enzymes and enhanced muscle protein breakdown; in Hörl, Heidland, Proteases: potential role in health and disease pp. 505–517 (Plenum Press, New York 1984).

12 Lundholm, K.; Bylund, A.-C.; Holm, J.; Scherstén, T.: Skeletal muscle metabolism in patients with malignant tumor. Eur. J. Cancer *12:* 465–473 (1976).

13 Millward, D. J.; Bates, P. C.; Brown, J. G.; Rosochacki, S. R.; Rennie, M. J.: Protein degradation and the regulation of protein balance in muscle. Ciba Fdn Symp. *75:* 307–329 (1979).

14 Lernau, O. Z.; Nissan, S.; Neufeld, B.; Mayer, M.: Myofibrillar protease activity in muscle tissue from patient in catabolic conditions. Eur. J. clin. Invest. *10:* 357–361 (1980).

15 Li, J. B.: Protein synthesis and degradation in skeletal muscle of normal and dystrophic hamsters. Am. J. Physiol. *239:* E401–E406 (1980).

16 Bird, J. W. C.; Carter, J. H.; Triemer, R. E.; Brooks, R. M.; Spanier, A. M.: Proteinases in cardiac and skeletal muscle. Fed. Proc. *39:* 20–25 (1980).

17 Guarnieri, G. F.; Toigo, G.; Situlin, R.; Del Bianco, A.; Crapesi, L.; Zanettovich, A.: Direct tissue analysis in vivo in hospital malnutrition. J. parent. ent. Nutr. (in press).

18 Griggs, R. C.; Rennie, M. J.: Muscle wasting in muscular dystrophy: decreased protein synthesis or increased degradation? Ann. Neurol. *13:* 125–133 (1983).

19 Barrett, A. J.: Lysosomal proteinases and their specificity; in Segal, Doyle, Protein turnover and lysosome function, pp. 295–298 (Academic Press, New York 1978).

20 Decker, R. S.; Wildenthal, K.: Lysosomal alterations in heart, skeletal muscle, and liver of hyperthyroid rabbits. J. Lab. Invest. *44:* 455–465 (1981).
21 Kay, J.: Degradation of myofibrillar proteins by neutral proteinases; in Ballard, Tomas, Ist Intern. Symp. on Protein Turnover, Growth and Muscle Wasting, Rottnest Island, August 11–15 (1982).
22 Newman, J. J.; Strome, D. R.; Goodwing, C. W.; Mason, A. D.; Pruitt, B. A.: Neutral proteinase activity in skeletal muscle from thermally injured rats. J. surg. Res. *35:* 515–519 (1983).
23 Hershko, A.; Ciechanover, A.: Mechanisms of intracellular protein breakdown. Annu. Rev. Biochem. *51:* 335–364 (1982).
24 Tischler, M. E.; Fagan, J. M.: Relationship of the reduction-oxidation state to protein degradation in skeletal and atrial muscle. Archs. Biochem. Biophys. *217:* 191–210 (1982).
25 Tischler, M. E.: Hormonal regulation of protein degradation in skeletal and cardiac muscle. Life Sci. *28:* 2569–2576 (1981).
26 Clowes, G. H. Jr.; George, B. C.; Villee, C. A. Jr.; Saravis, C. A.: Muscle proteolysis induced by a circulating peptide in patients with sepsis or trauma. New Engl. J. Med. *308:* 545–552 (1983).
27 Baracos, V.; Rodemann, H. P.; Dinarello, C. A.; Goldberg, A. L.: Stimulation of muscle protein degradation and prostaglandin E2 release by leukocytic pyrogen (interleukin-1). A mechanism for the increased degradation of muscle proteins during fever. New Engl. J. Med. *308:* 553–558 (1983).
28 Goldberg, A. L.; Baracos, V.; Rodemann, P.; Waxmann, L.; Dinarello, C.: Control of protein degradation in muscle by prostaglandins, Ca^{2+}, and leukocytic pyrogen (interleukin-1). Fed. Proc. *43:* 1301–1306 (1984).
29 Ruff, R.; Secrist, D.: Inhibitors of prostaglandin synthesis or cathepsin B prevent muscle wasting due to sepsis in the rat. J. clin. Invest. *73:* 1483–1486 (1984).
30 Scherstén, T.; Lundholm, K.: Lysosomal enzyme activity in muscle tissue from patients with malignant tumor. Cancer *30:* 1246–1251 (1972).
31 Rannels, D. E.; Kao, R.; Morgan, H. E.: Effect of insulin on protein turnover in heart muscle. J. biol. Chem. *250:* 1694–1701 (1975).
32 Sinnett-Smith, P. A.; Dumelow, N. W.; Buttery, P. J.: Protein turnover in sheep treated with trenbolone acetate and zeranol. Proc. Nutr. Soc. *42:* 58A (1983).
33 Salminen, A.; Vinko, V.: Effects of age and prolonged running on proteolytic capacity in mouse cardiac and skeletal muscle. Acta physiol. scand. *112:* 89–95 (1981).
34 Clark, A. F.; Vignos, P. J. Jr.: The role of proteases in experimental glucocorticoid myopathy. Muscle Nerve *4:* 219–222 (1981).
35 Decker, R. S.; Poole, A. R.; Crie, J. S.; Dingle, J. T.; Wildenthal K.: Lysosomal alterations in hypoxic and reoxygenated hearts. II. Immunohistochemical and biochemical changes in cathepsin D. Am. J. Path. *98:* 445–456 (1980).
36 Sellin, L. D.; Libelius, R.; Lundquist, I.; Tagerud, S.; Thesleff, S.: Membrane and biochemical alterations after denervation and during reinnervation of mouse skeletal muscle. Acta physiol. scand. *110:* 181–186 (1980).
37 Vernon, B. G.; Buttery, P. J.: The effect of the growth promoter trenbolone acetate, dexamethasone and thyroxine on skeletal muscle cathepsin D (EC 3.4.4.23) activity. Proc. Nutr. Soc. *40:* 13A (1980).

38 Pote, M. S.; Altekar, W.: Muscle aldolase: the stress-dependent modification of catalytic and structural properties by rat muscle lysosomal cathepsin B. Biochim. biophys. Acta *661:* 303–314 (1981).
39 Türk, V.; Lah, T.; Puisdar, V.; Locnikar, P.; Kregar, I.; Cotic, V.: Lysosomal aspartic and cysteine proteinases; in Ballard, Tomas, Ist Intern. Symp. on Protein Turnover, Growth and Muscle Wasting, Rottnest Island, August 11–15 (1982).
40 James, W. P. T.: Protein and energy metabolism after trauma: old concepts and new developments. Acta chir. scand. *507:* suppl. II, pp. 1–20 (1981).
41 Clague, M. B.; Keir, M. J.; Wright, P. D.; Johnston, I. D. A.: The effects of nutrition and trauma on whole-body protein metabolism in man. Clin. Sci. *65:* 165–175 (1983).
42 Long, C. L.; Birkhahn R. H.; Geiger, J. W.; Blakemore, W. S.: Contribution of skeletal muscle protein in elevated rates of whole body protein catabolism in trauma patients. Am. J. clin. Nutr. *34:* 1087–1093 (1981).
43 Rennie, M. J.; Millward, D. J.: 3-methylhistidine excretion and the urinary 3-methylhistidine/creatinine ratio are poor indicators of skeletal muscle protein breakdown. Clin. Sci. *65:* 217–225 (1983).
44 Rennie, M. J.; Bennegard, K.; Edén, E.; Emery, P. W.; Lundholm, K.: Urinary excretion and efflux from the leg of 3-methylhistidine before and after major surgical operation. Metabolism *33:* 250–256 (1984).
45 Rennie, M. J.; Harrison, R.: Effects of injury, disease, and malnutrition on protein metabolism in man. Unanswered questions. Lancet *i:* 323–325 (1984).
46 Trunkey, D. D.: Overview of trauma. Surg. Clins N. *62:* 3–7 (1982).
47 Iapichino, G.; Solca, M.; Radrizzani, D.; Zucchetti, M.; Damia, G.: Net protein utilization during total parenteral nutrition of injured critically ill patients: an original approach. J. parent. ent. Nutr. *5:* 317–321 (1981).
48 Edén, E.; Bennegård, K.; Bylund-Fellenius, A.-C.; Scherstén, T.; Lundholm, K.: Whole-body energy metabolism and metabolic capacity of skeletal muscles in malnourished patients before and after total parenteral nutrition. Human Nutr.: Clin. Nutr. *37C:* 185–196 (1983).
49 King, R. F. G. A.; MacFie, J.; Hill, G.: Activities of hexokinase, phosphofructokinase, fructose biophosphatase and 2-oxoglutarate dehydrogenase in muscle of normal subjects and very ill surgical patients. Clin. Sci. *60:* 451–456 (1981).
50 Newmann, J. J.; Strome, D. R.; Goodwin, C. W.; Mason, A. D.; Pruitt, B. A., Jr.: Altered muscle metabolism in rats after thermal injury. Metabolism *31:* 1229–1233 (1982).
51 Millward, D. J.; Brown, J. G.; Odedra, B.: Protein turnover in individual tissues with special emphasis on muscle; in Waterlow, Stephen, Nitrogen metabolism in man, pp. 475–494 (Applied Science Publishers, London 1981).
52 Chua, B.; Kao, R. L.; Rannels, D. E.; Morgan, H. E.: Inhibition of protein degradation by anoxia and ischemia in perfused rat hearts. J. biol. Chem. *254:* 6617–6623 (1979).

G. Guarnieri, M.D., Istituto di Patologia Medica, Università di Trieste,
Ospedale di Cattinara, I-34149 Trieste (Italy)

Dietze, Grünert, Kleinberger, Wolfram (eds.), Clinical Nutrition and Metabolic Research. Proc. 7th Congr. ESPEN, Munich 1985, pp. 40–53 (Karger, Basel 1986)

Metabolic Response of Muscle to Trauma: Altered Control of Protein Turnover

M. E. Tischler, E. Leng, M. Al-Kanhal, J. Mnichowicz, J. Reiser, L. W. Norton

Department of Biochemistry, University of Arizona, Tucson, Ariz., USA

Introduction

After the period of stabilization ('ebb' phase) following injury, the excretion of total nitrogen in the urine continues to increase during the catabolic or 'flow' phase [1, 2]. Hence, this phase is characterized by the net breakdown of body proteins which, because of its total mass, is largely contributed to by skeletal muscle [3–5]. This net breakdown reflects a negative balance between the rates of protein degradation and synthesis. Several situations can bring about negative protein balance including: (a) decreased synthesis with increased degradation, (b) a large decrease in synthesis with no change or even a fall in breakdown, or (c) no change in synthesis with accelerated degradation. The relevance of these scenarios to a number of physiological states has been reviewed recently [6].

Generally the numerous studies using traumatized or stressed animals or man can be assigned basically to two groups: (a) muscle protein synthesis decreases below the rate of protein degradation, or (b) protein breakdown accelerates above the synthesis rate. The assignment of these studies has been summarized by Rennie [6]. Of relevance to our study are the results obtained for the response to traumatic injury. Studies with patients or animals subjected to such trauma seem best to fit the second pattern [3, 4, 7–10]. Some studies on trauma due to thermal injury also seems to fit this pattern [11, 12], while studies by Clowes et al. and by Shangraw and Turinsky [3, 13] showed no increase in proteolysis.

Other studies have concerned the possible mechanism(s) for increased muscle proteolysis in response to trauma. Clowes et al. [5] have identified a circulating peptide in patients with sepsis or trauma which can increase protein degradation in isolated rat muscle relative to treatment with normal plasma or no plasma. It is possible that this peptide is a degradation product of interleukin-1, which can promote protein breakdown in isolated muscles [14, 15]. This effect may be related to acceleration of the production of prostaglandins which accelerate muscle proteolysis in the lysosome [16]. Accordingly, treatment of burned rats with EP 475, an inhibitor of lysosomal proteases [14–16], diminished protein degradation in epitrochlearis muscle from burned rats but not from unburned animals [11]. However, in vitro treatment of muscle with indomethacin, to block prostaglandin production, did not abolish the difference in protein breakdown [11].

In a previous study from this laboratory using blunt trauma to the rat as a model, we showed a diminished response to insulin of protein degradation in isolated muscles [9]. Work presented here has examined further this problem. One aspect of particular interest is whether circulating adrenal hormones might lead to this diminished response. This consideration was based on previous studies showing an interaction of glucocorticoids and insulin in their effects on muscle protein breakdown [17, 18].

Materials and Methods

Trauma Procedure

While under ether anesthesia, rats (male albino Sprague-Dawley, 70–80 g, bred by the University of Arizona) had the posterior portion of their left lower hind leg shaved. Blunt trauma was administered by automatically dropping a reflex hammer head (28.2 g) a distance of 7 mm on to the shaved leg. The hammer was padded to prevent cuts of the skin. Blows were delivered for 21 min at 72 blows/min. Further details are given elsewhere [9, 19].

Adrenalectomy and Cortisol Treatment

Animals were subjected to bilateral adrenalectomy 4 days prior to any other manipulations. In vivo subcutaneous injection of cortisol acetate (Sigma Chemical Co, St. Louis, MO) was performed as described in the legends to tables. Cortisol acetate (4 mg/ml) was suspended in 0.9% saline. Control animals received injections of 0.5 ml of 0.9% saline.

Muscle Incubations

Rats were killed by cervical dislocation and muscles were dissected out and weighed. The standard buffer for incubations at 37 °C was Krebs-Ringer bicarbonate buffer containing 5 mM glucose and equilibrated with 95% O_2 : 5% CO_2. Where provided plasma amino acid concentrations were normal values reported for the rat [20]. In experiments where muscles were not treated in vitro with cortisol, the tissues were preincubated for 30 min prior to the 2 h incubation. In other experiments, cortisol treatment replaced this 30 min preincubation period, as indicated.

Protein Metabolism

Protein synthesis and degradation were measured simultaneously [9, 21]. Protein degradation was calculated as the sum of protein synthesis and net protein breakdown. Net protein breakdown was taken as the appearance of tyrosine in the medium [22], which was heated in boiling water for 3 min after removal of the muscle, centrifuged at 2000 × g for 15 min, and saved for measurement of tyrosine. Incubation of soleus, extensor digitorum longus, and diaphragm muscles of traumatized rats for 1 or 2 h all showed a linear release of tyrosine into the medium when incubated with glucose and amino acids [9]. Protein synthesis was determined by measuring the incorporation of [^{14}C]phenylalanine (0.5 mM, 0.1 mCi/mmol) (ICN, Irvine, CA) into muscle protein after 2 h incubation. After incubation, skeletal muscles were homogenized in 3 ml of 10% trichloroacetic acid and then centrifuged at 2000 × g for 10 min. The protein pellet was washed once in 3 ml of 10% trichloroacetic acid and then twice with 3 ml of ethanol : ether (1 : 1). The final protein pellet was solubilized by addition of 0.05 ml H_2O and, after mixing, 0.25 ml Protosol (New England Nuclear, Boston, MA). Radioactivity in the solubilized pellet was counted in 5 ml Cytoscint (West Chem Products) in a Beckman LS250 liquid scintillation counter. Protein synthesis was expressed in terms of tyrosine units by multiplying the rate of phenylalanine incorporation by the ratio of tyrosine/phenylalanine incorporated into muscle protein. Previous results showed this ratio to average 0.77 in muscles from fed, fasted, traumatized, adrenalectomized, and cortisol-treated rats [9, 22]. Protein degradation was thus determined as the sum of the corrected value for protein synthesis (incorporation of [^{14}C]phenylalanine × 0.77) and the rate of net protein breakdown. When only degradation was determined, 0.5 mM cycloheximide was included to inhibit protein synthesis. The measured release of tyrosine under this condition provides a measurement of protein degradation and gives similar results to the calculated value [21]. Tyrosine is measured fluorometrically [23].

Results

In an earlier study [9, 19], we showed that the more negative protein balance of isolated skeletal muscles from traumatized rats was most evident with insulin provided in the incubation. Most of this catabolic response could be accounted for by faster protein degradation rather than slower protein synthesis. The maximal response for diaphragm occurred on the second day after traumatization whereas the uninjured soleus and extensor digitorum longus (EDL) muscles showed a peak on the third day. These patterns coincided with the rise in urinary nitrogen excretion which peaked for the 24 h collection between 48 to 72 h after traumatization.

As noted above, the greatest differences in protein balance were seen in the presence of insulin and seemed to result from a diminished inhibitory effect of insulin on protein degradation with apparently normal stimulation of protein synthesis (table I). Stimulation by insulin of the uptake of 2-deoxyglucose by the diaphragm and EDL muscles was also relatively normal, while this effect in the soleus was diminished to a small extent. Therefore, the only large diminution we observed for the effect of insulin was on protein degradation.

This finding was indicative of a post-receptor defect for insulin. To test this idea further, we carried out a dose-response curve for the inhibitory effect of insulin on protein degradation in diaphragm of normal and 2-day traumatized rats (fig. 1). Comparison of these curves supports the possibility of a post-receptor defect. Such a defect is characterized by a small difference in the response at low concentrations with a large difference at high concentrations that cannot be overcome at the highest amounts of insulin [24]. Accordingly, we found that even at 0.1 units

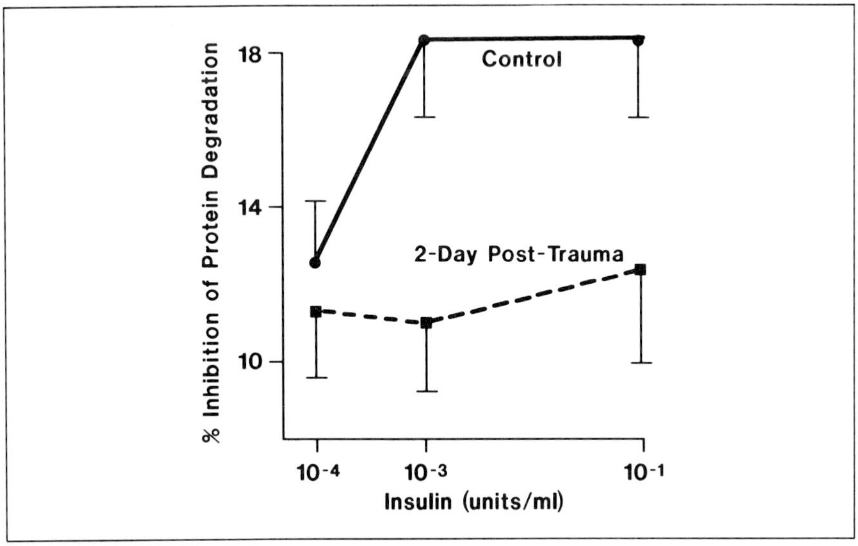

Fig. 1. Comparison of effect of varied insulin concentration on degradation of protein in diaphragms from normal and 2-day traumatized rats. Hemdiaphragms were incubated in Krebs-Ringer buffer containing glucose (5 mM), bovine serum albumin (1%), cycloheximide (0.5 mM) with or without insulin, at indicated amounts.

Table I. Effect of insulin on protein metabolism in muscles of normal and traumatized rats

Days after injury	Diaphragm	Soleus	EDL
	Percent effect on protein synthesis		
0	+ 18	+ 69	+ 87
2	+ 24	+ 66	+ 77
3	—	+ 71	+ 60
	Percent effect on protein degradation		
0	− 19	− 23	− 34
2	− 8	− 12	− 25
3	− 12	0	− 14

Muscles were incubated in the absence or presence of insulin (0.1 U/ml) in Krebs-Ringer buffer containing 5 mM glucose and 1 × plasma amino acids. Except for protein degradation in the diaphragm, all other data are calculated from [9]. EDL = extensor digitorum longus

Table II. Effect of preincubation with cortisol in the absence or presence of insulin on muscle protein metabolism

Preincubation treatment	Protein balance	(nmol tyrosine/mg muscle/2 h)	
		synthesis	degradation
	Soleus		
None	− 0.180 ± 0.017	0.057 ± 0.003	0.237 ± 0.015
Cortisol	− 0.216 ± 0.014*	0.044 ± 0.004**	0.260 ± 0.010*
Cortisol + insulin	− 0.170 ± 0.013	0.058 ± 0.003	0.228 ± 0.014
	Extensor digitorum longus		
None	− 0.186 ± 0.005	0.033 ± 0.002	0.219 ± 0.005
Cortisol	− 0.228 ± 0.008**	0.025 ± 0.002**	0.253 ± 0.007**
Cortisol + insulin	− 0.204 ± 0.016	0.028 ± 0.002*	0.233 ± 0.014

* $p < 0.05$; ** $p < 0.005$: significance of difference from none

Muscles were removed from adrenalectomized animals deprived of food for 24 h. The muscles were treated in gassed, stoppered flasks for 9 h in 4 ml of Krebs-Ringer buffer containing 10 mM glucose (10 mM) 5 × plasma amino acids and cortisol (1 mM) and insulin (0.1 U/ml) as indicated. Protein metabolism was measured subsequently following incubation for 2 h in Krebs-Ringer buffer containing glucose (5 mM) and ^{14}C-phenylalanine (0.5 mM; 0.1 mCi/mmol) insulin/ml the inhibitory effect on protein breakdown in the diaphragm of traumatized rats reached only 67% of the normal maximum response.

One circulating factor which seems to interact with insulin action in muscle is glucocorticoids. Mayer and Shafrir showed that the rise of muscle proteolysis in insulin-deficient animals may reflect a greater response to these hormones [18]. In an earlier study, Griffin and Wildenthal found that hydrocortisone had a catabolic effect on metabolism of fetal mouse hearts in culture in the absence of insulin but had an anabolic effect when insulin was provided [17]. We also have tested the effects of cortisol on isolated muscles. Following treatment of leg muscles for 9 h with cortisol hemisuccinate, overall protein balance became more negative as a result of both slower protein synthesis and faster protein degradation (table II). Diaphragms from either normal or traumatized rats treated with cortisol for only 6 h also showed increased protein degradation (table III). While this inhibitory effect of cortisol on synthesis is well-established [25–29], its effect on proteolysis has been less clear, with some investigators finding enhancement [27, 30, 31] and others no effect [32–36].

Table III. Effect of insulin on protein degradation in diaphragms from normal or traumatized, adrenalectomized rats pretreated with cortisol

Rats	Preincubation treatment	Insulin in incubation	Protein degradation (% of control)
Normal (control)	none	no	100
	none	yes	90 ± 2*
	cortisol	no	136 ± 5**
	cortisol	yes	120 ± 6*, **
Trauma (control)	none	no	100
	none	yes	98 ± 2
	cortisol	no	125 ± 9***
	cortisol	yes	123 ± 6***

* $p < 0.005$: significance of effect of insulin; ** $p < 0.005$; *** $p < 0.05$: significance of effect of cortisol

Hemidiaphragms from normal or 2-day traumatized, adrenalectomized rats were either not treated or treated for 6 h with cortisol hemisuccinate (1 uM), while attached to the ribs, in Krebs-Ringer buffer containing glucose (5 mM) and 5 × plasma amino acids. The muscles were then dissected from the ribs, bisected and incubated with or without insulin (0.1 U/ml) in Krebs-Ringer buffer containing glucose (5 mM) and cycloheximide (0.5 mM)

When insulin was provided during the treatment of leg muscles with cortisol, the catabolic effects of cortisol were generally abolished (table II). However, insulin did not improve the protein balance relative to nontreated muscles. When insulin effects were tested subsequent to treatment of normal diaphragm with cortisol (table III), it was found to be equally effective on a percentage basis (10% versus 12% in nontreated and treated muscles, respectively). However, insulin could not lower protein degradation down to the control value following cortisol treatment. In this experiment, insulin had no significant effect on proteolysis in diaphragm of 2-day traumatized rats and cortisol treatment did not alter this observation.

We also tested the effects of cortisol in vivo (table IV). Treatment of adrenalectomized rats with cortisol acetate (2 mg/100 g body wt) for 3 days resulted in slower in vitro protein degradation in the soleus and no effect in the EDL. Generally, physiological doses [30] of cortisol did not accelerate proteolysis and even caused a diminution when fed rats were

Table IV. Effect on protein degradation of cortisol treatment and trauma of adrenalectomized rats

Rat	Treatment	Muscle	Protein degradation
	(nmol tyrosine/mg muscle/2 h)		
Adx	saline	soleus	0.254 ± 0.012
Adx	saline	EDL	0.209 ± 0.026
	(% difference from control)		
Adx	cortisol	soleus	− 15*
Adx-trauma	saline		+ 11*
Adx-trauma	cortisol		+ 24*
Adx	cortisol	EDL	NS
Adx-trauma	saline		+ 20*
Adx-trauma	cortisol		+ 24*

* $p < 0.05$: significance of difference from adx, saline-treated
NS = not significant; EDL = extensor digitorum longus; Adx = adrenalectomized

Four days after adrenalectomy, rats were either injected with saline (0.9%) solution or cortisol acetate (2 mg/100 g body wt) for 3 days. Animals were traumatized immediately prior to injection. Protein degradation was measured in muscles incubated in Krebs-Ringer buffer containing glucose (5 mM), insulin (0.1 U/ml) and 1 × plasma amino acids (except tyrosine)

Table V. Comparison of effects of cortisol treatment on protein degradation in muscles from fed and fasted rats

Treatment	Nutritional state	Muscle	Protein degradation
Saline	*(nmol tyrosine/mg muscle/2 h)*		
	fed	diaphragm	0.26 ± 0.01
	fed	EDL	0.37 ± 0.03
	fasted	diaphragm	0.28 ± 0.02
	fasted	soleus	0.30 ± 0.02
	fasted	EDL	0.32 ± 0.01
Cortisol	*(% difference from saline-treated)*		
(5 mg/100 g)	fed	diaphragm	− 7*
(5 mg/100 g)	fed	EDL	NS
(1 mg/100 g)	fasted	diaphragm	+ 21**
(1 mg/100 g)	fasted	soleus	+ 30**
(1 mg/100 g)	fasted	EDL	+ 34**

* $p < 0.05$; ** $p < 0.01$: significant of difference from saline-treated
NS = not significant; EDL = extensor digitorum longus

Animals were adrenalectomized 4 days prior to treatment for 2 days with saline or cortisol acetate, at the doses indicated. Deprivation of food was carried out for the 24 h after the last injection. Protein degradation was measured in muscles incubated for 2 h in Krebs-Ringer buffer containing glucose (5 mM) and 1 × plasma amino acids (except for tyrosine)

used (tables IV, V). This finding fits with observations made using cultured fetal mouse hearts [17]. However, when adrenalectomized animals fasted for 24 h were tested, even a low dose (1 mg/100 g body wt) effectively led to faster protein breakdown in muscles taken from these animals (table V).

Protein degradation was also measured in muscles from saline- or cortisol-treated, adrenalectomized, traumatized rats. Despite the lack of circulating adrenal hormones, we still saw faster in vitro protein degradation in the soleus and EDL muscles. Administration of cortisol to these animals led to a greater difference in protein degradation for the soleus but not for the EDL. These results suggest that circulating adrenal hormones are probably not responsible for subsequent faster in vitro protein degradation, in the presence of insulin, in muscles of traumatized rats.

Although adrenal hormones do not seem to be responsible for the diminished response of protein degradation to insulin in vitro, it is possible that some other systemic factor might be important. Indeed, Clowes et al.

[5] have shown that a peptide from plasma of trauma patients can accelerate in vitro muscle protein degradation. Therefore, we determined whether some factor in plasma of trauma patients could diminish the effect of insulin on protein metabolism (table VI). Plasma was filtered to remove proteins greater than 50,000 daltons. In the presence of no plasma, normal plasma, or trauma plasma, insulin stimulation of protein synthesis did not differ. This stimulation by insulin was 20%, 23%, and 17% in the soleus and 45%, 39%, and 45% in the EDL, respectively. On the other hand, provision of trauma plasma seemed to diminish the effect of insulin on protein degradation. With no plasma or normal plasma, insulin inhibited degradation by 15–19% in the soleus and by 13% in the EDL. With trauma plasma, this value was 9% inhibition in the soleus and no significant effect in the EDL. This preliminary study suggests that some

Table VI. Effect of insulin on protein metabolism in skeletal muscles incubated in the absence or presence of plasma from normal or traumatized humans

Plasma	Insulin	(nmol tyr/mg muscle/2 h)	
		Protein synthesis	Protein degradation
	+	0.110 ± .006 (+ 20%)*	0.274 ± .008 (– 19%)*
Normal	–	0.094 ± .006	0.341 ± .031
	+	0.116 ± .006 (+ 23%)*	0.290 ± .029 (– 15%)*
Trauma	–	0.092 ± .005	0.335 ± .009
	+	0.108 ± .005 (+ 17%)*	0.307 ± .017 (–9%)**
		Extensor digitorum longus	
None	–	0.069 ± .005	0.386 ± .020
	+	0.100 ± .007 (+ 45%)*	0.336 ± .016 (– 13%)*
Normal	–	0.072 ± .006	0.380 ± .023
	+	0.100 ± .005 (+ 39%)*	0.330 ± .028 (– 13%)**
Trauma	–	0.064 ± .004	0.388 ± .014
	+	0.093 ± .002 (+ 45%)*	0.360 ± .023 (NS)

* $p < 0.005$; ** $p < 0.05$: significance of effect of insulin
NS = not significant; () = percent effect of insulin

Leg muscles were incubated for 2 h in the absence or presence of insulin (0.1 U/ml) with glucose (5 mM) and 1 × plasma amino acids (except for no tyrosine and 0.5 mM ^{14}C-phenylalanine; 0.1 mCi/mmol). Filtered plasma (0.25 ml), with > 50,000 dalton proteins excluded, was added to 2.75 ml of medium. Trauma plasma was taken the third morning after patients were admitted for injury. 12 each of overnight fasted normal and trauma volunteers were used

Table VII. Effects of fasting and trauma on protein metabolism in leg muscles

Rat	Muscle	Protein synthesis	Protein degradation
		nmol tyrosine/mg muscle/2 h	
Normal	soleus	0.139 ± 0.006	0.236 ± 0.006
Normal	EDL	0.154 ± 0.007	0.227 ± 0.011
		% difference from fed normal	
Fasted	soleus	− 20**	+ 32**
Trauma		NS	+ 13***
Fasted	EDL	− 39*	+ 58*
Trauma		NS	+ 10***
		% difference from fed trauma	
Fasted + trauma	soleus	NS	NS
Fasted + trauma	EDL	− 45*	+ 59*
		% difference from fasted	
Fasted + trauma	soleus	+ 10***	NS
Fasted + trauma	EDL	NS	+ 11***

* $p < 0.001$; ** $p < 0.005$; *** $p < 0.05$: significance of % difference
NS = not significant; EDL = extensor digitorum longus

Muscles from normal or 3-day traumatized animals, either fed or deprived of food for 48 h, were incubated in Krebs-Ringer buffer with glucose (5 mM), 1 × plasma amino acids (except for tyrosine), ^{14}C-phenylalanine (0.5 mM; 0.1 mCi/mmol) and insulin (0.1 U/ml)

factor in human trauma plasma might diminish the effect of insulin on protein degradation in vitro.

Since in this trauma model, an altered influence of insulin on protein degradation might be important, we carried out some studies with rats which were fasted to lower blood insulin. Soleus and EDL muscles from normal, fasted rats incubated with insulin, showed slower protein synthesis and greater protein degradation than these muscles of normal, fed animals (table VII). Although the incubated EDL muscle from fed and fasted, 3-day traumatized rats showed the same relative differences in protein synthesis and degradation, the soleus of traumatized rats seemed to be unaffected by fasting. In this experiment, as in others, trauma led to faster protein degradation with no change in protein synthesis. This same pattern was also found for the EDL of fasted rats. In contrast, for the soleus, trauma of fasted rats led to no change in degradation and a somewhat faster synthesis of protein in vitro. These results suggest that while the EDL muscle may respond to trauma in the same manner irrespective of the animal's nutritional status, the soleus response to trauma may be diminished in the face of other stress (e.g., fasting) in the animal.

Discussion

This study has investigated further those factors which may account for the diminished effect of insulin on protein degradation in muscle of traumatized rats. Additional data further support the idea that this probably is a post-receptor defect which seems to be restricted primarily to protein breakdown (fig. 1). Hence it was possible that some systemic factor might be taken into muscle in vivo and subsequently alter control of proteolysis by insulin in vitro. Our experiment with human plasma supports such an idea, since provision of trauma plasma seemed to diminish insulin's effect on protein degradation but not on synthesis (table VI). This finding agrees with that of Clark et al. [12] that the increase in protein catabolism induced by thermal injury was not mediated by these hormones. Future studies will examine if the factor in human trauma plasma responsible for altering the response to insulin might be interleukin-1, which promotes proteolysis [15, 16].

Another finding in the experiments described here was a differential response between the soleus and EDL under certain condition. In previous work, we reported that the pattern of the response of skeletal muscles to trauma may depend, to some extent, on their physiological and biochemical characteristics [9]. A differential response of the soleus and EDL to fasting has also been reported [37]. Furthermore, the soleus muscle is exquisitely more sensitive to reduced activity than is the EDL [38]. In this study, some other differential responses were noted. For instance, even though insulin prevented the inhibitory effect of cortisol on protein synthesis in the soleus, it was only partially effective in the EDL (table II). With adrenalectomized, traumatized rats, cortisol did not lead to a further increase in protein degradation in the EDL but did cause greater protein degradation in the soleus (table IV). This increase of proteolysis in response to cortisol seen in the soleus of fed, adrenalectomized, traumatized rats was not observed with fed, adrenalectomized, normal animals (table IV). Finally, the effects of fasting and trauma on subsequent measurement of protein degradation were additive for the EDL but not in the soleus (table VII). In the EDL, fasting led to a fall in protein synthesis of 0.06 nmol tyrosine/mg muscle/2 h, trauma had no effect and the combined conditions showed a decrease of 0.07 nmol tyr/mg muscle/ 2 h. Also in this muscle, fasting caused protein breakdown to increase by 0.132 nmol tyr/mg muscle/2 h, trauma increased it by 0.023 and their combined effect was 0.171. For the soleus, even though protein degradation rose by 0.076 nmol tyr/mg muscle/2 h with fasting and by 0.031 nmol tyr/mg muscle/2 h with trauma, the fasted trauma group showed an intermediate increase of 0.049 nmol tyr/mg muscle/2 h. Hence, in the soleus, fasting and trauma may, to some extent, override the effects of each other.

Acknowledgments

This work was carried out under the tenure of an established investigatorship from the American Heart Association to M. E. Tischler and was supported by grants from: Merck Sharp & Dohme Research Laboratories, National Aeronautics and Space Administration (NAGW-227), and USPHS Grant #T35 HL07479.

References

1 Cuthbertson, D. P.: Observations on the disturbance of metabolism produced by injury to the limbs. Q. Jl. Med. *1:* 233–246 (1932).
2 Cuthbertson, D. P.: Post-shock metabolic response. Lancet *i:* 433–437 (1942).
3 Clowes, G. H. A.; Randall, H. T.; Cha, C. J.: Amino acid and energy metabolism in septic and traumatized patients. J. parent. ent. Nutr. *4:* 195–205 (1980).
4 Long, C. L.; Birkhahn, R. H.; Geiger, J. W.; Betts, J. E.; Schiller, W. R.; Blakemore, W. S.: Urinary excretion of 3-methylhistidine: An assessment of muscle protein catabolism in adult normal subjects and during malnutrition, sepsis and skeletal trauma. Metabolism *30:* 765–776 (1981).
5 Clowes, G. H. A.; George, B. C.; Villee, C. A.; Saravis, C. A.: Muscle proteolysis induced by a circulating peptide in patients with sepsis or trauma. New Engl. J. Med. *308:* 545–552 (1983).
6 Rennie, M. J.: Muscle protein turnover and the wasting due to injury and disease. Brit. med. Bull. *41:* 257–264 (1985).
7 Birkhahn, R. H.; Long, C. L.; Fitkin, D.; Geiger, J. W.; Blakemore, W. S.: Effects of major skeletal trauma on whole body protein turnover in man measured by L-[1-^{14}C]leucine. Surgery *88:* 294–299 (1980).
8 Shangraw, R. E.; Turinsky, J.: Effect of disuse and thermal injury on protein turnover in skeletal muscle. J. surg. Res. *33:* 345–355 (1982).
9 Tischler, M. E.; Fagan, J.: Response to trauma of protein, amino acid, and carbohydrate metabolism in injured and uninjured rat skeletal muscles. Metabolism *32:* 853–868 (1983).

10 Tischler, M. E.; Cammisa, H.: Metabolism of protein, amino acids and glucose and their response to insulin in atria and cardiac myocytes of traumatized rats. Metabolism *33:* 515–520 (1984).
11 Odessey, R.; Paar, B.: Effect of insulin and leucine on protein turnover in rat soleus muscle after burn injury. Metabolism *31:* 82–87 (1982).
12 Clark, A. S.; Kelly, R. A.; Mitch, W. E.: Systemic response to thermal injury in rats. Accelerated protein degradation and altered glucose utilization in muscle. J. clin. Invest. *74:* 888–897 (1984).
13 Shangraw, R. E.; Turinsky, J.: Altered protein kinetics in vivo after single-limb burn injury. Biochem. J. *223:* 747–753 (1984).
14 Baracos, V.; Rodemann, H. P.; Dinarello, C. A.; Goldberg, A. L.: Stimulation of muscle protein degradation and prostaglandin E_2 release by leukocytic pyrogen (interleukin-1). A mechanism for the increased degradation of muscle proteins during fever. New Engl. J. Med. *308:* 553–558 (1983).
15 Goldberg, A. L.; Baracos, V.; Rodemann, P.; Waxman, L.; Dinarello, C.: Control of protein degradation in muscle by prostaglandins, Ca^{2+}, and leukocytic pyrogen (interleukin-1). Fed. Proc. *43:* 1301–1306 (1984).
16 Rodemann, H. P.; Goldberg, A. L.: Arachidonic acid, prostaglandin E_2 and F_2 influence rates of protein turnover in skeletal and cardiac muscle. J. biol. Chem. *257:* 8716–8723 (1982).
17 Griffin, E. E.; Wildenthal, K.: Regulation of cardiac protein balance by hydrocortisone: Interaction with insulin. Am. J. Physiol. *234:* E 306–E 313 (1978).
18 Mayer, M.; Shafrir, E.: Glucocorticoid- and insulin-mediated regulation of skeletal muscle protein catabolism; in Shafrir, Lessons from animal diabetes, pp. 235–239 (John Libbey, London 1984).
19 Tischler, M. E.: Metabolic response of muscle to trauma; in Adibi, Branched chain amino and keto acids in health and disease, pp. 361–383 (Karger, Basel 1984).
20 Mallette, L. E.; Exton, J. H.; Park, C. R.: Control of glucose from amino acids in the perfused rat liver. J. biol. Chem. *244:* 5713–5723 (1969).
21 Tischler, M. E.; Desaultels, M.; Goldberg, A. L.: Does leucine, leucyl tRNA or some metabolite of leucine regulate protein synthesis and degradation in skeletal and cardiac muscle? J. biol. Chem. *257:* 1613–1621 (1982).
22 Fulks, R. M.; Li, J. B.; Goldberg, A. L.: Effects of insulin, glucose and amino acids on protein turnover in rat diaphragm. J. biol. Chem. *250:* 290–298 (1975).
23 Waalkes, T. P.; Udenfriend, S.: A fluorometric method for the estimation of tyrosine in plasma and tissues. J. Lab. clin. Med. *50:* 733–736 (1957).
24 Olefsky, J. M.: Insulin resistance and insulin action. An in vitro and in vivo perspective. Diabetes *30:* 148–162 (1981).
25 Wool, I. G.; Weinshelbaum, E. I.: Incorporation of C^{14}-amino acids into protein of isolated diaphragms: Role of the adrenal steroids. Am. J. Physiol. *197:* 1089–1092 (1959).
26 Shimizu, C. S. N.; Kaplan, S. A.: Effects of cortisone on in vitro incorporation of glycine into protein of rat diaphragm. Endocrinology *74:* 709–713 (1964).
27 Goldberg, A. L.: Protein turnover in skeletal muscle. J. biol. Chem. *244:* 3223–3229 (1969).
28 Kostyo, J. L.; Redmond, A. F.: Role of protein synthesis in the inhibitory action of

adrenal steroid hormones on amino acid transport by muscle. Endocrinology *79:* 531–540 (1966).
29 Rannels, S. R.; Rannels, D. E.; Pegg, A. E.; Jefferson, L. S.: Glucocorticoid effects on peptide-chain initiation in skeletal muscle and heart. Am. J. Physiol. *235:* E 134–E 139 (1978).
30 Tomas, F. M.; Munro, H. N.; Young, V. R.: Effect of glucocorticoid administration on the rate of muscle protein breakdown in vivo in rats as measured by urinary excretion of N-methylhistidine. Biochem. J. *178:* 139–146 (1979).
31 Santidrian, S.; Moreyra, M.; Munro, H. N.; Young, V. R.: Effect of corticosterone and its route of administration on muscle protein breakdown, measured in vivo by urinary excretion of N-methylhistidine in rats: Response to different levels of dietary protein and energy. Metabolism *30:* 798–804 (1981).
32 Shoji, S.; Pennington, R. J. T.: The effect of cortisone on protein breakdown and synthesis in rat skeletal muscle. Mol. cell. Endocrinol. *6:* 159–169 (1977).
33 Millward, D. J.; Garlick, P. J.; Nnanyelugo, D. O.; Waterlow, J. C.: The relative importance of protein synthesis and breakdown in the regulation of muscle mass. Biochem. J. *156:* 185–188 (1976).
34 Rannels, S. R.; Jefferson, L. S.: Effects of glucocorticoids on muscle protein turnover in perfused rat hemicorpus. Am. J. Physiol. *238:* E 564–E 572 (1980).
35 McGrath, J. A.; Goldspink, J. F.: Glucocorticoid action on protein synthesis and protein breakdown in isolated skeletal muscles. Biochem. J. *206:* 641–645 (1982).
36 Odedra, B. R.; Millward, D. J.: Effect of cortisone treatment on muscle protein turnover in adrenalectomized rats and diabetic rats maintained on insulin. Biochem. J. *204:* 663–672 (1982).
37 Li, J. B.; Goldberg, A. L.: Effects of food deprivation on protein synthesis and degradation in rat skeletal muscles. Am. J. Physiol. *231:* 441–448 (1976).
38 Jaspers, S. R.; Tischler, M. E.: Atrophy and growth failure of rat hind-limb muscles in tail-cast suspension. J. appl. Physiol. *57:* 1472–1479 (1984).

M. E. Tischler, Ph.D., Dept. of Biochemistry, Arizona Health Sciences Center, Tucson, AZ 85724 (USA)

Dietze, Grünert, Kleinberger, Wolfram (eds.), Clinical Nutrition and Metabolic Research. Proc. 7th Congr. ESPEN, Munich 1985, pp. 54–65 (Karger, Basel 1986)

Effect of Nutritional Substrates on Muscle Amino Acid and Protein Metabolism in Surgical Patients

P. D. Greig, A. E. Grote, J. Askanazi, Ch. B. Michelsen, D. H. Elwyn, J. M. Kinney

Departments of Surgery and Anesthesiology, Columbia University, New York, N.Y., USA, and the Department of Surgery, University of Toronto, Ontario, Canada
In collaboration with J. Bergström, P. Fürst, E. Vinnars

Introduction

Skeletal muscle protein metabolism plays a vital role in the metabolic response to starvation, injury, and sepsis. There is an efflux of amino acids from skeletal muscle resulting from net protein catabolism which are mobilized for use as energy substrate, either directly or through gluconeogenesis, or as substrates for the synthesis of more 'vital' proteins (fig. 1). As a result, skeletal muscle undergoes net protein breakdown with loss of muscle mass and a decline in skeletal muscle function. This muscle protein breakdown probably occurs in all muscle beds including diaphragm and cardiac muscle [1]. In the surgical patient skeletal muscle protein catabolism contributes to the increased negative nitrogen balance. As a result of injury, sepsis and burns, the increased need for amino acids increases the rate of amino acid mobilization and muscle protein loss [2].

With the development of total parenteral nutrition (TPN) and more sophisticated enteral nutrition, it is possible to achieve zero nitrogen and energy balance in virtually all patients. The mechanism of achieving nitrogen equilibrium is, however, not clear. With injury and sepsis there are increases in whole body protein synthesis and degradation rates which increase further with TPN [3]. Since skeletal muscle contributes considerably to this turnover, muscle protein synthesis and degradation may respond in a similar manner. In critically ill patients receiving TPN, 3-methylhistidine excretion remains elevated suggesting that skeletal

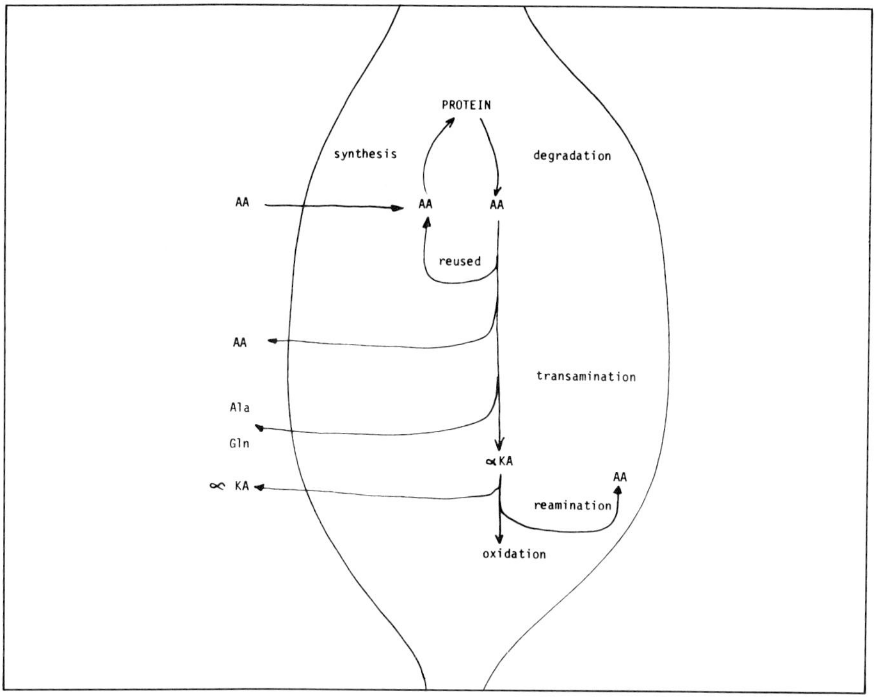

Fig. 1. Major metabolic pathways of intramuscular free amino acids.

muscle protein catabolism continues and that zero nitrogen balance is achieved through increases in protein synthesis rates [4]. A more recent study of acutely ill patients has reported a decrease in 3-methylhistidine excretion with TPN [5]. In-vitro studies have shown that skeletal muscle protein synthesis and degradation rates are sensitive to alterations in amino acids and glucose availability and hormonal changes [6]. In vivo, however, changes in protein synthesis rates appear to be primarily responsible for the dietary induced changes in protein metabolism [7].

Two questions arise: (1) What are the mechanisms responsible for the loss of skeletal muscle protein in man? and (2) How do nutritional substrates alter these mechanisms to achieve nitrogen equilibrium?

The ability to study skeletal muscle protein metabolism in man has been limited. Measurement of substrate balance across the forearm or leg are confounded by the contribution of other tissues of the limb and can only indicate the net balance of that substrate. Measurement of 3-methylhistidine excretion is confounded by the non-skeletal muscle protein contribution to this amino acid [8]. The development of in-vivo measurement of muscle protein synthesis rates using ^{13}C-leucine infusions represents an important breakthrough in this field [9]. This technique has been used to show that human muscle protein synthesis is highly sensitive to the effects of starvation and has suggested that it contributes to more than half of the whole body protein synthesis rate.

However, since these techniques cannot measure synthesis of proteins with rapid turnover times, and assume equilibration of isotope concentrations of precursors in cells and plasma, they severely underestimate the rates of protein synthesis on organs such as gut and liver.

We have used two techniques for the study of skeletal protein metabolism: (1) Measurement of intracellular free amino acid concentrations and (2) measurements of in-vitro protein synthesis and degradation rates.

Intramuscular Amino Acids

Plasma amino acid concentrations have been used to study the effect of injury and nutritional support on whole body protein metabolism [10]. The published results, however, have been highly variable. In general, with injury and sepsis there is an increase in circulating levels of phenylalanine and a decrease in alanine. Glutamine is often decreased, and the other amino acids, including the branched chain amino acids, tend to be unchanged. These levels are in general increased with the provision of amino acids or TPN. The significance of these changes, with respect to muscle protein metabolism, is not clear.

There is considerably more free amino acid intracellularly than in the extracellular fluid [10]. It is estimated that 80% of the free total amino acid pool is in skeletal muscle. There is a significant amino acid concentration gradient across the skeletal muscle cell ranging from approximately 25 for glutamate and glutamine to less than 2 for valine, leucine, isoleucine, phenylalanine, and tyrosine. Most other amino acids have an intracellular to extracellular ratio of between 5 and 10. It is not surprising, therefore, that circulating amino acid levels are relatively resistant to changes in nutritional state or the presence of surgical stress.

Intramuscular amino acid concentrations are more sensitive than plasma levels to the effects of trauma, injury, and sepsis. Moreover, there appears to be a complex interaction between the nutritional state, degree of activity, and the presence of surgical stress on free intracellular amino acids. In the postoperative state the total amount of free amino acid in skeletal muscle is decreased [11]. This results predominantly from decreases in the nonessential amino acids with an approximate 50% decrease in glutamine and smaller decreases in arginine, lysine, proline, and glutamic acid. There are significant increases in the branched chain amino acids – valine, isoleucine, and leucine – and increases in methionine and the aromatic amino acids, phenylalanine, and tyrosine. The same pattern is seen following severe trauma [12] and with the developement of sepsis, further increases in the branched chain and aromatic amino acids occur [13].

Total Hip Replacement as a Model for Operative Injury

To investigate the interaction of nutritional substrates and operative injury and the implications of these changes on intramuscular amino acids, the operation of total hip replacement was chosen as a model. This is an operation of moderate severity with a relatively consistent operative time, blood replacement, and degree of tissue injury from the dissection. In a series of prospective, randomized studies patients were recruited who were scheduled for elective total hip replacement. None had diabetes or liver disease and all were free from other significant illness. To study the different mechanisms by which amino acids and glucose effect skeletal muscle metabolism and attenuate the negative nitrogen balance in the postoperative state, patients were randomized to receive either 90 g of dextrose as 5% dextrose in water (D5W) or 70 g of 7% amino acids as their sole postoperative nutritional support. These diets were isocaloric. In some studies a combination of dextrose and amino acids was also used. Patients underwent a percutaneous skeletal muscle biopsy from the quadriceps femoris muscle preoperatively and again on the fourth postoperative day. Venous blood was drawn at the same time. These studies were approved by the Institutional Review Board at Columbia University and all patients gave informed written consent.

There was no difference in the nitrogen balance between those who received amino acids, D5W, or a combination of the two [14]. The resting energy expenditure on 5% dextrose was unchanged from the preoperative level but with 7% amino acids there was a 15% increase in REE. In the groups receiving amino acids only, this was associated with a significant increase in norepinephrine excretion.

Associated with these whole body changes there were significant changes in muscle composition. There were increases in muscle water, sodium, and chloride with a slight reduction in potassium. These changes were present regardless of the nutritional intake [15].

Intramuscular Amino Acids Following Hip Replacement

The free intramuscular amino acids demonstrated the pattern characteristic of injury in the postoperative state [16]. With 5% dextrose there were increases in the branched chain and aromatic amino acids, and decreases in glutamine, histidine, and ornithine (fig. 2). With isocaloric amino acids the pattern of change was essentially the same. The plasma concentrations of the branched chain and aromatic amino acids were increased postoperatively with D5W and were elevated further with isocaloric amino acids.

Some of these changes in muscle amino acid can be attributed to inactivity [17]. In normal volunteers with bed rest and 5% dextrose, there are modest increases in the branched chain amino acids and phenylalanine; however, the increases are not as great as those seen postoperatively. In addition, the postoperative increases in tyrosine and methionine and decrease in glutamine do not occur in the normal controls. Thus there appears to be an interaction between operative injury and inactivity on intramuscular levels of amino acids.

In normal subjects, unlike postoperative patients, intramuscular free amino acid levels are sensitive to nutritional control [18]. The intracellular levels of the branched chain amino acids are elevated to a greater extent with 7% amino acids than with isocaloric 5% dextrose. In the postoperative patient, however, it appears that the increases in these amino acids resulting from injury mask the effect of the different intravenous diets.

Similarly in the acutely ill patient, total parenteral nutrition has little effect on the free intracellular amino acid pattern [10]. The changes that are characteristic of trauma and sepsis are essentially unchanged with the administration of total parenteral nutrition.

This 'pattern of trauma' appears to be maintained irrespective of nutritional support. Moreover, the increased branched chain and aromatic amino acids are also increased in simple semistarvation or bed rest. Since

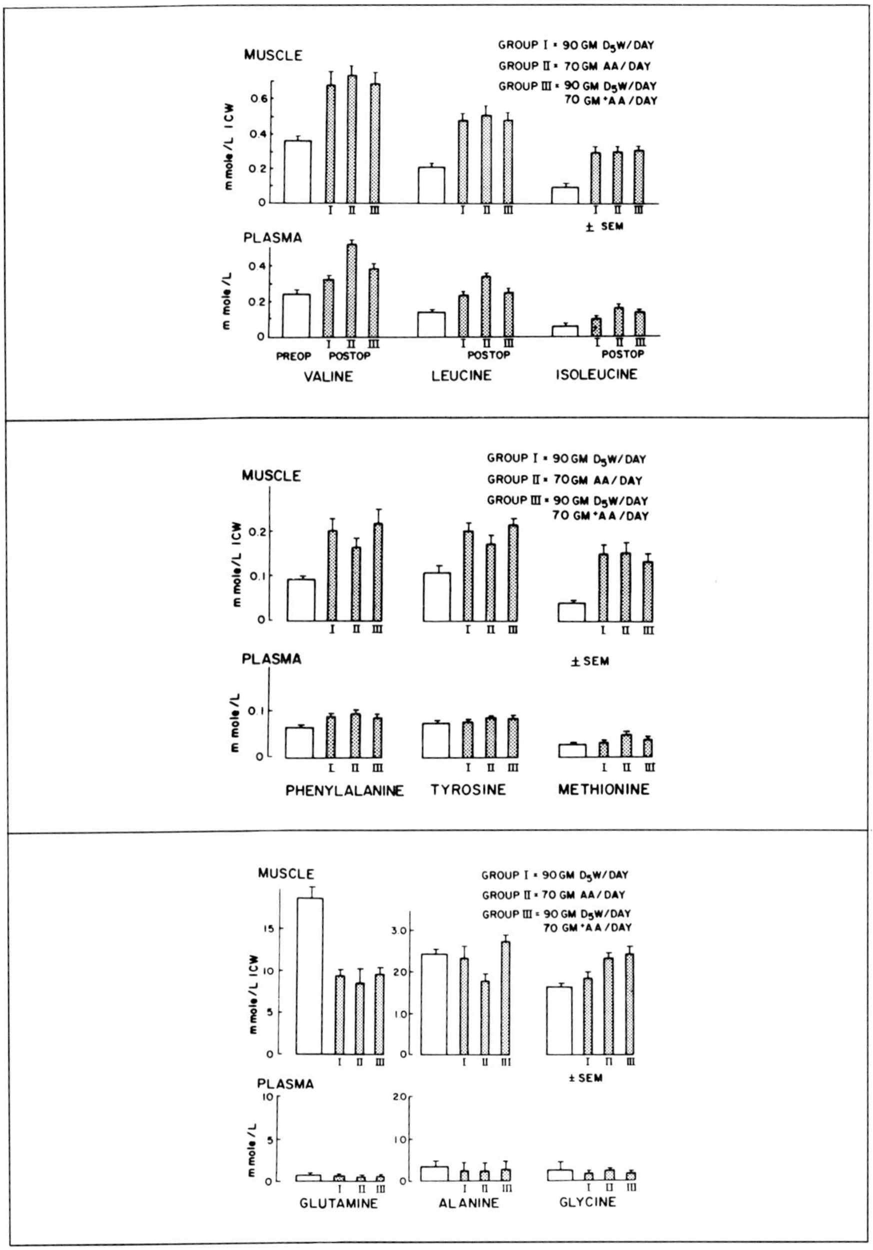

Fig. 2. Effect of glucose and amino acids on plasma and intramuscular free amino acids following total hip replacement [16].

it is likely that there are considerable differences in the muscle protein synthesis rate of each of these states, it is unlikely that intracellular amino acid levels regulate protein synthesis. These levels may, however, be the result of an increased rate of protein degradation. Alternatively, they may be the result of changes in muscle membrane transport mechanisms responsible for maintaining the extra- to intracellular gradient [31].

In-Vitro Studies of Skeletal Muscle Protein Metabolism

Skeletal muscle protein metabolism can also be studied by directly measuring the rates of protein synthesis and degradation. In incubations of isolated, intact rat muscles, the rates of in-vitro protein synthesis and degradation are constant for up to 3 h [1]. These in-vitro rates are sensitive to substrate and hormonal changes in the incubation medium [6, 19] and to the effects of starvation [1], burn injury [20], and trauma [21].

Lundholm et al. have extended this technique to studies of protein metabolism in fibers of human skeletal muscle [22, 23]. The in-vitro synthesis and degradation rates in tissue from surgical muscle biopsies were constant for 4 h and, like the intact rat muscles, were sensitive to changes in the incubation medium. Clowes et al. have also used this technique in man to identify increases in the in-vitro protein synthesis and degradation rates that occur in muscle fibers from septic patients [24].

We wished to study skeletal muscle protein synthesis and degradation rates using the muscle tissue obtained with the Bergstrom muscle biopsy needle [25]. In an experimental rat model we have determined that a 20–30 mg biopsy of skeletal muscle tissue can be used in a manner similar to that of the intact muscle to identify changes in protein synthesis and degradation rates that result from changes in the nutritional status of the animal [26].

The in-vitro protein synthesis rate of a biopsy taken from the gastrocnemius was constant for 3 h and was 39% and 32% for the extensor digitorum longus (EDL) and soleus muscles, respectively. The in-vitro protein degradation rate was intermediate between the rates of these two muscles. With starvation there was a 42% decrease in the synthesis rate and a 53% increase in degradation rate. These changes were intermediate between the changes measured in the EDL and soleus.

In-vitro protein synthesis was measured as the rate of incorporation of radioactively labeled tyrosine into protein during incubations in oxygen-ated Krebs-Ringer bicarbonate buffer, pH 7.4, with glucose (10 mM), insulin (0.1 IU/ml), and 23 amino acids at ten times rat plasma levels. The specific activity (SA) of the incubation medium was used as the SA of the precursor. Tyrosine was chosen as the tracer amino acid as it is neither synthesized nor degraded in skeletal muscle. The rate of degradation was measured as the rate of release of tyrosine from protein into the medium during incubations in buffer with glucose (10 mM) and cycloheximide (0.5 mM), an inhibitor of protein synthesis, to prevent re-utilization of the released tyrosine.

Caution must be exercised in the interpretation of in-vitro synthesis and degradation rates of biopsies of skeletal muscle tissue. The rate of protein degradation is considerably greater than that of in-vitro protein synthesis indicating a net catabolic state of the tissue during incubation. Moreover, the incubation medium does not reproduce in-vivo conditions but was designed to maximize both synthesis and degradation rate in vitro. Paired clinical studies have been used in an attempt to identify changes in the intramuscular synthesis or degradation mechanisms that occur in the postoperative period. The changes that are identified in vitro may be modified in vivo by the circulating hormone/substrate profile of the patient.

Protein Synthesis and Degradation Following Hip Replacement

Using the same model of operative injury as the previous human studies, we randomized 20 patients to receive either 5% dextrose (90 g/day, n = 10) or 7% amino acids (70 g/day, n = 10) for the first 4 postoperative days as their sole nutritional intake. Percutaneous suction needle biopsies of the vastus lateralis muscle [27] were taken preoperatively, in the postabsorptive state following the induction of anesthesia, and again on the morning of the fourth postoperative day under local anesthesia. Protein synthesis rate was measured in triplicate as the incorporation of ^{3}H-tyrosine into protein during 2-h incubations of 15–40 mg biopsies. In separate incubations the protein degradation rate was measured in triplicate as a release of tyrosine into the incubation medium.

There was no change in muscle protein content in either the amino acid or glucose group (table I). With glucose there was a significant 13% decrease in the RNA content. With the administration of isocaloric amino acids the 6% decline in RNA was not statistically significant.

Table I. Effect of dextrose or amino acids on muscle composition following total hip replacement

n	Dextrose 10		Amino acids 10	
	pre	post	pre	post
Protein mg/µg DNA	0.38 0.02	0.33 ± 0.02	0.36 ± 0.02	0.33 ± 0.02
RNA mg/µg DNA	2.0 ± 0.2	1.7* ± 0.2	1.9 ± 0.2	1.7 ± 0.1

p < 0.05

Associated with the decrease in RNA with 5% dextrose, there was a significant 20% decrease in the protein synthesis rate (fig. 3). The administration of amino acids attenuated this effect and the 5% decrease was not statistically significant. The in-vitro protein degradation rate with dextrose increased 11% ($p < 0.05$). With amino acids, the 12% decrease did not reach statistical significance (fig. 4).

With conventional postoperative support using 5% dextrose the net catabolism of skeletal muscle protein appears to be due in part to changes

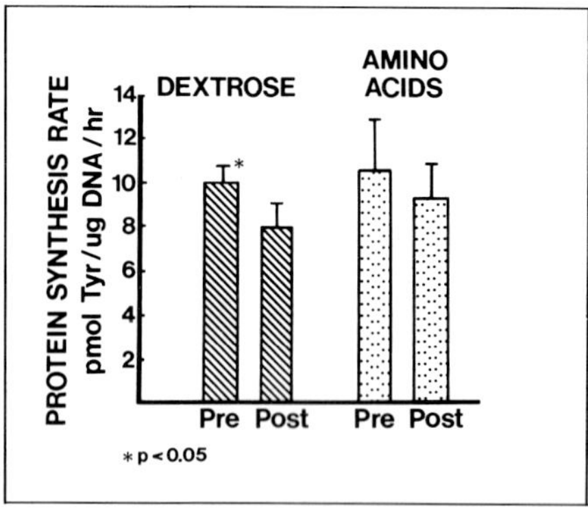

3

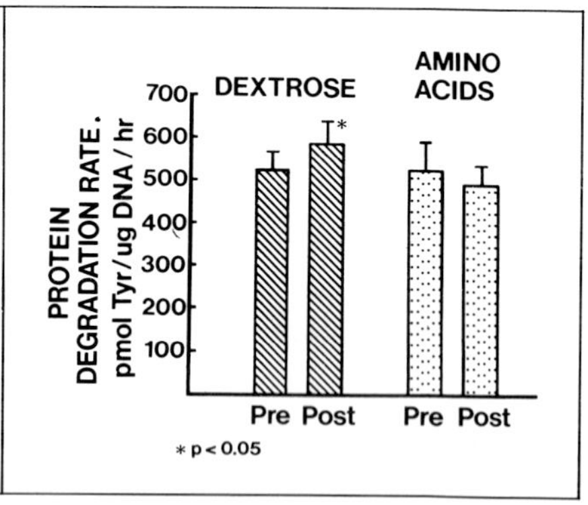

4

Fig. 3. Effect of dextrose or amino acids on in-vitro muscle protein synthesis rates following total hip replacement.

Fig. 4. Effect of dextrose or amino acids on in-vitro muscle protein degradation rates following total hip replacement.

in both protein synthesis and degradation. There are decreases in the total RNA content and in the ability of the skeletal muscle protein synthetic apparatus to incorporate amino acids into protein in vitro. In addition there is a significant increase of in-vitro protein degradation. Whether these changes of in-vitro protein metabolism reflect changes of in-vivo protein synthesis and degradation remains to be determined. There may be other in-vivo factors which are not present in the incubation media, including prostaglandins, interleukin-1 [28], and other circulating factors [24] and hormones, which are known to alter synthesis or degradation rates.

Although the same degree of nitrogen sparing can be achieved with the provision of isocaloric amino acids [14], this study demonstrates that this nutritional substrate has a different effect on skeletal muscle protein metabolism. There is an attenuation of the decrease of the RNA content and the changes in both synthesis and degradation that occur with glucose. Amino acids have been recognized to maintain RNA content and the integrity of ribosomal RNA and protein synthesis in liver [29]. It may be that the same mechanism is operative in skeletal muscle. These data suggest that either amino acids spare skeletal muscle protein at the expense of other protein in the body or that there are in-vivo changes in synthesis or degradation rates that cannot be identified with these in-vitro studies. Circulating factors which have been shown to increase the protein degradation rate [24, 28] may be particularly important here.

Combining these findings with the previous studies of intramuscular amino acid concentrations following hip replacement [16], it appears that the differences in RNA content and in-vitro protein synthesis and degradation rates occur in the setting of equivalent patterns of intracellular amino acids. If these changes in synthesis and degradation occur in vivo, this dissociation suggests that postoperative changes in free intramuscular amino acids are not related in a cause or effect manner to the changes in protein turnover, but may be more the net result of changes in a membrane transport that result from operative injury, inactivity or semistarvation.

The model of total hip replacement has also been used to study the effect of nutritional substrates on high energy phosphogens postoperatively [30]. With 5% dextrose no changes could be identified in ATP, ADP, PC, AMP, or free creatine. However, with isocaloric amino acids, significant decreases in ATP, ADP and PC were measured, with reciprocal increases in AMP and free creatine. These data suggest that both the characteristic pattern of postoperative intramuscular amino acids and the changes of in-vitro protein synthesis and degradation are independent of the high energy phosphate content of muscle.

References

1 Li, J. B.; Goldberg, A. L.: Effects of food deprivation on protein synthesis and degradation in rat skeletal muscles. Am. J. Physiol. *231:* 441–448 (1976).

2 Aulick, L. H.; Wilmore, D. W.: Increased peripheral amino acid release following burn injury. Surgery *85:* 560–565 (1979).

3 Kinney, J. M.; Elwyn, D. H.: Protein metabolism and injury. Ann. Rev. Nutr. *3:* 433–466 (1983).

4 Shenkin, A.; Neuhauser, M.; Bergstrom, J.; Chao, L.; Larsson, J.; Liljedahl, S.-O.; Schildt, B.; Fürst, P.: Biochemical changes associated with severe trauma. Am. J. clin. Nutr. *33:* 2119–2127 (1980).

5 Iapichino, G.; Radrizzani, D.; Solca, M.; Bonetti, G.; Leoni, L.; Ferro, A.: Influence of total parenteral nutrition on protein metabolism following acute injury: assessment by urinary 3-methylhistidine excretion and nitrogen balance. J. parent. ent. Nutr. *9:* 42–46 (1985).

6 Fulks, R. M.; Li, J. B.; Goldberg, A. L.: Effects of insulin, glucose and amino acids on protein turnover in rat diaphragm. J. biol. Chem. *250:* 290–298 (1975).

7 Waterlow, J. C.; Garlick, P. J.; Millward, D. J.: The effects of nutrition and hormones on protein turnover in muscle; in Protein turnover in mammalian tissues and the whole body, pp. 625–696 (North-Holland Pub. Co., Amsterdam 1985).

8 Millward, D. J.; Bates, P. C.; Grimble, G. K.; Brown, J. G.: Quantitative importance of non-skeletal-muscle sources of Nt-methyl-histidine in urine. Biochem. J. *190:* 225–228 (1980).

9 Rennie, M. J.; Edwards, R. H. T.; Halliday, D.; Matthews, D. E.; Wolman, S. L.; Millward, D. J.: Muscle protein synthesis measured by stable isotope techniques in man: the effects of feeding and fasting. Clin. Sci. *63:* 519–523 (1982).

10 Vinnars, E.; Fürst, P.; Liljedahl, S.-O.; Larsson, J.; Schildt, B.: Effect of parenteral nutrition on intracellular free amino acid concentration. J. parent. ent. Nutr. *4:* 184–187 (1980).

11 Vinnars, E.; Bergstrom, J.; Fürst, P.: Influence of the postoperative state in intracellular free amino acids in human muscle tissue. Ann. Surg. *182:* 665–671 (1975).

12 Milewski, P. J.; Threlfall, C. J.; Heath, D. F.; Holbrook, I. B.; Wilford, K.; Irving, M. H.: Intracellular free amino acids in undernourished patients with or without sepsis. Clin. Sci. *62:* 83–91 (1982).

13 Askanazi, J.; Carpentier, Y. A.; Michelsen, C. B.; Elwyn, D. H.; Fürst, P.; Kantrowitz, L. R.; Gump, F. E.; Kinney, J. M.: Muscle and plasma amino acids following injury. Influence of intercurrent infection. Ann. Surg. *192:* 78–85 (1980).

14 Askanazi, J.; Carpentier, Y. A.; Jeevanandam, M.; Michelsen, C. B.; Elwyn, D. H.; Kinney, J. M.: Energy expenditure, nitrogen balance, and norepinephrine excretion after injury. Surgery *89:* 478–484 (1981).

15 Bergstrom, J.; Fürst, P.; Holmstrom, B.; Vinnars, E.; Askanazi, J.; Elwyn, D. H.;

Michelsen, C. B.; Kinney, J. M.: Influence of injury and nutrition on muscle water and electrolytes. Effect of elective operation. Ann. Surg. *193:* 810–816 (1981).

16 Askanazi, J.; Fürst, P.; Michelsen, C. B.; Elwyn, D. H.; Vinnars, E.; Gump, F. E.; Stinchfield, F. E.; Kinney, J. M.: Muscle and plasma amino acids after injury. Hypocaloric glucose vs. amino acid infusion. Ann. Surg. *191:* 465–472 (1980).

17 Askanazi, J.; Elwyn, D. H.; Kinney, J. M.; Gump, F. E.; Michelsen, C. B.; Stinchfield, F. E.: Muscle and plasma amino acids after injury. The role of inactivity. Ann. Surg. *188:* 797–803 (1978).

18 Gil, K. M.; Fürst, P.; Wood, J.; Askanazi, J.; Elwyn, D. H.; Kinney, J. M.: Muscle and plasma amino acids during semistarvation in normal subjects: hypocaloric glucose vs. amino acid infusions. Clin. Nutr. *4:* 21–27 (1985).

19 Hedden, M. P.; Buse, M. G.: Effects of glucose pyruvate, lactate, and amino acids on muscle protein synthesis. Am. J. Physiol. *242:* E 184–E 192 (1982).

20 Shangraw, R. E.; Turinsky, J.: Effect of disuse and thermal injury on protein turnover in skeletal muscle. J. Surg. Res. *33:* 345–355 (1982).

21 Tischler, M. E.; Fagan, J. M.: Response to trauma of protein, amino acid, and carbohydrate metabolism in injured and uninjured rat skeletal muscles. Metabolism *32:* 853–868 (1983).

22 Lundholm, K.; Schersten, T.: Protein synthesis in human muscle tissue: influence of insulin and amino acids. Eur. J. clin. Invest. *7:* 531–536 (1977).

23 Lundholm, K.; Edstrom, S.; Ekman, L.; Karlberg, I.; Walker, P.; Schersten, T.: Protein degradation in human skeletal muscle tissue. The effect of insulin, leucine, amino acids, and ions. Clin. Sci. *60:* 319–326 (1981).

24 Clowes, G. H. A.; George, B. C.; Villee, C. A.; Saravis, C. A.: Muscle proteolysis induced by a circulating peptide in patients with sepsis or trauma. New Engl. J. Med. *308:* 545–552 (1983).

25 Bergstrom, J.: Muscle electrolytes in man. Scand. J. clin. Lab. Invest. *14:* suppl. 68, 1–110 (1962).

26 Greig, P. D.; Rozovski, S. J.; Elwyn, D. H.; Kinney, J. M.: Protein synthesis and degradation in biopsies of rat skeletal muscle. J. Surg. Res. (in press).

27 Greig, P. D.; Askanazi, J.; Kinney, J. M.: Needle biopsy of skeletal muscle using suction. Surgery Gynec. Obstet. *160:* 466–468 (1985).

28 Baracos, V.; Rodemann, H. P.; Dinarello, C. A.; Goldberg, A. L.: Stimulation of muscle protein degradation and prostaglandin E2 release by leucocytic pyrogen (interleukin-1). A mechanism for the increased degradation of muscle protein during fever. New Engl. J. Med. *308:* 553–558 (1983).

29 Flaim, K. E.; Liao, W. S. L.; Peavy, D. E.; Taylor, J. M.; Jefferson, L. S.: The role of amino acids in the regulation of protein synthesis in perfused rat liver. II. Effects of amino acid deficiency on peptide chain initiation, polysomal aggregation and distribution of albumin mRNA. J. Biol. Chem. *257:* 2939–2946 (1982).

30 Liaw, K. Y.; Askanazi, J.; Michelsen, C. B.; Fürst, P.; Elwyn, D. H.; Kinney, J. M.: Effect of postoperative nutrition on muscle high energy phosphates. Ann. Surg. *195:* 12–18 (1982).

P. D. Greig, MD, Department of Surgery? Toronto General Hospital,
Eaton Wing 9-237, 200 Elizabeth Street, Toronto, Ontario, M5G 1L7 (Canada)

Dietze, Grünert, Kleinberger, Wolfram (eds.), Clinical Nutrition and Metabolic Research. Proc. 7th Congr. ESPEN, Munich 1985, pp. 66–85 (Karger, Basel 1986)

Protein Synthesis after Trauma as Studied by Muscle Ribosome Profiles

J. Wernerman, A. von der Decken, E. Vinnars

Dept. of Anaesthesiology and Metabolic Research Laboratory, St. Erik's Hospital, Stockholm, and the Wenner-Gren Institute for Experimental Biology, University of Stockholm, Sweden

Background

The metabolic response to injury includes an increase in oxygen consumption and lipolysis, retention of sodium and water, and a phase of protein catabolism in which body proteins are degraded [30]. Since proteins have specific functions in the organism and the loss of protein can be considerable, protein catabolism will eventually lead to impairment of organ function. Normally there is a balance between protein synthesis and breakdown, but posttraumatically the degree of degradation becomes greater than that of synthesis. After surgery of moderate magnitude, there is a decrease in whole-body synthesis rather than an increase in degradation [11, 42]. In the case of larger trauma, both synthesis and degradation increase, the enhancement of degradation being the more pronounced [5, 29]. In the posttraumatic period, the nitrogen balance becomes negative as a result of an increase in urinary excretion of nitrogenous compounds, mainly urea [12, 13, 20]. A major part of the nitrogen excreted derives from skeletal muscle [13]. Protein loss from skeletal muscle causes muscular fatigue and, hence, trauma in a patient needs to be followed by a period of convalescence, the extent of which depends upon the amount of muscle protein lost [30]. Preservation of body proteins is, therefore, an important task in the management of posttraumatic patients.

Nutritional support has been instituted posttraumatically to counteract the catabolism and reverse the negative nitrogen balance [14, 30]. Enteral and parenteral feeding improve the negative nitrogen balance but not to a sufficient extent for it to attain equilibrium [14]. Several adjuvant therapies have been instituted in addition to postoperative nutrition; epidural blockade [9, 29], pharmacological doses of insulin [66], ornithine-alpha-ketoglutarate [32, 53], branched-chain amino acids [10], and growth hormone [65] are examples.

Skeletal muscle supplies the major part of the excreted nitrogen posttraumatically [13]. The muscle protein waste is greater than would be expected from immobilization alone [13, 48]. There is a postoperative efflux of amino acids from peripheral tissues [47, 50], and there are typical changes in the pattern of the intracellular concentrations of free amino acids in skeletal muscle following trauma [4, 54, 55]. Indirect calculations suggest that there is a decrease in muscle protein synthesis rather than an increase in degradation following uncomplicated surgery [11, 43]. Therefore, estimation of muscle protein synthesis in the posttraumatic period is necessary to understand the pathophysiology of trauma and for evaluation of nutritional support.

Analysis of Ribosomes

The formation of a polypeptide chain involves initiation, elongation, and termination phases in which the ribosomes are involved in a cyclic manner (fig. 1). Polyribosomes represent the active ribosome state of protein synthesis [1, 2, 39], and monoribosomes and subunits, the inactive state. The amount of polyribosomes in percent of the total ribosomes is positively correlated to the activity of protein synthesis [16–18, 22, 24, 34, 41, 67]. Monoribosomes and subunits which are not reutilized are successively degraded [23]. Isolation of ribosomes and analysis of their size distribution have been performed in animal studies for more than 20 years to assess protein synthesis. A ribosome profile should reproduce as closely as possible the size distribution of ribosomes in the intact cell in vivo. The ribosome profile and the percentage amount of polyribosomes in skeletal muscle have been used to study muscle dystrophy in human subjects [25, 37, 52]. The growth and development of muscle tissue in animals have been investigated by means of sucrose density gradient analysis of ribosomes [67]. The impact of different dietary proteins on protein synthesis in rat skeletal muscle has been elucidated from ribosome profiles [16]. The viability of muscle tissue close to shot wounds in pigs has also been assessed [22]. The effect of changes in nutrition condition upon

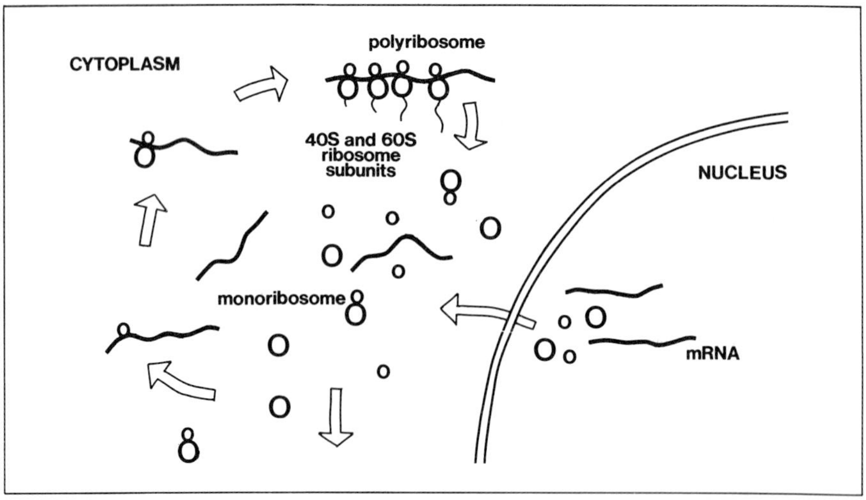

Fig. 1. The polyribosome-subunit cycle [24]. Translation of one molecule of protein is completed within a few minutes [39, 49]. Thereafter, ribosomes are present in the cytoplasm as monoribosomes and subunits. New ribosome subunits are produced from the nucleus and old ribosomes are degraded. When changes in protein synthesis activity occur, the relative distribution between polyribosomes, monoribosomes and subunits is altered [67]. The initiation of translation when a ribosome becomes attached to a mRNA molecule is thought to be the rate-limiting step [35], followed by elongation of the polypeptide chain and the termination of translation provided charged tRNAs and promoting factors are available. Figure from [59].

protein synthesis in the epaxial muscle in fish has also been studied by this method [34].

For harvesting of ribosomes, the biopsy material is gently homogenized and then centrifuged, and a postmitochondrial supernatant is obtained [64]. If the homogenization is too gentle, membrane-bound ribosomes will collect in the low-speed centrifugation pellet. On the other hand, too vigorous homogenization will disrupt the polyribosome complexes. The ribosome fraction is isolated from the postmitochondrial supernatant by ultracentrifugation through a layer of increased sucrose concentration. This facilitates washing of the ribosomes, and detergents accumulate in the top layer. The ribosomes sediment to a pellet. The RNase activity is confined to the postribosome supernatant but monoribosomes still tend to separate from the preparation unless the profile is spun quickly through the sucrose gradient after harvesting [45]. The size distribution is revealed by ultracentrifugation in a continuous sucrose gradient [64] which can be designed according to the purpose of the investigation.

The preparation of ribosomes from skeletal muscle was performed as described by Bullock et al. [8], Peters et al. [44], and von der Decken et al. [16], with several minor modifications [60]. Smaller tissue specimens than have been used in earlier animal studies were employed, and the spectrophotometer had a greater sensitivity than in the early investigations. The analytic procedure, including the isolation of ribosomes and their separation according to size, was carried out at 4 °C. All samples from the same subject were analyzed in parallel. The biopsy specimen was homogenized gently in a medium containing sucrose, an RNase inhibitor, and the detergent Nonidet P40. After a low-speed centrifugation, the ribosomes remained in the supernatant fraction while nuclei, mitochondria, and membrane fragments had sedimented. The pellet was saved for DNA analysis [61]. The addition of a detergent agent to the medium is essential for a good yield of ribosomes without too rough homogenization which would destroy the polyribosomes. Using this technique, 90% of the RNA was found in the low-speed supernatant as measured by the orcinol method [59], assuming that 10% of the DNA present in the pellet also reacted with orcinol [38]. No DNA or mitochondria that could have interfered with subsequent analyses were present in the supernatant. To separate the ribosomes from particles of lower molecular weight, the supernatant was layered onto a medium with an increased sucrose concentration and ultracentrifuged. The ribosome pellet thus obtained was suspended in medium and the ribosome concentration was measured as absorbance at 260 nm [38]. The concentration of ribosomes was expressed per g wet weight of muscle tissue, or per mg of DNA. Since the water content of muscle tissue varies in connection with starvation and trauma, a reference not subject to such changes was preferred. It is also shown that the DNA to protein ratio increases in depleted patients (Wernerman, Hultman, unpublished data).

The separation of ribosomes according to size was performed according to the method of von der Decken et al. [15, 16] with some modifications [60]. A part of the ribosome suspension was layered onto a sucrose density gradient of between 0.4 M and 1.5 M. After ultracentrifugation, the gradient was pumped through a continuous flow cuvette and the absorbance was monitored at 260 nm. The absorbance profile was recorded and the peaks were identified as corresponding to ribosome particles of different sedimentation values (fig. 2). The areas under the

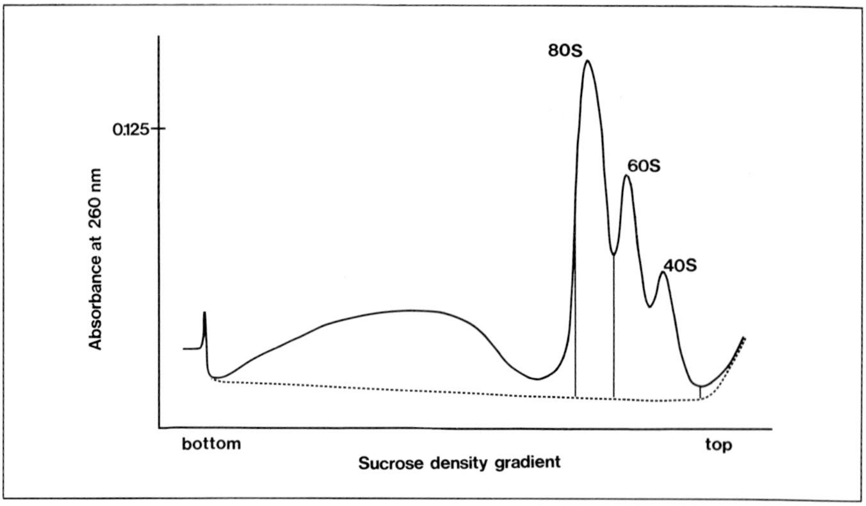

Fig. 2. The size distribution of ribosomes in a 50 mg specimen of human skeletal muscle as demonstrated by the absorbance at 260 nm. The ribosomes were isolated and then separated according to their mass by ultracentrifugation in a linear sucrose density gradient [60]. The 80S monoribosome peak and the peaks corresponding to the 40S and 60S ribosome subunits are indicated. Polyribosomes are distributed according to size left of the 80S peak. The relative abundance of the particles was calculated from the areas under the curve as percent of the total area. Figure from [59].

curve representing the amount of particles were determined. The content of polyribosomes was calculated as percentage of the total ribosome area including ribosome subunits, monoribosomes, and polyribosomes. The same separation technique and equal amounts of material from different species and from different tissues yielded ribosome profiles of slightly different appearances (fig. 3). The percentage proportion of polyribosomes is higher in human papillary muscle than in human skeletal muscle (fig. 3d; Wernerman, Sylvén, Jansson, von der Decken, Vinnars, unpublished results). Incubation of the ribosome suspension in the presence of RNase before the density gradient centrifugation transformed 85% of the polyribosomes into monoribosomes and subunits, indicating that true polyribosomes were being measured [7, 34].

Percutaneous muscle biopsies were taken from the lateral portion of the quadriceps femoris muscle after local anesthesia of the skin [3]. Muscle tissue specimens of 50 mg wet weight were obtained without difficulty and the procedure could be repeated 3 or 4 times in the same subject without causing more than minor discomfort. The biopsy was carefully dissected to remove visible fat and connective tissue, and weighed 5 times in 40 s; from these weights, the wet weight at time zero was extrapolated. The specimen was frozen in liquid nitrogen within 3 min and stored at – 80 °C for no longer than 2 weeks before analysis.

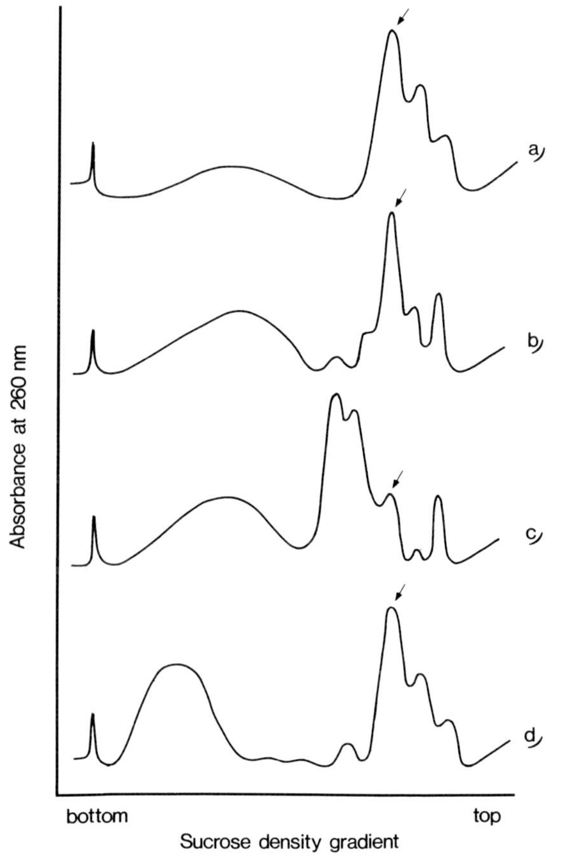

Fig. 3. The size distribution in a sucrose density gradient of ribosomes isolated from a 50 mg specimen of tissue from: (*a*) the lateral portion of the quadriceps femoris muscle in man, (*b*) the gastrocnemic muscle of the mouse hind leg, (*c*) the extensor digitorum longus muscle of the rat hind leg, and (*d*) human papillary muscle. The 80S monoribosome peaks are indicated by arrows. In some curves, there are peaks corresponding to ribosome dimers and trimers immediately to the left of the 80S peak followed by the polyribosome area. To the right are ribosome subunit peaks. Figure from [59].

Characterization of the Ribosome Method

A standardized hospital diet was given to 12 healthy male volunteers [62]. The total ribosome concentration per mg of DNA and the percentage proportion of polyribosomes were determined. No significant changes were recorded in either of these variables during the day (fig. 4). The results show that a muscle specimen taken in the morning after an overnight fast is representative of the ribosome concentration and size distribution during the day. This favors sampling in the morning which is a well-defined and easily reproducible point in time. Since there were no changes in the total ribosome concentration per mg of DNA and the percentage proportion of ribosomes during the day, the data from the above series of experiments were used to evaluate the reproducibility of the ribosome method. The mean value during the day for the former variable for each individual subject gave a coefficient of variation of 5.6% and for the latter variable 5.4%.

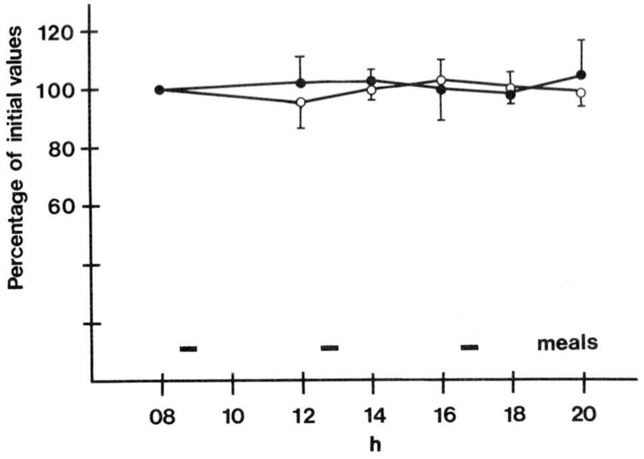

Fig. 4. The diurnal patterns of the concentration of ribosomes per mg of DNA (●——●) and the percentage of polyribosomes (○——○) expressed as percent of the initial value, determined at 08.00 h after an overnight fast in healthy volunteers [62]. The food intake was a standardized hospital diet and meals were given at 08.30, 12.30, and 16.30 h. Biopsies were taken either 3.5 h (experiment 1; n = 6) or 1.5 h (experiment 2; n = 6) following the start of a meal. No differences in either of the variables were detected during the day. Data are given as mean ± SEM. Figure from [59].

During 3 days of total starvation in 23 healthy volunteers, there was a decrease in the total concentration of ribosomes per g wet weight muscle tissue [60] and per mg of DNA [61] as compared with the prestarvation values (fig. 5). The percentage proportion of polyribosomes also decreased. On the first day of starvation, the decreases were only of a

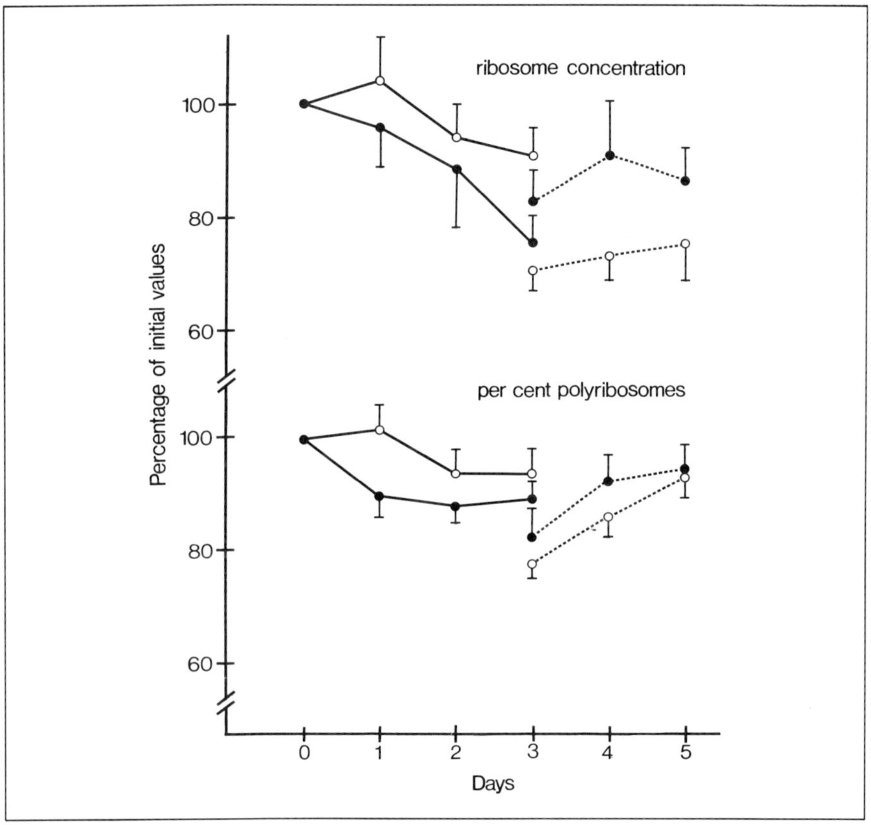

Fig. 5. The concentration of ribosomes per g wet weight or mg of DNA (upper curves) and the percentage proportion of polyribosomes (lower curves) expressed as percent of the initial values obtained on day 0 of the studies in healthy volunteers [60, 61]. The curves represent men (●——●; n = 6) and women (○——○; n = 5) who were starved for 3 days, and refeeding in male subjects after 3 days of starvation, either parenterally (●-----●; n = 6) or enterally (○-----○; n = 6). The two variables measured decreased significantly during starvation in all groups, and the percentage proportion of polyribosomes increased significantly during refeeding in both groups. There were no differences between the groups. Data are given as mean ± SEM. Figure from [59].

minor degree, but on the second and third days they became significant [60]. No sex-dependent differences were observed [60]. In 12 healthy subjects, 2 days of refeeding following 3 days of starvation caused a rise in the percentage proportion of polyribosomes and there was a slight increase in the ribosome concentration per mg of DNA. Refeeding was given parenterally or enterally but no differences were observed attributable to the route of food administration [61]. The refeeding experiment showed an increase in ribosome utilization attributable to the provision of nutrition after a period of starvation. The improvement was most pronounced in the percentage proportion of polyribosomes, corresponding to a more efficient use of available ribosomes. The total ribosome concentration responded more slowly to refeeding and the increase did not reach significance. This suggests that changes in protein synthesis activity are most readily reflected in the percentage of polyribosomes. It is noteworthy that the total ribosome concentration decreased after 2 days of starvation but did not increase on the second day of refeeding.

Comparison of the Ribosome Method and Incorporation Methods

Rats were used to compare 3 different methods of studying protein synthesis in skeletal muscle during changes in nutrition conditions [63]. The animals were starved for 3 days, followed by 2 days of refeeding. The extensor digitorum longus (EDL) muscles of both hind legs were used to study protein synthesis. The total ribosome concentration, the percentage proportion of polyribosomes and the incorporation of ^{14}C-leucine into protein in a cell-free system were determined. The incorporation of ^{14}C-phenylalanine into protein by the intact EDL muscle is a well-characterized method [51] and was also used for comparison. The total ribosome concentration per mg of DNA decreased during starvation (fig. 6), indicating a marked fall in the capacity for protein synthesis. After the 2 days of refeeding, no increase in the total ribosome concentration was observed. The percentage proportion of polyribosomes decreased after 1 day of starvation, was restored to the original level on the 3rd day of starvation, and lay above that level after 2 days of refeeding. The results suggest that the percentage proportion of polyribosomes became a measure of the changes in the activity of protein synthesis. The 2 methods, incorporation of amino acids into protein by cell-free systems or by intact muscle, showed similar results. During starvation, the incorporation

Fig. 6. The concentration of ribosomes per mg of DNA (○——○), the percentage proportion of polyribosomes (●——●), the incorporation of ^{14}C-leucine into protein in a cell-free system (○-----○), and that of ^{14}C-phenylalanine into protein in the intact muscle (●-----●) expressed as percent of the initial nonstarvation value [63]. Rats were starved for 3 days followed by 2 days of refeeding. The concentration of ribosomes decreased significanlty during starvation and was still low after refeeding. The percentage proportion of polyribosomes decreased significantly on the first day of starvation, returned to the nonstarvation level on the third day of starvation, and increased significantly over that level after refeeding. The values in the two incorporation assays decreased significantly during starvation and increased after refeeding as compared with the starvation values. Incorporation by the intact muscle increased significantly above the nonstarvation value after refeeding. Data are given as mean ± SEM. Figure from [59].

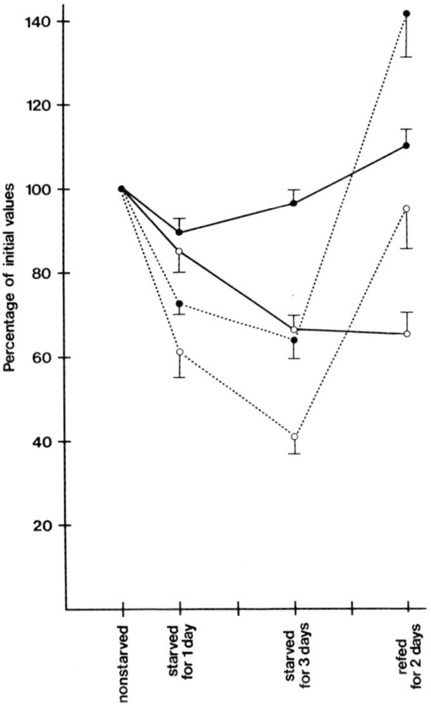

activities decreased to half the nonstarvation values and, after 2 days of refeeding, the original level was restored; and, in the case of incorporation by the intact muscle, that level was even exceeded. The results obtained in rats indicate that protein synthesis can be measured either by combining the results for the total ribosome concentration with the percentage proportion of polyribosomes, or by the incorporation studies.

The Effect of Elective Abdominal Surgery upon Muscle Protein Synthesis

Patients undergoing cholecystectomy (n = 16) were investigated [58]. Independent of nutritional support, the total ribosome concentration per mg of DNA and the percentage proportion of polyribosomes decreased on the first and third days postoperatively (fig. 7), suggesting that the operative trauma per se initiated the decrease in ribosome utilization. The decrease in the concentration of polyribosomes was of the same magnitude as that observed during total starvation, indicating that skeletal muscle was used as a source of nutritional substrates posttraumatically. Physical immobilization is not likely to contribute to the decrease in ribo-

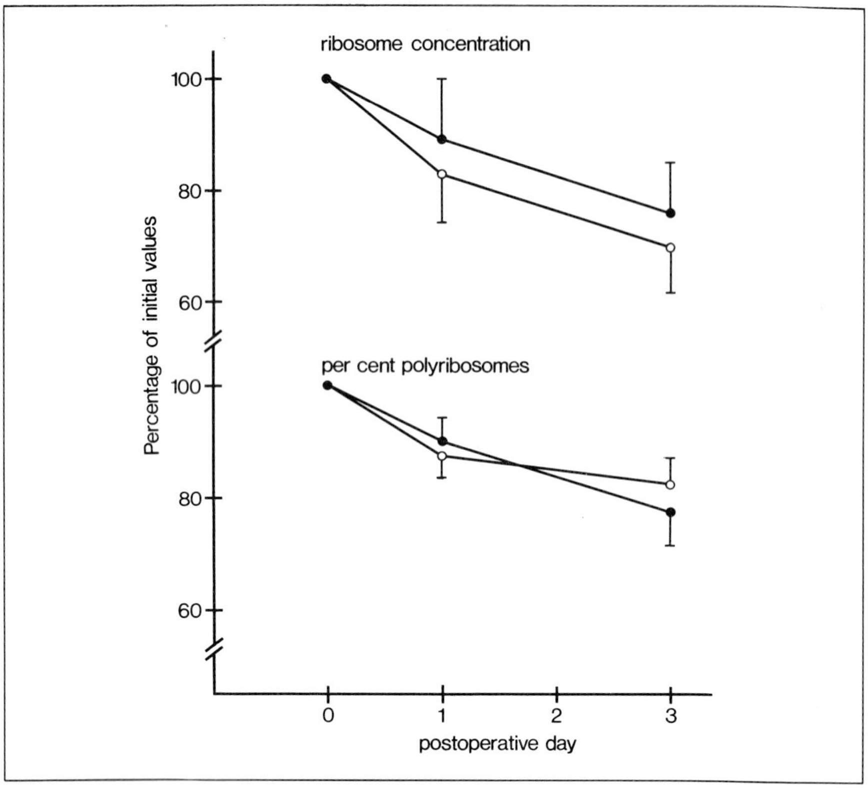

Fig. 7. The concentration of ribosomes per mg of DNA and the percentage proportion of polyribosomes as percent of the initial value obtained preoperatively in patients undergoing elective abdominal surgery [58]. Postoperatively the patients were given electrolyte solutions only (○——○; n = 7) or TPN (●——●; n = 9). The two variables decreased significantly in the immediate postoperative period in both groups. There were no differences between the groups, indicating that muscle protein synthesis did not benefit from postoperative TPN. Data are given as mean ± SEM. Figure from [59].

some function since it has been reported that a negative nitrogen balance is not observed until the 5th day of immobilization in a plaster of Paris splint [51]. Protein synthesis in skeletal muscle after surgery has not previously been estimated by tissue analysis. The results presented indicate a marked decrease in both the activity and the capacity of protein synthesis.

The Effect of Postoperative TPN upon Protein Synthesis in Skeletal Muscle

To evaluate the effect of nutritional support postoperatively, patients were given TPN after elective abdominal surgery [58]. The nitrogen balance was improved in the group receiving TPN ($n = 9$) for 3 days following surgery, as compared to the group given electrolyte solutions alone ($n = 7$). However, the nitrogen balance did not attain equilibrium. The 2 groups did not receive the same amount of calories and, therefore, the nitrogen balances were not quite comparable [69]. The marked difference in nitrogen balance was indicative of nitrogen retention in the TPN group, although the quantification must be interpreted with caution.

Protein synthesis in skeletal muscle, as determined by the ribosome method, did not respond to the administration of postoperative TPN. There were no differences in the total ribosome concentration and the percentage proportion of polyribosomes between the 2 groups (fig. 7). This finding is in accordance with the results obtained from measurements of the concentrations of intracellular free amino acids in skeletal muscle [55, 56] and of the efflux of tyrosine from the leg [47]. The distinct changes in muscle amino acids observed posttraumatically are not reversed by the provision of nutritional support.

The improvement in nitrogen balance in the TPN group as compared with the group receiving electrolyte solutions alone, combined with the unaltered state of protein synthesis in the skeletal muscle, indicates that other organs benefit from the nutritional support. This is also suggested by reports of an increase in the incorporation of labelled amino acids into whole-body protein in patients receiving postoperative TPN as compared with those maintained on 5% glucose solutions only [43]. The question in what tissues protein synthesis responds to nutritional support after surgery is still unanswered.

The Effect of Postoperative TPN Enriched with BCAA upon Muscle Protein Synthesis

BCAA are claimed to preserve muscle nitrogen when given after trauma [6]. Six patients were studied after elective abdominal surgery [21]. They were given a TPN program which was enriched with BCAA, 36% against 16% in the conventional TPN formula. The patients received 0.2 g N/kg body weight/day and 135 kJ/kg body weight/day,

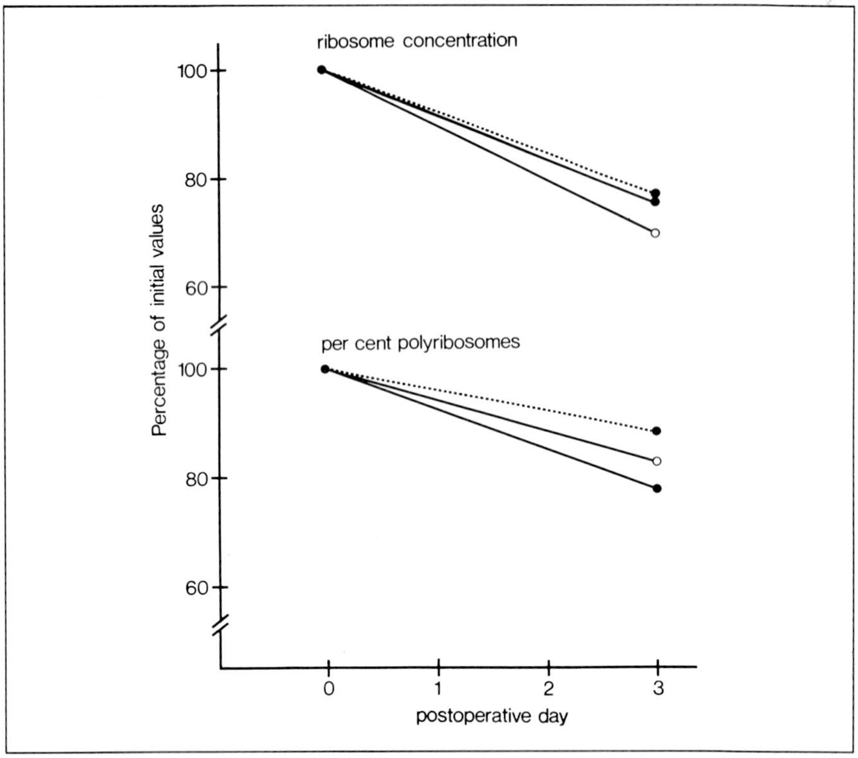

Fig. 8. The concentration of ribosomes per mg of DNA and the percentage proportion of polyribosomes as percent of the initial value obtained preoperatively in patients undergoing elective abdominal surgery [21, 58]. Postoperatively the patients were given electrolyte solutions only (○——○; n = 7), conventional TPN (●——●; n = 9), or a TPN formula enriched with BCAA (●-----●; n = 6). The two variables decreased significantly in the immediate postoperative period in all three groups. There were no differences between the groups, indicating that muscle protein synthesis did not benefit from postoperative TPN, enriched with BCAA or not. Data are given as mean ± SEM.

equal amounts of carbohydrate and fat. The results were compared to a group of patients receiving a conventional TPN program of the same nitrogen and energy content. Muscle biopsies were taken before surgery and on the third postoperative day. There was no difference in nitrogen balance. The concentration of ribosomes per g wet weight and the size distribution of ribosomes revealed no differences between the two groups attributable to the content of BCAA in the TPN formula (fig. 8).

Discussion

When the ribosome method was applied to a situation of starvation in human subjects, the polyribosome content showed a tendency to decrease before any reduction in the total ribosome concentration occurred [60]. In rats, there was an initial decrease in the percentage proportion of polyribosomes and restoration to normal on the third day of starvation, corresponding to a lower rate of ribosome degradation [63]. Upon refeeding, there was an increase in the percentage amount of polyribosomes in both rat and man, indicating efficient utilization of the available ribosomes [61, 63]. However, there was only a tendency towards an increase in the total ribosome population during the 2 days of refeeding studied.

The control of translation is regarded to lie at the level of initiation [31, 35]. The attachment of the mRNA molecule to the initiation complex seems to be the rate-limiting step [31]. This implies that the proportion of polyribosomes is a direct indicator of the activity of protein synthesis. An additional factor of importance is the total ribosome concentration [40]. This concentration and the percentage amount of polyribosomes together reflect the capacity and the activity of protein synthesis. In rapidly regenerating animal systems, it has been shown that available ribosomes are better able to incorporate radioactive amino acids as compared with control systems [26, 44]. This can be explained by a more intensive use of amino acids from exogenous sources for protein synthesis since the translation time has been found to be unaltered [49]. In addition, at least in rapidly regenerating systems, the individual ribosome seems to have a greater ability to form peptide bonds [27].

The findings during short-term starvation of healthy subjects [60, 61] are consistent with earlier reports [36]. Rennie et al. reported that the incorporation of ^{13}C-leucine into protein in skeletal muscle in vivo was doubled in the fed state compared with 18 h of fasting [46]. The effect on the polyribosome concentration was less marked [60, 61]. In vivo experiments require knowledge about the pool size of the amino acid which is used as the isotope and also about deamination and oxidation rates. The apparent discrepancy between the incorporation of ^{13}C-leucine in vivo and the polyribosome concentration cannot be explained at present. It is clear that there is a need to assess protein synthesis by several independent methods.

Elective abdominal surgery leads to a reduction of protein synthesis in skeletal muscle in the immediate postoperative period [58]. This finding is in accordance with earlier reports on muscle protein synthesis measured indirectly [11, 43], or as the efflux of tyrosine from the leg [47]. Physical immobilization was not considered to contribute to this decrease, considering the short period that elapsed from the time of operation until a negative nitrogen balance was recorded [48] and in view of the early mobilization of the patients. In addition, the capacity of key enzymes in the energy metabolism has been reported to be unaltered 3 days after elective surgery [64]. This is in accordance with the findings after 1 week of immobilization but in contrast to the decrease observed after 6 weeks (Sylvén, Eriksson, personal communication). The influence of starvation was ruled out by the finding that administration of TPN did not change either the total ribosome content or the size distribution of the ribosomes.

Complete postoperative nutritional support did not prevent the decrease in ribosome concentration and activity in skeletal muscle that have been shown to occur following surgery [58]. The results are consistent with the changes observed in muscle amino acid composition and concentration [55, 56], and the failure of the nitrogen balance to reverse and become positive by nutritional means [19]. The decrease in polyribosome concentration could not be attributed to immobilization since in healthy subjects this concentration increased during parenteral refeeding after 3 days of starvation [61], the physical activity of the volunteers and the cholecystectomy patients being comparable. Since the nitrogen balance was markedly improved by postoperative TPN, it was proposed that the protein synthesis in organs other than skeletal muscle was stimulated. This concept is supported by the increase in whole-body protein synthesis noted in response to postoperative nutritional support [43]. It was demonstrated that the depression of protein synthesis in skeletal muscle following trauma can neither be prevented nor reversed by nutritional means alone in the immediate postoperative period. This unresponsiveness has been suggested previously but has not, until now, been demonstrated by direct measurements in the actual tissue. The effects of providing an amino acid solution enriched with branched-chain amino acids following elective abdominal surgery was also studied, but this did not improve protein synthesis in skeletal muscle postoperatively as compared with a conventional TPN regimen [21]. New therapeutic approaches must be sought in order to prevent the muscle waste following surgery. The ribosome method of assessing muscle protein synthesis is a tool which can be used to evaluate the effect of different adjuvant therapies combined with total parenteral nutrition in posttraumatic patients.

Acknowledgments

The authors wish to acknowledge the skillful technical assistance of Mrs. H. Lundström and Mrs. C. Hebert. This work was supported by grants from the Swedish Medical Research Council (project B83-17X-04210-10C), the TRYGG-HANSA Research Fund, the PFRIMMER/MEDA Scholarship 1984, and the Swedish Nutrition Foundation.

References

1 Beecher, G. R.: Some practical applications of protein synthesis and muscle growth. J. Anim. Sci. *38:* 1071–1078 (1974).
2 Bergen, W. G.: Protein synthesis in animal models. J. Anim. Sci. *38:* 1079–1091 (1974).
3 Bergström, J.: Muscle electrolytes in man. Scand. J. clin. Lab. Invest. *14:* suppl. 168, pp. 11–13 (1962).
4 Bergström, J.; Fürst, P.; Noree, L.-O.; Vinnars, E.: The intracellular free amino acid concentration in human muscle tissue. J. appl. Physiol. *36:* 690–697 (1974).
5 Birkhahn, R. H.; Long, C. L.; Fitkin, D.; Geriger, J. W.; Blakemore, W. S.: Effects of major skeletal trauma on whole body turnover in man measured by L-(1,^{14}C)-leucine. Surgery *88:* 294–300 (1980).
6 Blackburn, G. L.; Moldawer, L. L.; Usui, S.; Bothe, A.; O'Keefe, S. J. D.; Bistrian, B. R.: Branched chain amino acid administration and metabolism during starvation, injury, and infection. Surgery *86:* 307–315 (1979).
7 Breuer, C. B.; Davies, M. C.; Florini, J. R.: Amino acid incorporation into protein by cell-free preparations from rat skeletal muscle. II. Preparation and properties of muscle ribosomes and polyribosomes. Biochemistry *3:* 1713–1719 (1964).
8 Bullock, G.; White, A. M.; Worthington, J.: The effect of catabolic and anabolic steroids on amino acid incorporation by skeletal muscle ribosomes. Biochem. J. *108:* 417–425 (1968).
9 Christensen, T.; Waaben, J.; Lindeburg, T.; Vesterberg, K.; Vinnars, E.; Kehlet, H.:

Epidural analgesia attenuates postoperative changes in muscle amino acids. 42nd Congr. Nordic Surg. Soc., 1985, p. 31 (1985).
10 Clauge, M. B.; Borzotta, A. P.; Johnston, I. D. A.: Leucine and protein kinetics following surgery in man given varying branched-chain amino acid concentrations in a parenteral nutrition regimen. Proc. Nutr. Soc. *413:* 19 (1985).
11 Crane, C. W.; Picou, D.; Smith, R.; Waterlow, J. C.: Protein turnover in patients before and after elective orthopedic operations. Br. J. Surg. *64:* 129–133 (1977).
12 Cuthbertson, D. P.: The disturbance of metabolism produced by bony and non-bony injury, with notes on certain abnormal conditions of bone. Biochem. J. *24:* 1244–1263 (1930).
13 Cuthbertson, D. P.: The distribution of nitrogen and sulfur in the urine during conditions of increased catabolism. Biochem. J. *25:* 236–244 (1931).
14 Cuthbertson, D. P.: Further observations on the disturbance of metabolism caused by injury, with particular reference to the dietary requirements of fracture cases. Br. J. Surg. *23:* 505–521 (1936).
15 Decken, A. von der: Activation in vitro of rat liver polyribosomes. J. Cell Biol. *43:* 138–147 (1969).
16 Decken, A. von der; Omstedt, P. T.: Protein feeding of rats after protein starvation: Incorporation of amino acid into polypeptide by skeletal muscle polyribosomes. J. Nutr. *100:* 623–630 (1970).
17 Decken, A. von der: Experimental studies on the quality of food proteins. Compar. Biochem. Physiol. *74B.* 213–220 (1983).
18 Enwonwu, C. O.; Stambaugh, R.; Sreebny, L.: Synthesis and degradation of liver ribosomal RNA in fed and fasted rats. J. Nutr. *101:* 337–346 (1971).
19 Ewerth, S.; Allgén, L.-G.; Fürst, P.; Holmström, B.; Odebäck, A.-C.; Schildt, B.; Vinnars, E.: Metabolic effects of four intravenous nutritional regimens after elective surgery. I. Clinical data and biochemistry. Clin. Nutr. *1:* 313–324 (1983).
20 Fleck, A.; Munro, H. N.: The determination of organic nitrogen in biological materials. Clin. Chem. *11:* 2–12 (1965).
21 Hammarkvist, F.; Wernerman, J.; Decken, A. von der; Vinnars, E.: The effect of branched chain amino acids (BCAA) on postoperative muscle protein synthesis and nitrogen balance. Clin. Nutr. *4:* spec. suppl., p. 68 (1985).
22 Hasselgren, P. O.; Almskog, B.; Lund, B.; Decken, A. von der; Nordström, G.; Seeman, T.: Leucine incorporation into skeletal muscle proteins in vitro and protein synthesis by isolated ribosomes from skeletal muscle around a high velocity missile injury. Acta chir. scand., suppl. 508, pp. 337–344 (1982).
23 Henshaw, E. C.; Hirsch, C. A.; Morton, B. E.; Hiatt, H. H.: Control of protein synthesis in mammalian tissues through changes in ribosome activity. J. biol. Chem. *246:* 436–446 (1971).
24 Henshaw, E. C.; Guiney, D. G.; Hirsch, C. A.: The ribosome cycle in mammalian protein synthesis. I. The place of monometric ribosomes and ribosomal subunits in the cycle. J. biol. Chem. *248:* 4367–4376 (1973).
25 Ionasescu, V.; Zellweger, H.; Conway, T. W.: Ribosomal protein synthesis in Duchenne muscular dystrophy. Archs Biochem. Biophys. *144:* 51–58 (1971).
26 Jones, G. H.: Protein synthesis in bupivacaine (marcaine)-treated, regenerating skeletal muscle. Muscle Nerve *5:* 281–290 (1982).

27 Jones, G. H.: Function of ribosomes and glutamyl-tRNA isoacceptors in protein synthesis in regenerating skeletal muscle. Biochim. biophys. Acta *824:* 324–329 (1985).
28 Kehlet, H.; Brandt, M. R.; Prange Hansen, A.; Alberti, K. G. M. M.: Effect of epidural analgesia on metabolic profiles during and after surgery. Br. J. Surg. *66:* 543–546 (1979).
29 Kien, C. L.; Young, V. R.; Rohrbaugh, D. K.; Burke, J. F.: Increased rates of whole body protein synthesis and breakdown in children recovering from burns. Ann. Surg. *187:* 383–391 (1978).
30 Kinney, J. M.: The metabolic response to injury; in Richards, Kinney, Nutritional aspects of care in the critically ill, pp. 95–133 (Churchill Livingstone, Edinburgh 1977).
31 Kramer, G.; Hardesty, B.: Regulation of eukaryotic protein synthesis; in Prescott, Goldstein, Cell biology: A comprehensive treatise. IV. Gene expression: Translation and the behavior of proteins, pp. 69–105 (Academic Press, New York 1980).
32 Leander, U.; Fürst, P.; Vesterberg, K.; Vinnars, E.: Nitrogen sparing effect of Ornicetil® in the immediate postoperative state: Clinical biochemistry and nitrogen balance. Clin. Nutr. *4:* 43–51 (1985).
33 Lied, E.; Lund, B.; Decken, A. von der: Protein synthesis in vitro by epaxial muscle polyribosomes from cod, Gadus Morhua. Compar. Biochem. Physiol. *72B:* 187–193 (1982).
34 Lied, E.; Rosenlund, G.; Lund, B.; Decken, A. von der: Effect of starvation and refeeding on in vitro protein synthesis in white trunk muscle of atlantic cod (Gadus Morhua). Compar. Biochem. Physiol. *76B:* 777–781 (1983).
35 Lodish, H. F.: Translational control of protein synthesis. Annu. Rev. Biochem. *45:* 39–72 (1976).
36 Meguid, M. M.; Collier, M. D.; Howard, L. J.: Uncomplicated and stressed starvation. Surg. Clins N. Am. *61:* 529–543 (1981).
37 Monckton, G.; Nihei, T.: A correlation of histology and amino acid incorporation studies in Duchenne muscular dystrophy. Neurology *19:* 415–418 (1969).
38 Munro, H. N.; Fleck, A.: The determination of nucleic acids. Meth. biochem. Analysis *14:* 113–176 (1966).
39 Munro, H. N.: A general survey of mechanisms regulating protein metabolism in mammals; in Munro, Mammalian protein metabolism, vol. IV, pp. 3–130 (Academic Press, New York 1970).
40 Munro, H. N.; Hubert, C.; Baliga, B. S.: Regulation of protein synthesis in relation to amino acid supply – A review; in Rothschild, Oratz, Schreiber, Alcohol and abnormal protein biosynthesis, biochemical and clinical, pp. 33–66 (Pergamon Press, Oxford 1975).
41 Nowak, T. S.; Carty, E. R.; Lust, W. D.; Passonneau, J. V.: An in vitro amino acid incorporation method for assessing the status of in vivo protein synthesis. Analyt. Biochem. *136:* 285–292 (1984).
42 O'Keefe, S. J. D.; Sender, P. M.; James, W. P. T.: 'Catabolic' loss of body nitrogen in response to surgery. Lancet *ii:* 1035–1038 (1974).
43 O'Keefe, S. J. D.; Moldawer, L. L.; Young, V. R.; Blackburn, G. L.: The influence of intravenous nutrition on protein dynamics following surgery. Metabolism *30:* 1150–1158 (1981).

44 Peters, R. F.; Richardson, M. C.; Small, M.; White, A. M.: Some biochemical effects of triamcinolone acetonide on rat liver and muscle. Biochem. J. *116:* 349–355 (1970).

45 Pronczuk, A. W.; Baliga, B. S.; Triant, J. W.; Munro, H. N.: Comparison of the effect of amino acid supply on hepatic polysome profiles in vivo and in vitro. Biochim. biophys. Acta *157:* 204–206 (1968).

46 Rennie, M. J.; Edwards, R. H. T.; Halliday, D.; Matthews, D. E.; Wolman, S. L.; Millward, D. J.: Muscle protein synthesis measured by stable isotope techniques in man: The effects of feeding and fasting. Clin. Sci. *63:* 519–523 (1982).

47 Rennie, M. J.; Bennegård, K.; Edén, E.; Emery, P. W.; Lundholm, K.: Urinary excretion and efflux from the leg of 3-methylhistidine before and after major surgical operation. Metabolism *33:* 250–256 (1984).

48 Schønheyder, F.; Heilskov, N. S. C.; Olesen, K.: Isotopic studies on the mechanism of negative nitrogen balance produced by immobilization. Scand. J. clin. Lab. Invest. *6:* 178–188 (1954).

49 Scornic, O. A.: In vivo rate of translation by ribosomes of normal and regenerating liver. J. biol. Chem. *249:* 3876–3883 (1974).

50 Stjernström, H.; Lund, J.; Vinnars, E.; Wiklund, L.: Peripheral turnover of amino acids during abdominal surgery. Clin. Nutr. *1:* spec. suppl., p. 100 (1984).

51 Svaninger, G.; Bennegård, K.; Ekman, L.; Ternell, M.; Lundholm, K.: Lack of evidence for elevated breakdown rate of skeletal muscles in weight-losing, tumor-bearing mice. J. natn. Cancer Inst. *71:* 341–346 (1983).

52 Trampé, P. O.; Buuren, K. J. H. van: A rapid procedure for the isolation of active human muscle polysomes. Archs Biochem. Biophys. *144:* 54–58 (1982).

53 Vesterberg, K.; Leander, U.; Fürst, P.; Vinnars, E.: Nitrogen sparing effect of Ornicetil® in trauma. II. Muscle and plasma amino acids. Clin. Nutr. *1:* spec. suppl., p. 138 (1982).

54 Vinnars, E.; Bergström, J.; Fürst, P.: Influence of the postoperative state on the intracellular free amino acids in human muscle tissue. Ann. Surg. *182:* 665–671 (1975).

55 Vinnars, E.; Fürst, P.; Liljedahl, S.-O.; Larsson, J.; Schildt, B.: The effect of parenteral nutrition on intracellular free amino acid concentration. J. parent. ent. Nutr. *4:* 184–187 (1980).

56 Vinnars, E.; Holmström, B.; Schildt, B.; Odebäck, A.-C.; Fürst, P.: Metabolic effects of four intravenous nutritional regimens in patients undergoing elective surgery. II. Muscle amino acids and energy-rich phosphates. Clin. Nutr. *2:* 3–11 (1983).

57 Wernerman, J.; Decken, A. von der; Vinnars, E.: The effect of short-term postoperative total parenteral nutrition upon the protein synthesis activity in skeletal muscle. ESPEN 6th Congress, Milan 1984 (not published).

58 Wernerman, J.; Magnusson, K.; Ekman, L.; Decken, A. von der; Vinnars, E.: Comparison of different techniques to measure protein synthesis in skeletal muscle. Clin. Nutr. *4:* spec. suppl., p. 91 (1985).

59 Wernerman, J.; Decken, A. von der; Vinnars, E.: Size distribution of ribosomes in biopsy specimen of human skeletal muscle during starvation. Metabolism *34:* 665–669 (1985).

60 Wernerman, J.; Decken, A. von der; Vinnars, E.: Polyribosome concentration in human skeletal muscle after starvation and parenteral or enteral refeeding. Metabolism (in press).

61 Wernerman, J.; Decken, A. von der; Vinnars, E.: The diurnal pattern of protein synthesis in human skeletal muscle. Clin. Nutr. (in press).

62 Wernerman, J.: Protein synthesis in skeletal muscle: Assessed by the concentration and size distribution of ribosomes; thesis Stockholm (1985).

63 Wernerman, J.; Sylvén, C.; Jansson, E.; Decken, A. von der; Vinnars, E.: Energy metabolism and protein synthesis in human skeletal muscle following abdominal surgery. Clin. Nutr. *4:* spec. suppl., p. 38 (1985).

64 Wettstein, F. O.; Staehlin, T.; Noll, H.: Ribosomal aggregate engaged in protein synthesis: Characterization of the ergosome. Nature *197:* 430–435 (1963).

65 Wilmore, D. W.; Moylan, J. A.; Briston, B. F.: Anabolic effects of human growth hormone and high caloric feeding following thermal injury. Surgery Gynec. Obstet. *138:* 875–884 (1974).

66 Woolfson, A. M. J.; Heatley, R. V.; Allison, S. P.: Insulin to inhibit protein catabolism after injury. New Engl. J. Med. *300:* 14–17 (1979).

67 Young, V. R.; Chen, S. C.; Newberne, P. M.: Effect of infection on skeletal muscle ribosomes in rats fed adequate or low protein. J. Nutr. *94:* 361–368 (1968).

68 Young, V. R.: The role of skeletal and cardiac muscle in the regulation of protein metabolism; in Munro, Mammalian protein metabolism, pp. 585–674 (Academic Press, New York 1970).

69 Young, V. R.; Robert, J. J.; Motl, K. J.; Matthews, D. E.; Bier, D. M.: Protein and energy intake in relation to protein turnover in man; in Waterlow, Stephen, Nitrogen metabolism in man, pp. 419–447 (Applied Science Publishers, London 1981).

J. Wernerman, Dept. of Anaesthesiology, St. Erik's Hospital. S-10691 Stockholm (Sweden)

Dietze, Grünert, Kleinberger, Wolfram (eds.), Clinical Nutrition and Metabolic Research. Proc. 7th Congr. ESPEN, Munich 1985, pp. 86–92 (Karger, Basel 1986)

Intestinal Motility in the Critically Ill – Influences on Enteral Feeding

R. C. Spiller

Gastroenterology Unit, Mayo Clinic, Rochester, Minn., USA

The conventional teaching that critically ill patients could not be fed by the enteral route because of the associated 'paralytic ileus' is currently under challenge. This challenge is based both on the practical experience of a number of enthusiasts [1–4] and on the results of a number of radiological studies of motility early in the postoperative period. These studies showed that although barium contrast remained in the hypomotile stomach if barium could be either induced to empty from the stomach or was instilled by tube directly into the jejunum, then passage through the small bowel was relatively normal [5, 6] as was absorption [7, 8]. However, transit of barium provides only a very crude assessment of motor activity and since these studies were done there have been very substantial advances in our understanding of small bowel motility. In particular, we now recognize that in normal fasting man, there is a recurring cyclical pattern, the interdigestive migrating motor complex [9, 10]. This comprises three phases which migrate in sequence down the jejunum and proximal ileum [11] about once every 90 min. Phase I comprises a period of quiescence lasting for about one-third to one-half of the cycle. This is followed by a period of increasing but irregular activity, phase II, which ends in phase III, a period of rapid (7–12 cpm), uniform, high amplitude, phasic pressure waves, lasting 5–10 min in the jejunum. Although in the dog these migrating complexes invariably reach the ileocolonic junction [12], in man most fade out in the distal ileum [13]. The significance of such migrating complexes is that they effectively propel small bowel contents distally [14, 15] and this acceleration of transit may reduce absorption [16]. Thus, in the dog jejunum absorption is reduced during phase III compared with phases I and II. Feeding by either the oral [17], gastric

[18], or intrajejunal [19] route promptly abolishes this cyclical pattern replacing it with more continuous irregular pressure waves which resemble those seen in phase II. This fed pattern is associated with a significantly greater absorption of water and electrolytes [16]. The implication of this appears to be that to maximize absorption a fed pattern should be induced. This can most easily be achieved with intrajejunal feeding if some fat is included in the diet, as calorie for calorie this is the most potent nutrient for abolishing the fasting motility pattern [19].

Turning now from studies of normal physiology to the critically ill patient who may be hypoxic, shocked, traumatized, in pain, and is often under the influence of opiate analgesia. All these factors are known to delay gastric emptying by a combination of pylorospasm and antral hypomotility [20–23]. However, the effect of such stimuli on small bowel motility is much less well documented perhaps because until recently the recording techniques have been considered too invasive to be used in such patients. Modern studies have therefore been largely confined to patients recovering from elective major abdominal surgery. In these patients, serosal electrodes can be attached to the small bowel and the leads taken out via the drain site to recording devices allowing documentation of small bowel myoelectric patterns. Such studies [24] have demonstrated that the myoelectric equivalent of phase III recurs regularly soon after surgery. Less invasively, pressure wave activity in the upper small intestine can be monitored using a perfused nasoduodenal manometry tube [25] or if electrodes are placed on such a tube, it can be modified to provide a recording of small bowel myoelectric activity [26]. Using these techniques, it has been shown that whereas the motor and myoelectric activity of the stomach is disrupted for 1–2 days following surgery, regular phase III activity can be detected in the duodenum [25] and jejunum [26] within 2 h of closing the abdomen. Compared with normal subjects [11], these patients showed rather frequent cycles (intercycle time 40–60 min) which often had very short or absent phase II activity. Part of this increased frequency appears to be related to the administration of morphine which causes an abrupt increase in cycle frequency [25] but this is not the only factor since a similar frequency was noted when opiates were withheld [26]. It may reflect in part the release of endogenous opiates such as β-endorphin which are released in such stressed patients and have been shown to induce frequent phase IIIs in man [27]. When comparing these few human studies with the more analytical studies on experimental animals, it becomes apparent that there may be important species differences. Thus, in both dogs and rats [28, 29], laparotomy and intestinal handling tends to disrupt the fasting pattern in the first 24 h, replacing it with irregular spiking, whereas similar procedures in sheep inhibit only phase II, leaving phase III relatively unchanged. Increasing the amount of trauma inflicted on the canine intestine by rubbing it with a dry sponge [30], or resecting part of the colon [28], prolongs this disruption to 1–3 days and delays transit of plastic particles through the small bowel [30]. Interestingly, splanchnic nerve section [28, 29] prevented this disruption of motility but alpha and beta blockade with high doses of phentolamine and propranolol [30] did not, suggesting that the effects of laparotomy are mediated via non-adrenergic inhibitory pathways in the splanchnic nerves. There is no ready explanation why the pattern observed in man after surgery differs from some of the experimental animals but in the normal case, when routine postoperative analgesia is provided, opiates undoubtedly do stimulate the frequent occurrence of phase III-like activity. The effect of morphine has been most extensively analyzed in dogs in which species it stimulates MMCs in both the fasting and fed state. These morphine-induced phase IIIs are of normal duration and frequency but migrate more rapidly down the jejunum slowing up in the ileum [31]. The dose required to produce phase IIIs is larger (0.1 μg/kg) in the fed state than during fasting (0.05 μg/kg) and part of its effect may depend upon inhibition of gastric emptying. Thus, if food is presented intrajejunally, morphine induces for the most part, non-migrating phase IIIs which, unlike normal phase IIIs, do not appear to accelerate transit and enhance rather than impair absorption [32]. Thus, we can conclude that the use of opiates as postoperative analgesia, though it decreases tolerance for oral food, will not interfere with nasojejunal feeding and may aid its absorption.

Opiates are also known to exert variable inhibitory [33, 34] effects on colonic motility which is also independently depressed by laparotomy [35], especially if the surgery involves retroperitoneal trauma [36]. The earlier recovery of propulsive motility by the small bowel means that 2–3 days following surgery, secretions and gas propelled from the small intestine will enter an immobile colon. The effect of this is cecal distension which is seen so commonly on plain abdominal films [35] in the first 3–4 days. The significance of this distension lies not only in the abdominal discomfort experienced, but also in the possibility that it may activate inhibitory intestino-intestinal reflexes [37] which are known to inhibit small bowel motor activity [38]. This may account for the disruption in regular fasting pattern noted by Pouyet et al. [26] 1–3 days after laparotomy. This disruption, which lasted only about 12 h, was terminated by the first passage of flatus indicating the return of colonic motility. Such a sequence lends support to the idea that a distended colon may exert deleterious inhibiting effects on small bowel motility and, unless otherwise contraindicated, should be avoided by efficient esophagogastric aspiration of secretions and swallowed air [39] and by the use of an enema if no colonic movements have occurred within 3–4 days after surgery or trauma.

Most of the data considered so far has dealt with the effects of uncomplicated surgery. Studies on small bowel motility relevant to other types of critically ill patients are very limited and have often used very crude assessments of motor patterns. However, it does appear that severe hemorrhage inhibits small bowel movements [40] as does hypoxia [41]. Another early paper also described delayed small bowel transit caused by hypoproteinemia [42] which was also associated with defective water and electrolyte [43] absorption and may be of importance in severely malnourished patients. None of these early works considered the effect of such stresses on the normal fasting pattern and there is plainly a need for many of the studies to be repeated using modern methods of recording and analysis.

Conclusion

While many critically ill patients will have altered gastrointestinal motility, impairment of gastric emptying and colonic movements is likely to be greater than the corresponding impairment of small bowel motility. Data in the immediate postoperative period indicate that regular fasting-type motor patterns continue immediately after surgery and this may in part reflect the stimulating effect of opiate analgesics. If food is introduced directly into the jejunum then opiate-induced phase III activity usually retards rather than accelerates transit and thus facilitates absorption. Delayed recovery of movement of colonic contents in the face of relatively normal small bowel motility may give rise to cecal distension a few days after surgery and this can exert an inhibitory effect on the small bowel. Decreased blood flow and oxygen delivery to the small intestine impairs its motor and absorptive function as will marked hypoalbuminemia. The logical deduction from the evidence presented is that, providing the small bowel is otherwise normal, most seriously ill patients could be fed enterally if a means were available to bypass the stomach. Obviously, correction of shock, hypoxia, and hypoalbuminemia would also be advisable as would avoidance of colonic distension by efficient esophagogastric aspiration and the judicious use of an enema if no stools have been produced after 3–4 days of feeding. There is little evidence from these studies that alpha or beta adrenergic receptor blockers will significantly improve small bowel motor function. Finally, the use of opiates for analgesia appears both humane and likely to aid rather than inhibit normal absorption by the intestine.

References

1 McDonald, A. A.: Intrajejunal drip in gastric surgery. Lancet *i:* 1007 (1954).

2 Delaney, H. M.; Carnevale, N.; Garvey, J. W.; Moss, C. M.: Postoperative nutritional support using needle catheter feeding jejunostomy. Ann. Surg. *186:* 165–170 (1977).

3 Page, C.; Carlton, P.; Andrassy, R.; Feldtman, R.; Shield, C.: The safety of needle catheter jejunostomy for administration of defined formula diet. Acta chir. scand., suppl. 494, pp. 233–235 (1979).

4 Sagar, R.; Harland, P.; Shields, R.: Early postoperative feeding with elemental diet. Br. Med. J. *1:* 293–295 (1979).

5 Rothnie, N. G.; Harper, R. A. K.; Catchpole, B. N.: Early postoperative gastrointestinal activity. Lancet *ii:* 64–67 (1963).

6 Nachlas, M. N.; Younis, M. T.; Roda, C. P.; Wityk, J. J.: Gastrointestinal motility studies as a guide to postoperative management. Ann. Surg. *175:* 510–522 (1972).

7 Cox, A. G.: Small intestinal absorption before and after vagotomy in man. Lancet *ii:* 1075–1077 (1962).

8 Shoemaker, C. P.; Wright, H. K.: Rate of water and sodium absorption from the jejunum after abdominal surgery in man. Am. J. Surg. *119:* 62–63 (1970).

9 Wingate, D. L.: Backwards and forwards with the migrating motor complex. Dig. Dis. Sci. *26:* 641–666 (1981).

10 Vantrappen, G.; Janssens, J.; Hellemans, J.; Ghoos, Y.: The interdigestive motor complex of normal subjects and patients with bacterial overgrowth of the small intestine. J. clin. Invest. *59:* 1158–1166 (1977).

11 Kerlin, P.; Phillips, S. F.: Variability of motility of the ileum and jejunum in healthy man. Gastroenterology *82:* 694–700 (1982).

12 Szurszewski, J. A.: A migrating electric complex of the canine small intestine. Am. J. Physiol. *217:* 1757–1763 (1969).

13 Quigley, E. M. M.; Borody, T. J.; Phillips, S. F.; Wienbeck, M.; Tucker, R. L.; Haddad, A. C.: Motility of the terminal ileum and ileocecal sphincter in healthy humans. Gastroenterology *87:* 857–866 (1984).

14 Kerlin, P.; Zinsmeister, A. R.; Phillips, S. F.: Relationship of motility to flow of contents in the human small intestine. Gastroenterology *82:* 701–706 (1982).

15 Code, C. F.; Schlegel, J. R.: The gastrointestinal interdigestive housekeeper: Motor correlates of the interdigestive myoelectric complex of the dog; in Daniel, Proc. of the Fourth International Symp. on Gastrointestinal Motility, pp. 631–634 (Mitchell Press, Vancouver 1973).
16 Sarr, M. G.; Kelly, K. A.; Phillips, S. F.: Canine jejunal absorption and transit during interdigestive and digestive motor states. Am. J. Physiol. *239:* G 167–G 172 (1980).
17 DeFilippi, C.; Valenzuela, J. E.: Sham feeding disrupts the interdigestive motility complex in man. Scand. J. Gastroent. *16:* 977–979 (1981).
18 Code, C. F.; Marlett, J. A.: The interdigestive myoelectric complex of the stomach and small bowel of dogs. J. Physiol. *246:* 289–309 (1975).
19 Schang, J.-C.; Angel, F.; Lambert, F.; Crenner, F.; Aprahamian, A.; Grenier, J. F.: Inhibition of canine duodenal interdigestive myoelectric complexes by nutrient perfusion of jejunal and ileal Thiry-Vella Loops. Gut *22:* 738–743 (1981).
20 Szabo, J. S.; Stonestreet, B. S.; Oh, W.: Effects of hypoxemia on gastrointestinal blood flow and gastric emptying in the newborn piglet. Pediat. Res. *19:* 466–471 (1985).
21 Zaricznyi, B.; Rockwood, C. A.; O'Donoghue, D. H.; Ridings, G. R.: Relationship between trauma to the extremities and stomach motility. J. Trauma *17:* 920–930 (1977).
22 Stanghellini, V.; Malagelada, J.-R.; Zinsmeister, A. R.; Go, V. L. W.; Kao, P. C.: Stress-induced gastroduodenal motor disturbances in humans: Possible humoral mechanisms. Gastroenterology *85:* 83–91 (1983).
23 Ingrams, D. M.; Sheiner, H. J.: Postoperative gastric emptying. Br. J. Surg. *68:* 572–576 (1981).
24 Stoddard, C. J.; Smallwood, R. H.; Duthie, H. L.: Migrating myoelectric complexes in man; in Duthie, Gastrointestinal motility in health and disease, pp. 9–15 (MTP Press, Lancaster 1978).
25 Catchpole, B. N.; Duthie, H. L.: Postoperative gastrointestinal complexes; in Duthie, Gastrointestinal motility in health and disease, pp. 33–41 (MTP Press, Lancaster 1978).
26 Pouyet, M.; Denavit, M.; Roche, M.; Achard, F.: Profit electromyographic du jejunum humain apres chirurgie abdominale. Gastroentérol. clin. biol. *9:* 412–416 (1985).
27 Camilleri, M.; Malagelada, J.-R.; Stanghellini, V.; Zinsmeister, A. R.; Kao, P. C.; Li, C. H.: Dose-related effects of synthetic human β-endorphin and naloxone on fed gastrointestinal motility. Am. J. Physiol. (in press).
28 Bueno, L.; Fioramonti, J.; Ruckebusch, Y.: Postoperative intestinal motility in dogs and sheep. Dig. Dis. Sci. *23:* 682–689 (1978).
29 Bueno, L.; Ferre, J.-P.; Ruckebusch, Y.: Effects of anesthesia and surgical procedures on intestinal myoelectric activity in rats. Dig. Dis. Sci. *23:* 690–695 (1978).
30 Smith, J.; Kelly, K. A.; Weinshilboum, R. M.: Pathophysiology of postoperative ileus. Archs Surg. *112:* 203–209 (1977).
31 Sarna, S. K.; Landon, R. E.: Morphine-initiated migrating myoelectric complexes in the fed state in dogs. Gastroenterology *86:* 662–669 (1984).
32 Loo, F. D.; Sarna, K. H.; Soergel, K. H.; Cunningham, J. A.; Wood, C. M.; Cowles, V. E.: Effect of morphine on human jejunal motility and flow in the fed state. Gastroenterology *84:* 1233 (1983).
33 Ekbom, G.; Schulte, W. J.; Condon, R. E.; Woods, J. H.; Cowles, V.: Effects of

narcotic analgesics on bowel motility in subhuman primates. J. Surg. Res. *28:* 293–296 (1980).

34 Adler, H. F.; Atkinson, A. J.; Ivy, A. C.: Effect of morphine and dilaudid on the ileum and of morphine, dilaudid, and atropine on the colon of man. Archs intern. Med. *69:* 974–985 (1942).

35 Wilson, J. P.: Postoperative motility of the large intestine in man. Gut *16:* 689–692 (1975).

36 Woods, J. H.; Erickson, L. W.; Condon, R. E.; Schulte, W. J.; Sillin, L. F.: Postoperative ileus: A colonic problem? Surgery *84:* 527–532 (1978).

37 Bayliss, W. M.; Starling, E. H.: The movement and innervation of the small intestine. J. Physiol. *24:* 99–143 (1899).

38 Kock, N. G.: An experimental analysis of mechanisms engaged in reflex inhibition of intestinal motility. Acta physiol. scand. *47:* suppl. 164, pp. 5–54 (1959).

39 Moss, G.: Maintenance of gastrointestinal function after bowel surgery and immediate enteral full nutrition. J. parent. ent. Nutr. *5:* 215–220 (1981).

40 Wakim, K. S.; Mason, J. W.: The influence of hemorrhage and of depletion of plasma proteins on intestinal activity. Gastroenterology *4:* 92–101 (1945).

41 Meissner, A.; Bowes, K. L.; Sarna, S. K.: Effects of ambient and stagnant hypoxia on the mechanical and electrical activity of the canine upper jejunum. Can. J. Surg. *19:* 316–321 (1976).

42 Barden, R. P.; Thompson, W. D.; Ravdin, I. S.; Frank, I. L.: The influence of the serum proteins on the motility of the small intestine. Surgery Gynec. Obstet. *66:* 814–821 (1938).

43 Moss, G. S.: Plasma albumin and postoperative ileus. Surg. Forum *18:* 333–336 (1967).

Dr. R. C. Spiller, MRCP, Department of Gastroenterology & Nutrition, Central Middlesex Hospital, London NW10 7NS (UK)

Dietze, Grünert, Kleinberger, Wolfram (eds.), Clinical Nutrition and Metabolic Research. Proc. 7th Congr. ESPEN, Munich 1985, pp. 93–100 (Karger, Basel 1986)

Exocrine Pancreatic Function in the Critically Ill: Effect of Enteral and Parenteral Feeding

U. R. Fölsch

Division of Gastroenterology and Metabolism, Dept. of Medicine, University of Göttingen, FRG

A variety of endogenous and exogenous conditions have been altered in the critically ill patient compared to normal man which may affect the control of pancreatic exocrine function (table I). Whereas only limited information is available to which extent endogenous factors (i.e., 'stress', anemia, pancreatitis, etc.) may influence pancreatic exocrine secretion and/or composition of enzymes, the effects of exogenous factors such as enteral or parenteral feeding or drugs have been quite extensively investigated in animal and man although mostly under healthy conditions only. In the following, these interactions will be discussed in more detail.

Endogenous Factors Which May Affect Pancreatic Function in the Critically Ill

No studies are available investigating the pancreatic function in the critically ill patient. Therefore only experimental information exists which

Table I. Factors which may influence pancreatic function in the critically ill state

Endogenous
– Stress
– Inflammation of the pancreas (pancreatitis)
– Neural or hormonal changes caused by different diseases
Exogenous
– Enteral feeding of elemental diets
– Parenteral feeding (and withdrawal of enteral feeding)
– Drugs

may indirectly point to the conditions in the critically ill. It is rather difficult to define specifically the neural or hormonal changes which might occur in the critically ill patient since different diseases are responsible for the critical state. A common feature of these patients is a stressfull situation. Thompson et al. [1] investigated the effect of ice water cold stress on postprandial gastric, duodenal, and pancreatic function in 9 healthy adult volunteers. Cold pain produced a biphasic alteration in both gastric secretion and pancreatic trypsin output with an initial reduction during the response to the stress followed by an increase during the post-stress period. An increased release of catecholamines could be observed in response to cold stress [2]; furthermore, both beta-endorphins and enkephalins are known to be released in response to experimental stress in animals [3, 4]. Both substances – catecholamines and endorphins/enkephalins – have inhibitory effects on pancreatic flow and enzyme secretion [5–7]. On the other hand, somewhat different observations have been made from experiments with hens exposed to intermittent periods of 4 h heating at 42 °C [8]. The initial exposure to heat brought about a significant increase of amylase in the duodenum and jejunum indicating an augmented pancreatic enzyme secretion. This increased amylase output vanished after 3 days of heating at which time the duodenal amylase levels fell back to control values.

A special situation might occur when the critically ill patient is suffering from an attack of acute pancreatitis. It has been described in animal studies that pancreatic volume and enzyme secretion is considerably lowered during the acute inflammation and that stimulation with caerulein remains ineffective upon this secretory response [9].

It is concluded from these studies that heat or cold stress as well as acute pancreatitis in animal and man may result in quite different responses from the pancreas so that it is not possible to transform general data on pancreatic function during various types of experimental stress and disease to the situation in the critically ill.

Exogenous Factors Which May Affect Pancreatic Function in the Critically Ill

More detailed information exists about the influence of enteral and parenteral feeding on pancreatic exocrine function although again these data are mostly gained from studies in healthy man or dog. For descriptive purposes it is convenient to divide the pancreatic secretory response to a meal into three different phases:

(i) cephalic phase (sight and smell of food stuff); (ii) gastric phase (gastric distention, acid, gastric emptying, gastrin (?)); and (iii) the most important intestinal phase in which different initiators such as protein, amino acids, and fat could stimulate pancreatic volume, bicarbonate and enzyme secretion [10]. By giving an elemental diet through an intestinal feeding tube, the cephalic and gastric phase of pancreatic exocrine secretion are bypassed which will reduce the overall response. Furthermore, it has been reported from comparative studies in normal human subjects that the stimulative effect on pancreatic enzyme secretion in response to jejunal perfusion of a complex nutritional solution is greater than to an elemental solution [11]. It has been known for a long time that peptides and amino acids, the products of digestion of dietary protein, initiate pancreatic enzyme secretion when infused into the intestine [12–14]. Go et al. (1970) described that only enteral infusion of essential amino acids stimulated pancreatic secretion [12]. Of these, only methïonin, valine, and phenylalanine were effective stimulants when given alone. And it appears furthermore that the pancreatic response to intestinally perfused amino acids and peptides is related to the perfused load (amount per unit time) rather than to concentration of amino acids [14]. One has to be aware of considerable species differences as far as the different initiators of pancreatic enzyme secretion are concerned, particularly when one tries to extrapolate from a study in animals to conditions in man (table II). From this table it is noticeable that in rats only intact protein evoke pancreatic enzyme secretion, whereas all other initiators such as peptides or amino acids do not.

Fat digestion products are another major initiator of the intestinal phase of pancreatic secretion. Whereas intact triglycerides do not stimu-

Table II. Initiators of the intestinal phase of pancreatic enzyme secretion in different species

	Protein	Peptides	Amino acids				
			Meth	Val	Phe-al	Try	Ly
Man	+	+	+	+	+	–	–
Dog	–	+	+	–	+	+	+
Rat	+	–	–	–	–	–	–

late pancreatic secretion, fatty acids with a chain length of C_8, C_{12}, and C_{18} and monoglycerides are effective stimulants of enzyme secretion in humans [15, 16] and dogs [17]. The magnitude of pancreatic enzyme secretion in response to fatty acids has been described to be nearly equal to the maximal response to exogenous CCK [15].

Recently, convincing evidence has been accumulated that pancreatic enzyme secretion evoked by intraluminal amino acids or fat is mediated by the release of CCK from the intestinal mucosa. The simultaneous application of proglumide, a specific competitive cholecystokinin (CCK)/gastrin receptor antagonist, during intraluminal infusion of amino acids or fat resulted in a virtually complete inhibition to all doses of intraduodenal amino acids or fat, supporting the concept that CCK is the major mediator of the intestinal phase of exocrine pancreatic secretion [18].

In contrast to amino acids and fat, carbohydrates, both starch (own unpublished observation), dextrose and glucose, do not stimulate pancreatic enzyme secretion in human or animal [12, 19].

So far, I have only listed the effects which may occur and have been demonstrated in acute studies in animal and man. No conclusive data are available so far about the pattern of pancreatic secretion during or after long-term enteral feeding. Recently, Emde et al. [20] investigated possible adaptive effects of the exocrine pancreas in response to a diet which consisted of 76 cal.% carbohydrates, 10 cal.% fat (more than 90% C_{18} fatty acids), and 14 cal.% protein (11.8 g nitrogen per day) which has been given as a 10-day continuous intraduodenal infusion. This diet, rich in carbohydrates and low in fat, did not cause an increase of amylase or decrease of lipase as could be concluded from studies in rats [21, 22]. In this study, an increase of stimulated protease output could be observed though the protein content of the diet was in the physiological range.

In contrast to intraduodenal infusion, the effect of intravenous application of digestive end products such as amino acids, fat, or glucose on exocrine pancreatic secretion are only poorly understood and still a matter of controversy. Some authors described a stimulatory effect of fat and amino acids on pancreatic secretion [23–26]. This is, however, contrasted by other studies which did not find any effect of these substances [27–29]. In a recent investigation, Niederau et al. [30] studied 31 healthy male volunteers with regard to an intravenous infusion of amino acids, fat, and glucose on basal pancreatic secretion. Whereas glucose (10%) and fat (10%) had no effect, amino acids (10%) stimulated the release of chymotrypsin and trypsin only but left the amylase and lipase levels unaffected. High glucose concentration (20%) caused in this and another study [31] an overall inhibition of pancreatic secretion (all enzymes, bicarbonate and volume). But all in all, total parenteral nutrition has no major effect on overall pancreatic secretion and should be particularly the nutrient therapy of choice in relapsing acute pancreatitis.

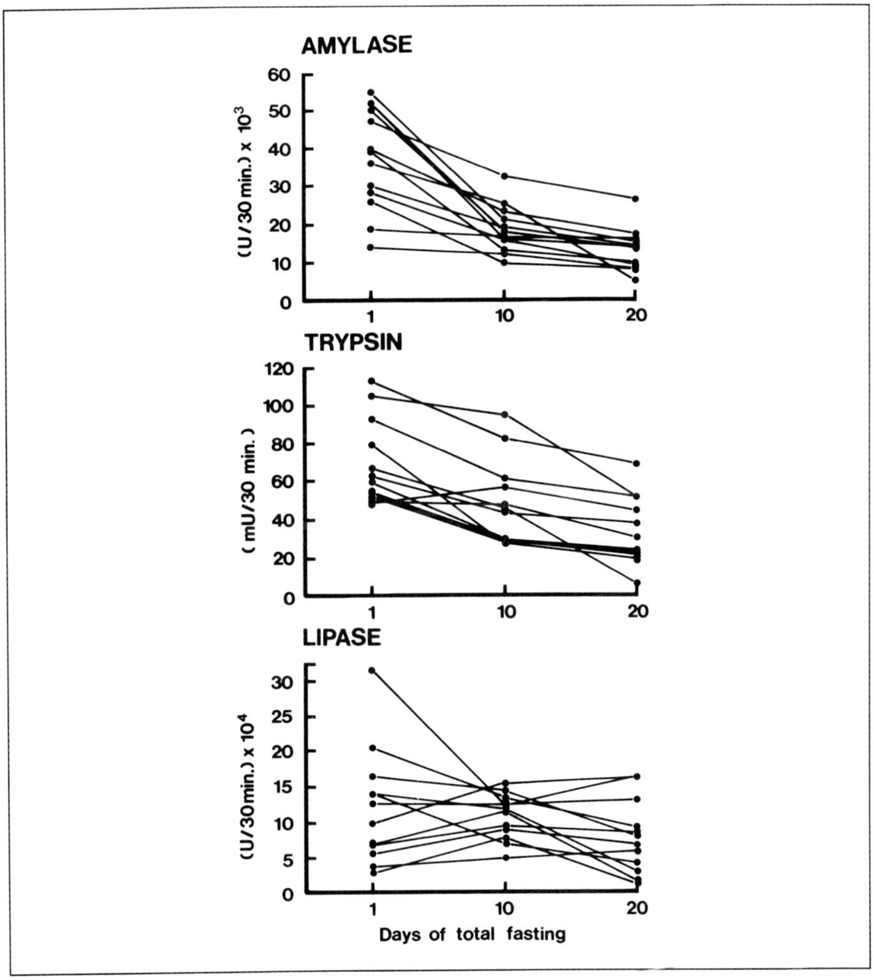

Fig. 1. Output of amylase, trypsin, and lipase in response to 1 IU CCK/kg i.v. in 12 obese subjects at the 1st, 10th, and 20th day of total fasting. The values of each individual patient are depicted (from [32]).

However, one important point has to be considered at this stage. It is well established that prolonged withdrawal of enteral feeding by total fasting [32, 33] or parenteral nutrition [34, 35] causes hypotrophy of the exocrine pancreas [33, 34] or pancreatic hyposecretion in animal and man [32, 35] (fig. 1) which is however reversible [35]. Starvation up to 72 h causes a parallel fall in intestinal CCK content and pancreatic DNA synthesis [33] so that it could be concluded from this that CCK is physiologically a trophic hormone for the pancreas which is released in sufficient amounts during enteral feeding to maintain the trophic state of this organ [36].

References

1 Thompson, D. G.; Richelson, E.; Malagelada, J.-R.: Perturbation of upper gastrointestinal function by cold stress. Gut *24:* 277–283 (1983).

2 Lovallo, W.: The cold pressor test and autonomic function: A review and integration. Psychophysiology *12:* 268–282 (1975).

3 Gullemin, R.; Vargo, T.; Rossier, J. et al.: Beta endorphin and adrenocorticotrophin are secreted concomitantly by the pituitary gland. Science *197:* 1367–1369 (1977).

4 Viveros, O. H.; Diliberto, E. J.; Hazum, E.; Chang, K.: Enkephalins as possible adrenomedullary hormones: Storage, secretion and regulation of synthesis; in Costa, Trabucchi, Neural peptides and neuronal communication, pp. 191–204 (Raven Press, New York 1980).

5 Mann, F. C.; McLachlin, L. C.: The action of adrenaline in inhibiting the flow of pancreatic secretion. J. Pharmac. exp. Ther. *10:* 251–259 (1917).

6 Harper, A.; Vass, C.: The control of the external secretion of the pancreas in cats. J. Physiol. *99:* 415–435 (1941).

7 Konturek, S. J.; Tasler, J.; Cieszkowski, M.; Mikos, E.; Coy, D. H.; Schally, A. V.: Inhibition of pancreatic secretion by enkephalin and morphine in dogs. Gastroenterology *74:* 851–855 (1978).

8 Osman, A. M.; Tanios, N. I.: The effect of heat on the intestinal and pancreatic levels of amylase and maltase of laying hens and broilers. Compar. Biochem. Physiol. *75 A:* 563–567 (1983).

9 Evander, A.; Hederström, E.; Hultberg, B.; Ihse, I.: Exocrine pancreatic secretion in acute experimental pancreatitis. Digestion *24:* 159–167 (1982).

10 Solomon, T. E.: Regulation of pancreatic secretion. Clin. Gastroenterol. *13*(3): 657–678 (1984).

11 Vidon, N.; Hecketsweiler, P.; Butel, J.; Bernier, J. J.: Effect of continuous jejunal perfusion of elemental and complex nutritional solutions on pancreatic enzyme secretion in human subjects. Gut *19:* 194–198 (1978).

12 Go, V. L. W.; Hofmann, A. F.; Summerskill, W. H. J.: Pancreozymin bioassay in man based on pancreatic enzyme secretion: Potency of specific amino acids and other digestive products. J. clin. Invest. *49:* 1558–1564 (1970).

13 Meyer, J. H.; Kelly, G. A.; Jones, R. S.: Canine pancreatic response to intestinally perfused oligopeptides. Am. J. Physiol. *231:* 678–681 (1976).
14 Meyer, J. H.; Kelly, G. A.; Spingola, L. J.; Jones, R. S.: Canine gut receptors mediating pancreatic responses to luminal L-amino acids. Am. J. Physiol. *231:* 669–677 (1976).
15 Malagelada, J. R.; Go, V. L. W.; DiMagno, E. P.; Summerskill, W. H. J.: Interactions between luminal bile acids and digestive products on pancreatic and gallbladder function. J. clin. Invest. *52:* 2160–2165 (1973).
16 Malagelada, J. R.; DiMagno, E. P.; Summerskill, W. H. J.; Go, V. L. W.: Regulation of pancreatic and gallbladder function by intraluminal fatty acids and bile acids in man. J. clin. Invest. *58:* 493–499 (1976).
17 Meyer, J. H.; Jones, R. S.: Canine pancreatic responses to intestinally perfused fat and products of fat digestion. Am. J. Physiol. *226:* 1178–1187 (1974).
18 Stubbs, R. S.; Stabile, B. E.: Role of cholecystokinin in pancreatic exocrine response to intraluminal amino acids and fat. Am. J. Physiol. *248:* G 347–G 352 (1985).
19 Sum, P. T.; Preshaw, R. M.: Intraduodenal glucose infusion and pancreatic secretion in man. Lancet *ii:* 340–341 (1967).
20 Emde, C.; Liehr, R.-M.; Gregor, M.; Pleul, O.; Riecken, E. O.; Menge, H.: Lack of adaptive changes in human pancreatic amylase and lipase secretion in response to high-carbohydrate, low-fat diet applied by a 10-day continuous intraduodenal infusion. Digestive Diseases and Sciences *30:* 204–210 (1985).
21 Grossman, M. I.; Greengard, H.; Ivy, A. C.: On the mechanism of the adaptation of pancreatic enzymes to dietary composition. Am. J. Physiol. *141:* 38–41 (1944).
22 Fölsch, U. R.; Wormsley, K. G.: The pancreatic secretion of enzymes in rats treated with soybean diet. Scand. J. Gastroent. *9:* 679–683 (1974).
23 Froehlich, C.; Locher, M.; Olderhausen, H. F.: Die Beeinflussung des exokrinen Pankreas durch die intravenöse Infusion einer Nährlösung. Klin. Wschr. *51:* 1207–1209 (1973).
24 Stastna, R.; Skala, I.; Hruba, F.; Shlygin, G. K.; Sysoev, Y.: The effect of some N-solutions for parenteral nutrition on gastric and pancreatic secretion. Nutr. Metab. *23:* 349–356 (1979).
25 Konturek, S. J.; Tasler, J. T.; Cieszkowski, M.; Jaworek, J.; Konturek, J.: Intravenous amino acids and fat stimulate pancreatic secretion. Am. J. Physiol. *236:* E 678–E 684 (1979).
26 Klein, E.; Shnebaum, S.; Ben-Ari, H.; Dreiling, D. A.: Effects of total parenteral nutrition on exocrine pancreatic secretion. Am. J. Gastroent., N. Y. *78:* 31–33 (1983).
27 Stabile, B. E.; Borzatta, M.; Stubbs, R. S.; Debas, H. T.: Intravenous mixed amino acids and fat do not stimulate exocrine pancreatic secretion. Am. J. Physiol. *246:* G 274–G 280 (1984).
28 Fried, G. M.; Ogden, W. D.; Rhea, A.; Greeley, G.; Thompson, J. C.: Pancreatic protein secretion and gastrointestinal hormone release in response to parenteral amino acids and lipid in dogs. Surgery *92:* 902–905 (1982).
29 Edelmann, K.; Valenzuela, J. E.: Effect of intravenous lipid on human pancreatic secretion. Gastroenterology *85:* 1063–1066 (1983).
30 Niederau, C.; Sonnenberg, A.; Erckenbrecht, J.: Effect of intravenous infusion of

amino acids, fat, or glucose on unstimulated pancreatic secretion in healthy humans. Digestive Diseases and Sciences *30:* 445–455 (1985).

31 Saito, Y.; Tokutake, K.; Matsuno, S.; Noto, N.; Honda, T.; Sato, T.: Effects of hypertonic glucose and amino acid infusions on pancreatic exocrine function. Tohoku J. exp. Med. *124:* 99–115 (1978).

32 Fölsch, U. R.; Dreessen, U.-W.; Talaulicar, M.; Willms, B.; Creutzfeldt, W.: Effect of long-term fasting of obese patients on pancreatic exocrine function, gastrointestinal hormones and bicarbonate concentration in plasma. Z. Gastroenterologie *22:* 357–364 (1984).

33 Brand, S. J.; Morgan, R. G. H.: The influence of starvation on intestinal cholecystokinin-like activity and pancreatic growth. J. Physiol. *321:* 469–482 (1981).

34 Johnson, L. R.; Copeland, E. M.; Dudrick, S. J.; Lichtenberger, L. M.; Castro, G. A.: Structural and hormonal alterations in the gastrointestinal tract of parenterally fed rats. Gastroenterology *68:* 1177–1183 (1975).

35 Kotler, D. P.; Levine, G. M.: Reversible gastric and pancreatic hyposecretion after long-term total parenteral nutrition. New Engl. J. Med. *300:* 241–242 (1979).

36 Fölsch, U. R.: Regulation of pancreatic growth. Clin. Gastroenterol. *13:* 679–699 (1984).

Prof. Dr. med. U. R. Fölsch, Medizinische Klinik und Poliklinik der Georg-August-Universität, Robert-Koch-Str. 40, D-3400 Göttingen (FRG)

Dietze, Grünert, Kleinberger, Wolfram (eds.), Clinical Nutrition and Metabolic Research. Proc. 7th Congr. ESPEN, Munich 1985, pp. 101–118 (Karger, Basel 1986)

Intestinal Absorption of Fat and Fat-Soluble Vitamins[1]

W. Stremmel

Medical Clinic D, University of Dusseldorf, FRG

Introduction

Fat absorption is a multistep process involving the coordinated participation of several organs and can be considered as being composed of a luminal and a mucosal phase. The marked efficiency of the entire process of fat absorption can be judged by the fact that under normal conditions less than 5% of ingested fat is recovered in the stool.

Luminal Phase of Fat Absorption (Fig. 1)

The luminal phase of fat absorption is characterized by 3 sequential steps:

(1) the mechanical dispersion of bulk fat globules into finely divided emulsion particles; (2) the enzymatic hydrolysis of fatty acid esters at the emulsion-water interface; (3) solubilization of the insoluble products of lipolysis into a water-soluble, absorbable form.

The first step in fat absorption is the formation of a crude emulsion by the chewing of food and the mixing and churning action of the stomach. To some extent this crude emulsion is stabilized by peptic digestion of dietary proteins, polysaccharides, and phospholipids, all acting as emulsi-

[1] Supported by Grant STR 216/2-2 from the Deutsche Forschungsgemeinschaft, Bonn, FRG

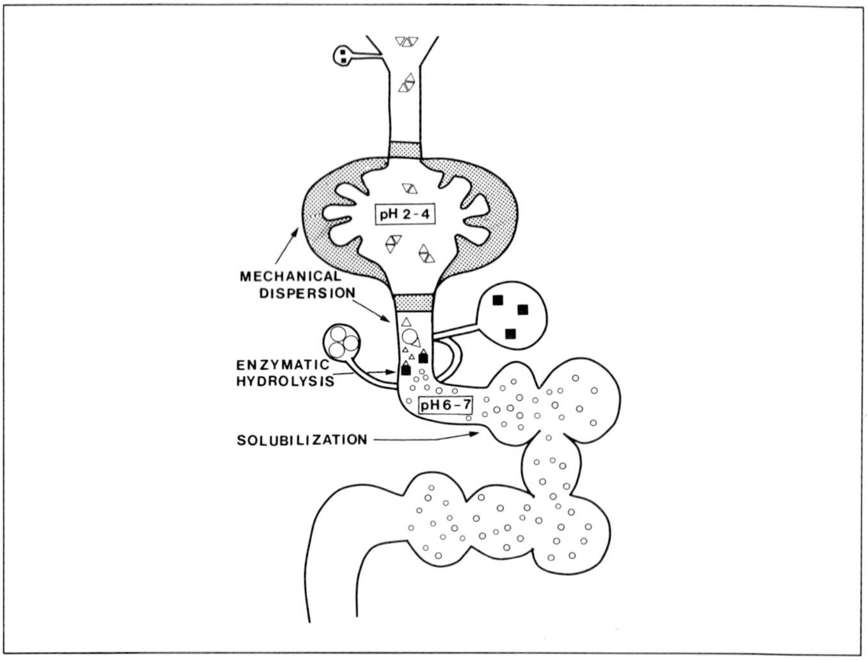

Fig. 1. Luminal phase of fat absorption.

fiers. During the 2–4 h fat is present in the stomach, some hydrolysis of triglycerides already begins due to the action of lingual lipase originating from serous glands of the tongue, which is active at gastric pH and does not require bile salts [1, 2]. As the crudely emulsified lipids at low pH are ejected from the stomach into the duodenum, the contents meet duodenal fluid arising from the pancreas, gallbladder, and small intestine. Secretin, released from the duodenal mucosa by gastric acid, stimulates the pancreas to secrete bicarbonate and water which considerably increase the pH in the duodenum compared to the stomach. This facilitates the physicochemical process for further emulsification of the fat droplets and provides the milieu for the action of pancreatic lipase. Simultaneously cholecystokinin-pancreozymin (CCK-PZ) is released from duodenal epithelial cells in response to the presence of free fatty acids, certain essential amino acids, and acid itself. CCK-PZ induces the ejection of biliary lipids from the gallbladder in form of mixed micelles (fig. 2). They collide with the fat emulsion particles coming from the stomach and transfer to their surface.

The detergent properties of ionized fatty acids, biliary lipids, and particularly bile salts markedly increase the surface of the lipid droplets and, in concert with the mechanical emulsification due to the peristaltic and segmental contractions in the duodenum, they create smaller stabilized particles [3, 4]. This finely dispersed emulsion system with its large surface area serves as suitable substrate for the essential step of fat digestion, the hydrolysis by pancreatic lipase/colipase as well as for the action of phospholipase A_2 and other nonspecific esterases, also released by CCK-PZ.

Hydrolysis of the major class of dietary fat, the triglycerides, is accomplished by the combined action of pancreatic lipase and trypsin-activated colipase. Colipase binds first to the bile salt-covered triglycerides. Then lipase tightly anchors to colipase by electrostatic bonding, bringing it in a suitable configuration to hydrolyze the substrate. This enzyme system hydrolyzes triglycerides very efficiently at the 1,3 positions, leaving β-monoglyceride, diglycerides, and free fatty acids [5]. The generated mass of lipolytic products creates an increasing surface pressure in the emulsion coat and consequently buds off fragments in form of

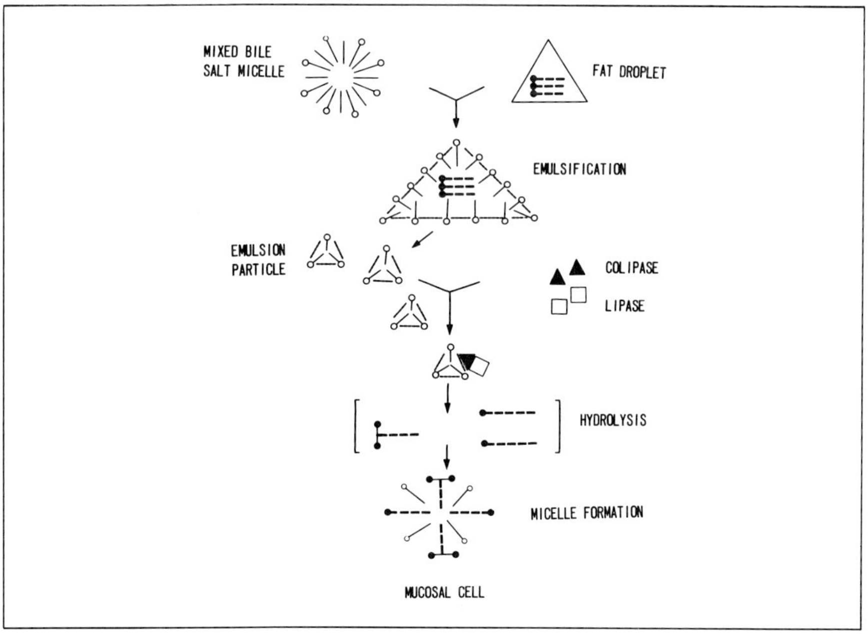

Fig. 2. Enzymatic hydrolysis.

mixed bile salt micelles or – in absence of a sufficient concentration of bile salts – unilamellar liposomal particles [6]. Both, containing lipolytic products such as fatty acids, monoglyceride, cholesterol, or lysophospholipids as well as fat-soluble vitamins, separate into the aqueous suspension and are ready to be absorbed by the mucosal cell.

Mucosal Phase of Fat Absorption

Uptake of solute molecules from the intestinal lumen into the mucosal cell is determined by the rates of penetration across two barriers, an unstirred water layer and the cell membrane of the enterocyte (fig. 3). The unstirred water layer is believed to be an unequilibrated area along the luminal surface of the small intestine with a thickness estimated to be in the range of 100–600 μm [7]. The products of intraluminal lipid hydrolysis are presented to the mucosal surface mainly as an aqueous suspen-

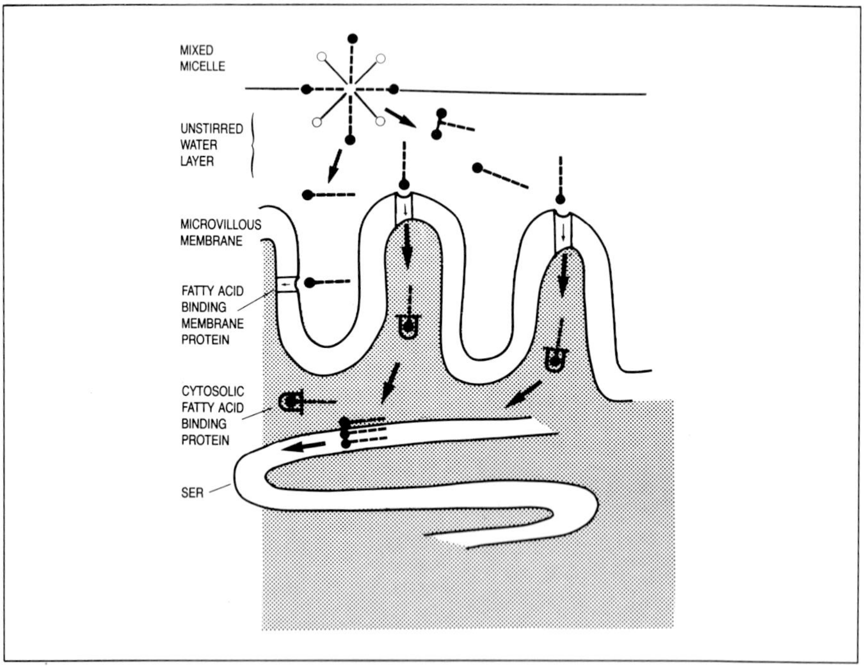

Fig. 3. Schematic representation of fatty acid uptake by the mucosal cell.

sion of mixed bile salt micelles. However, since the lipolytic products are absorbed in the proximal intestine, whereas bile salts are absorbed by the distal ileum [8, 9], dissociation of the mixed bile salt micelles has to occur. It was suggested that the unstirred water layer may mediate this dissociation by generating an acidic microclimate, which was attributed to mucosal cell hydrogen secretion [10]. Using a microelectrode technique, it was shown that the pH in the area adjacent to the cell membrane indeed had a lower pH than the bulk phase, facilitating micellar diffusion as well as micellar dissociation [11].

The next step in mucosal uptake of fatty acids and other lipolytic products represents penetration across the microvillous membrane of the mucosal cell, which was long considered as a passive diffusional process. However, this common opinion was recently challenged by the observation that long chain fatty acids bind to high-affinity binding sites of microvillous membranes [12]. Furthermore, a specific fatty binding protein was identified and isolated from these membranes [12]. Immunofluorescence studies of various parts of the rat gastrointestinal tract revealed the presence of this protein in the upper ileum, but predominantly in the jejunum, the major site of fatty acid absorption. The finding of a specific microvillous membrane protein with high affinities for long chain fatty acids suggests that the protein might serve as a general acceptor for long chain fatty acids in the gut and is compatible with the hypothesis that intestinal absorption of long chain fatty acids represents a carrier-mediated transport system. Whether other lipolytic products might also be absorbed by a carrier-mediated transport system is unknown.

After entering the cytoplasma of the enterocyte, long chain fatty acids bind to a low molecular weight cytosolic fatty acid binding protein, which serves as intracellular transport protein, directing fatty acids to the smooth endoplasmatic reticulum, the site of triglyceride synthesis [13] (fig. 4). From there reesterified triglycerides move together with cholesterol, phospholipids, and fat-soluble vitamins through the profiles of the endoplasmatic reticulum to the Golgi apparatus [14]. Here they interact with apolipoproteins to form chylomicrons and very low density lipoproteins [15]. Of particular importance is the incorporation of apolipoprotein B, since it is essential for synthesis and secretion of intestinal lipoproteins. Golgi vesicles then migrate towards the lateral cell membrane where they appear to fuse with the membrane and discharge their contents into the intercellular space by reverse pinocytosis. Thereafter chylomicrons move as a result of the pumping action of contracting villi through the lamina

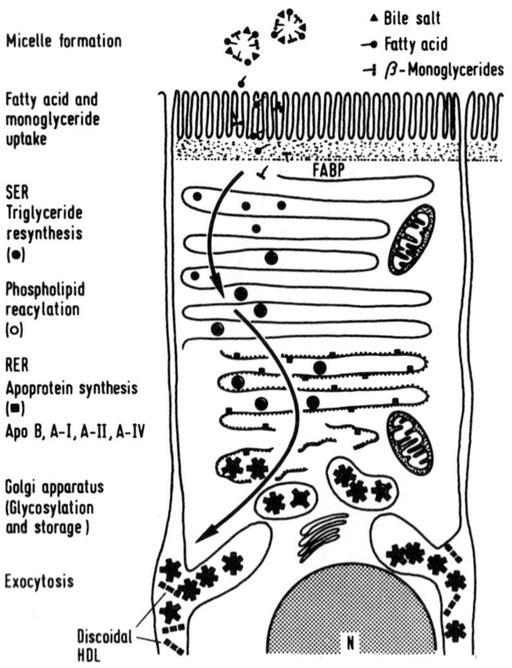

Fig. 4. Schematic representation of events within the mucosal cell during fat absorption [15].

propria to the lacteal and further via the lymphatic system to the systemic circulation.

The absorption of short and medium chain fatty acids is different from the absorption of long chain fatty acids. Triglycerides which contain short and medium chain fatty acids are more water soluble, more rapidly hydrolyzed by lingual and pancreatic lipase, and do not require bile salt micelles for absorbing the products of hydrolysis [16]. The mechanism by which those fatty acids enter the enterocyte is not completely understood. It was suggested that they compete with long chain fatty acids for some membrane compound [17], possibly the membrane fatty acids-binding protein involved in the mucosal uptake of fatty acids. In contrast to long chain fatty acids, short and medium chain fatty acids are not esterified and consequently not incorporated into chylomicrons [18]. After release at the basolateral membrane of the enterocyte, they are bound to albumin and transported by the portal vein to the liver for further metabolism.

The absorption of the fat-soluble vitamins A, D, K, and E is closely connected with the pathways of dietary lipid absorption. It includes the formation of small fat globules containing the fat-soluble vitamins, emulsification of the lipid droplets, and incorporation of the fat-soluble vitamins into the mixed micelles. After uptake by the mucosal cell, the lipid-soluble vitamins are accumulated in the chylomicrons and reach via the lymphatic system the circulation. Vitamin A is mainly ingested in form of long chain fatty acid esters, predominantly retinyl palmitate, whereas vitamin D_3 fatty acid esters may occur in minor amounts in the diet. Foodstuffs fortified with vitamin E chiefly contain tocopheryl acetate or other esters of this vitamin. All vitamin esters are hydrolyzed by the pancreatic ester hydrolase. The various fat-soluble vitamins reveal different absorption efficiencies [19]. Whereas the average absorption of the vitamins A and K amounts to about 80%, vitamin D is only absorbed to about 50%, and vitamin E absorption is as low as 20–30%. The reason for this different behavior of fat-soluble vitamins during intestinal absorption is not fully understood. Due to their different chemical structures and lipid solubility, it can be assumed that they differ in regard to their capacities for incorporation into mixed micelles, their transport mechanism across the mucosal cell membrane, and for limitations in their enveloping in carrier lipoproteins [19].

Diseases with Impaired Absorption of Fat and Fat-Soluble Vitamins

Patients with impaired absorption of fat and fat-soluble vitamins suffer from disorders affecting organs directly involved in the absorption process of fat (fig. 5). In the following diseases which affect the various levels of fat absorption will be discussed.

Digestive Defects

Disorders of the luminal phase of fat absorption (digestive defects) include emulsification problems, lack of triglyceride hydrolysis, and impaired mixed micelle formation.

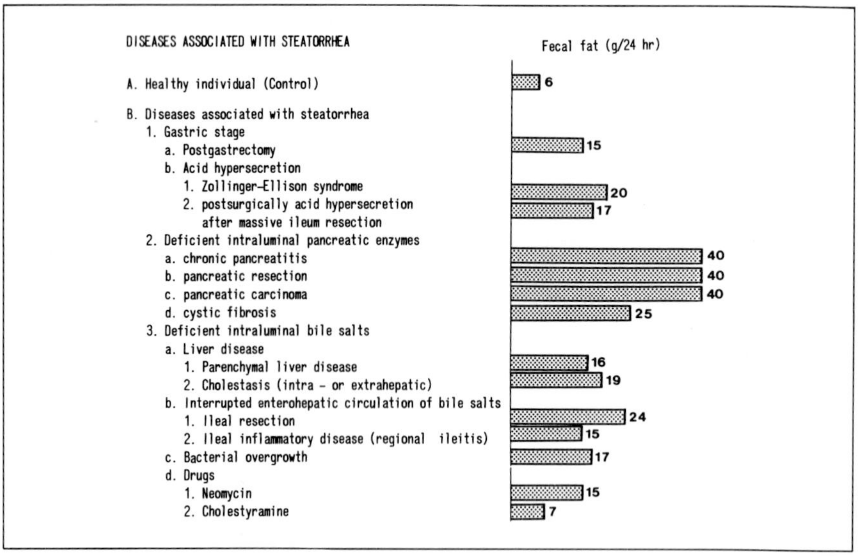

Fig. 5. Fecal fat excretion in various diseases associated with steatorrhea.

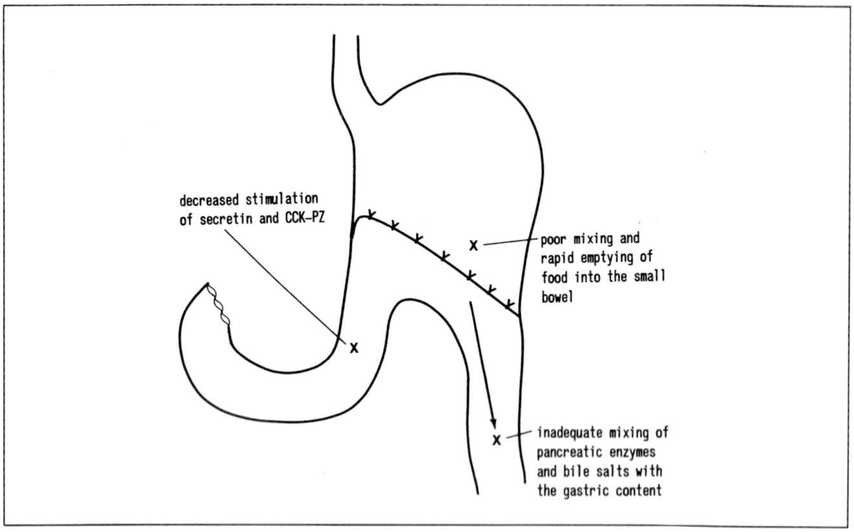

Fig. 6. Steatorrhea after subtotal gastrectomy billroth II anastomosis.

Postgastrectomy Malabsorption

The presence of a malabsorption syndrome has been documented frequently in patients after subtotal gastrectomy [20]. Steatorrhea is more common with a Billroth II than Billroth I type of anastomosis (fig. 6). Usually the fat loss is minimal, ranging from 7 to 10 g per 24 h. This malabsorption is caused partially by poor mixing and emulsification within the stomach and rapid emptying of the gastric content into the small bowel by the loss of the pylorus. Furthermore with a Billroth II anastomosis the duodenum is bypassed and there is a decreased entry of food and acid into the proximal duodenum. This leads to a decreased stimulation of the mucosal cell to release the hormones, secretin and cholecystokinin-pancreozymin (CCK-PZ), resulting in insufficient secretion of pancreatic enzymes and bile salts. There may also be inadequate mixing of the pancreatic enzymes and bile salts secreted into the afferent loop with the gastric contents entering the efferent loop. In some patients frequent smaller meals, together with pancreatic replacement enzymes, may lead to a significant improvement of the observed steatorrhea.

Zollinger-Ellison Syndrome

Steatorrhea is one of the clinical features of this gastrin producing tumor of the pancreas [21]. Excess acid secretion by the stomach lowers the pH of the luminal contents of the duodenum and jejunum, and leads to major disturbances in fat digestion and absorption. Impaired emulsification by ionized fatty acids and inactivation of pancreatic lipase are probably the major factors in the production of steatorrhea. Other factors contributing to fat malabsorption in this disorder include precipitation of glycine-conjugated bile salts and alteration of the intestinal mucosa with ulceration and metaplasia. In this condition reduction of gastric acid by H_2-receptor antagonists or surgery should reduce fat malabsorption.

Pancreatic Insufficiency

Impaired triglyceride hydrolysis caused by a lack of sufficient pancreatic lipase, colipase, and bicarbonate secretion is a well-recognized cause of steatorrhea [22]. Such pancreatic insufficiency may be caused by chronic pancreatitis, pancreatic resection, or pancreatic duct obstruction. Therapy is directed toward replacement of lacking enzymes and H_2-receptor antagonists as an adjunct to reduce or neutralize gastric acid.

Deficient Intraluminal Bile Salt Concentration

Fat maldigestion may occur when the excretion, intraluminal functioning, or ileal reabsorption of the conjugated bile salts is abnormal so that the enterohepatic circulation of bile salts is not efficient (fig. 7). Regardless of whether the primary defect is caused by impaired synthesis of bile salts in the liver, their excretion via the common bile duct, their deconjugation by intestinal bacteria to free bile acids, or by failure of the reabsorption at the ileal level, the final effect is reduction of the intraluminal concentration of bile salts below the critical micellar concentration important for the solubilization of fat and fat-soluble vitamins. Therefore steatorrhea has been described in patients with acute viral hepatitis, postnecrotic or nutritional cirrhosis, chronic extrahepatic biliary tract

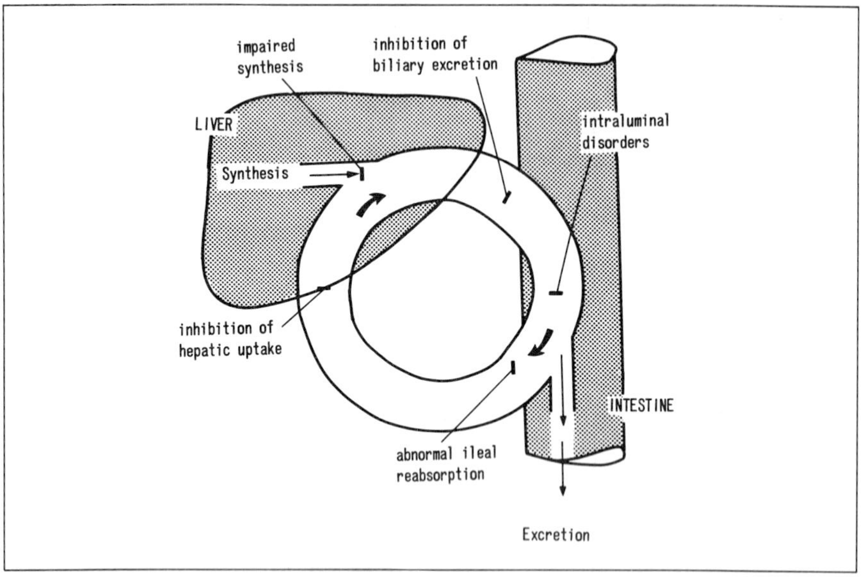

Fig. 7. Deficient intraluminal bile salt concentration due to disturbance of their enterohepatic circulation.

obstruction, primary biliary cirrhosis, distal ileal resection (> 100 cm), surgical ileal bypass, or severly diseased terminal ileum. Patients with these disorders are able to absorb some ionized fatty acids, but little cholesterol or fat-soluble vitamins A, D, or K. However, fat malabsorption in these patients is often only minimal, suggesting that a lack of bile salts may be compensated by other emulsification processes and mucosal absorption occurs via formation of non-micellar liposomes [6, 23]. Severe steatorrhea should be treated by substituting medium chain triglycerides in the diet. Because of the better water solubility of medium chain fatty acids, bile salts are not necessary for their efficient absorption.

Bacterial Overgrowth of the Small Bowel

Because of the acid milieu of the stomach, intestinal motility, and secretion of immunoglobulins, the proximal small intestine is usually bacteriologically sterile. Since the major mechanism limiting the growth of bacteria is normal peristalsis, any disorder leading to impaired intestinal motility may result in abnormal stasis. This in turn may cause bacterial overgrowth, which is accompanied by impaired lipid absorption. There are a number of conditions leading to bacterial overgrowth and steatorrhea

Table I. Causes of intestinal bacterial overgrowth

Due to impairment of
1. Acid milieu of the stomach
pernicious anemia
2. Secretion of immunoglobulins
hypogammaglobulinemia
3. Intestinal hypomotility
scleroderma
amyloidosis
diabetes mellitus
hypothyroidism
vagotomy
intestinal pseudoobstruction
4. Fistulas
5. Structural abnormalities
diverticula
strictures
afferent loop syndrome

including blind loops that do not empty, e.g., small bowel diverticula; surgically created pouches; strictures; impaired muscular contractibility of the small bowel wall caused by scleroderma, amyloid, or diabetes mellitus; or fistulas (table I). When high numbers of bacteria are present in the upper small intestine (10^8–10^{10}/ml), bile salt molecules are altered to become less polar and much less capable of forming micelles [24]. Certain bacteria deconjugate the glycine or taurine portion of the bile salt molecule or remove a hydroxyl group in the 7 position. The deconjugated bile salts are more readily absorbed by the upper small intestine but more important, they precipitate out of solution at the luminal pH (6.5) of the small bowel. The net effect is impaired formation of mixed micelles and decreased fat absorption leading to steatorrhea. Therapy is directed toward surgically removing the cause of bacterial overgrowth, or, if caused by general stasis, long-term therapy with antibiotics.

Absorptive Defects

Most diseases, whose principal disorder is of the intestinal mucosa itself, result in panmalabsorption, although fat malabsorption is often prominent.

Disorders of Intestinal Mucosal Cells

Celiac disease (nontropical sprue) [25] and tropical sprue [26] impair fat uptake by an overall decrease in the absorptive area of the bowel wall caused by villous atrophy and loss of the microvilli. Jejunal biopsies of both diseases classically reveal blunting and flattening of the mucosal surface, with villi either absent or broad and short. The crypts are elongated, and there is generally a dense infiltration of inflammatory cells in the lamina propria. In addition the fatty acid transport into the mucosal cells and triglyceride resynthesis seem to be impaired. Celiac disease is treated by removal of gluten from the diet. Tropical sprue responds well to tetracycline and folic acid.

Extensive morphologic damage of the small intestinal mucosa often follows abdominal irradiation [27]. These changes include a decrease in crypt mitoses, marked shortening of the villi, megalocytosis of epithelial cells, and inflammatory cell infiltration of the lamina propria. In this condition steatorrhea has been frequently observed, ranging from 10–40 g/die. However, restoration of normal intestinal architecture and function is usually complete within 2 weeks after cessation of therapy. Late complications may occur in form of intestinal strictures and intestinal lymphangiectasia due to lymphatic obstruction, resulting in malabsorption which may be refractory to methods of management.

Similar alteration of the intestinal mucosal, where crypt-cell division is inhibited due to impaired DNA-synthesis, is observed in severe folate deficiency, pernicious anemia, or methotrexate sodium therapy.

Disorders of Chylomicron Formation

Abetalipoproteinemia is a rare familial disease, characterized by the inability of absorptive cells to synthesize apolipoprotein B [28]. Consequently, resynthesized triglycerides accumulate in the absorptive cell and are unable to pass out of the lateral cell wall into the lacteals of the lymphatic system. A similar phenomenon is observed in patients with protein caloric malnutrition or after chemotherapeutic regimens leading to impaired protein synthesis, particularly of apolipoproteins [29, 30]. Although studies of chylomicron apoprotein synthesis have not been carried out in various human malabsorptive disorders, it is probable that mucosal destructive diseases, such as sprue or other conditions associated with intestinal repair or regeneration, which are characterized by functionally immature (less differentiated) epithelial cells, perhaps also reveal a limited capacity for chylomicron formation. Treatment consists of substituting medium chain triglycerides in the diet, which are rapidly hydrolyzed to fatty acids in the intestinal lumen. The absorbed medium chain fatty acids are able to pass directly into the portal system, and chylomicron formation is not needed.

Defective Transport of Fat to the Systemic Circulation

In another group of mucosal diseases causing malabsorption of fat, the principal manifestation is an infiltrative process of the lamina propria or lamina submucosa. Impaired fat transport by the lymphatic system has been implicated in some of these patients as a mechanism of steatorrhea, since on small bowel biopsy specimens, there are dilated fat-filled lacteals.

Whipple's disease is one of these disorders with appreciable steatorrhea characterized by an infiltrate of unusual macrophages beneath the lining epithelium of the intestine and the finding of bacillary bodies in those lesions [31]. Antibiotics such as penicillin, tetracyclines, ampicillin, and chloramphenicol can produce long remissions that may even constitute cure of this disease.

Intestinal lymphangiectasia, either congenital or aquired as a result of retroperitoneal disease causing mesenteric lymphatic obstruction, also may cause steatorrhea. In these circumstances, fat absorption may be improved by treating the patient with medium chain triglycerides as a source of calories.

There are a number of other diseases associated with infiltration of the submucosa which may also cause lymphatic obstruction and possibly damage of the mucosal epithelium. These include Crohn's disease, tuberculosis, intestinal lymphoma, carcinomatosis, or amyloidosis.

Comment on Treatment of Steatorrhea

Although most of the disorders of fat absorption can be treated according to the underlying cause, some instances require supplement of fat or fat-soluble vitamins. Medium chain triglycerides were shown to be particularly useful in steatorrhea, because they are very efficiently hydrolyzed, do not require bile salt micelles for absorption of the products of hydrolysis, and because the products are not absorbed into the lymphatics but directly into the systemic circulation. However, there are also problems with the use of medium chain triglycerides. Their caloric content is about 20% less than that of long chain triglycerides and they may cause in large amounts diarrhea, owing to the toxic effect of medium chain fatty acids on the mucosa. Nevertheless, medium chain triglycerides can deliver a small, but perhaps important, addition of calories to a marginal diet. Moreover, since they are detergent-like, they can help to solubilize fat-soluble vitamins and enhance their absorption.

When steatorrhea is present, fat-soluble vitamins also may need to be replaced. These are offered as water-miscible preparations, i.e. with detergent added. When the vitamins enter the intestinal tract, they still require bile acid micelles for absorption; hence, if fat malabsorption is caused by impaired mixed micelle formation, large doses of these vitamins will be needed to achieve some absorption. The exception is vitamin K, which is available in a water-soluble form. Supplement of vitamin E is normally not necessary, since it is present in virtually all dietary fats in sufficient quantities. When the vitamins A and D are given in large therapeutic doses, the patients must be watched for toxicity.

Supplement of Fat in the Enteral Nutrition of the Critically Ill

Supplement of fat and fat-soluble vitamins is essential during enteral nutrition in the critically ill, particularly when associated with multi-organ failure. This inhomogeneous group consists of patients with polytrauma, sepsis, thermal injuries, or patients in the early postoperative stage, etc. Since these patients have increased energy requirements due to hypermetabolism, it is essential to provide them with sufficient nutrients. It was clearly demonstrated that enteral feeding is the preferential route of nutrient administration is those patients [32]. The enteral diets employed should contain a well-balanced amount of fat and fat-soluble vitamins, serving as energy source and essential biologic constituents. Experimentally it was shown that in the presence of fat the nitrogen balance is markedly improved compared to the absence of dietary fat [33]. However, in some of the critically ill patients intestinal absorption of fat is impaired due to e.g., gastric acid hypersecretion, hypomotility (ileus), bacterial overgrowth, drugs, or the underlying disorder itself. Furthermore, much of the malabsorption problems observed in those patients (e.g., diarrhea, delayed gastric emptying) is thought to be initiated by excess high fat content in the diet. Therefore it was recommended to use medium chain triglycerides in addition to long chain triglycerides. These are better tolerated due to their efficient hydrolysis and absorption, and serve as solubilizers in the absorption process of fat-soluble vitamins. Newly developed substitutes containing so-called 'structural lipids' seem to be even more efficient in promoting weight gain, positive nitrogen balance, and improved serum albumin concentration [34, 35].

Another consideration in enteral nutrition, particularly in regard to the absorption of fat and fat-soluble vitamins, is the positioning of the feeding tube. According to the physiology of fat absorption, placement in the proximal GI tract provides more efficient absorption of fat than in the distal intestine. However, positioning of the feeding tube in the stomach may bear the risk of aspiration in those bedridden patients often revealing delayed gastric emptying. Therefore it is often preferred to place the tube in the duodenum or proximal jejunum [36]. In contrast, distal jejunostomy feeding [37] appears to be of only limited value in the enteral application of fat since hydrolysis and mucosal absorption of long and medium chain triglycerides seems to be less efficient.

Conclusion

The multistep process of the absorption of fat and fat-soluble vitamins involves the participation of several organs. Since the complex mechanism of fat absorption can be disturbed at various levels, there are a number of specific disorders which may lead to steatorrhea. According to the various pathophysiological mechanisms of this syndrome, treatment of diseases associated with fat malabsorption has to be individually tailored. The application of medium chain triglycerides can serve in several instances of steatorrhea as suitable substitute for long chain triglycerides since they are efficiently hydrolyzed and absorbed even in the absence of bile salts and do not require reesterification in the mucosal cell prior to their transport to the systemic circulation. Since they are detergent like, they facilitate absorption of fat-soluble vitamins. Medium chain triglycerides were shown to be particularly useful as supplement in the enteral nutrition regimen of critically ill patients.

References

1 Hamosh, M.; Scow, R. O.: Lingual lipase and its role in the digestion of dietary lipid. J. clin. Invest. *52:* 88 (1973).
2 Hamosh, M.; Klaeneman, H. L.; Wolf, R. O.; Scow, R. O.: Pharyngeal lipase and digestion of dietary triglyceride in man. J. clin. Invest. *55:* 908 (1975).
3 Senior, J. R.: Intestinal absorption of fat. J. Lipid Res. *5:* 495 (1964).
4 Dasher, G. F.: Surface activity of naturally occurring emulsifiers. Science *116:* 660 (1952).
5 Borgström, B.: On the interactions between pancreatic lipase and colipase and the substrate, and the importance of bile salts. J. Lipid Res. *16:* 411 (1975).
6 Carey, M. C.; Small, D. M.; Bliss, C. M.: Lipid digestion and absorption. Annu. Rev. Physiol. *45:* 651 (1983).
7 Smithson, K. W.; Millar, D. B.; Jacobs, L. R.; Gray, G. M.: Intestinal diffusion barrier: Unstirred water layer of membrane surface mucous coat? Science *214:* 1241 (1981).
8 Borgström, B.; Lundh, G.; Hofmann, A. F.: The site of absorption of conjugated bile salts in man. Gastroenterology *45:* 229 (1963).

9 Gordon, S. G.; Kern, Jr., F.: The absorption of bile salts and fatty acids by hamster small intestine. Biochim. biophys. Acta *152:* 372 (1968).
10 Shiau, Y. F.; Levine, G. M.: pH dependence of micellar diffusion and dissociation. Am. J. Physiol. *239:* G 177 (1980).
11 Lucas, M. L.; Schneider, W.; Haberich, F. J.; Blair, J. A.: Direct measurement by pH microelectrode of the pH microclimate in rat proximal jejunum. Proc. R. Soc. London Ser. B. *192:* 39 (1975).
12 Stremmel, W.; Lotz, G.; Strohmeyer, G.; Berk, P. D.: Identification, isolation, and partial characterization of a fatty acid binding protein from rat jejunal microvillous membranes. J. clin. Invest. *75:* 1068 (1985).
13 Ockner, R. K.; Manning, J. A.: Fatty acid binding protein: Role in esterification of absorbed long chain fat in rat intestine. J. clin. Invest. *58:* 632 (1976).
14 Cardell, Jr., R. R.; Badenhausen, S.; Porter, K. P.: Intestinal triglyceride absorption in the rat. An electron microscopical study. J. Cell Biol. *34:* 125 (1967).
15 Glickman, R. M.: Fat absorption and malabsorption. Clin. Gastroenterol. *12:* 1202 (1983).
16 Clark, S. B.; Holt, P. R.: Rate-limiting steps in steady state intestinal absorption of trioctanoin I-^{14}C. J. clin. Invest. *47:* 612 (1968).
17 Clark, S. B.; Holt, P. R.: Inhibition of steady-state intestinal absorption of long-chain triglyceride by medium-chain triglyceride in the unanesthetized rat. J. clin. Invest. *48:* 2235 (1969).
18 Greenberger, N. J.; Skillman, T. G.: Medium chain triglycerides. Physiological considerations and clinical implications. New Engl. J. Med. *280:* 1045 (1969).
19 Weber, F.: Absorption mechanism for fat-soluble vitamins and the effect of other food constituents; in Harper, Dav, Nutrition in Health and Disease and International Development: Symposia from the XII. International Congress of Nutrition, pp. 119–135 (Alan R. Liss, New York 1981).
20 Corsini, G.; Gandolfi, E.; Bonechi, E.; Cerri, B.: Postgastrectomy malabsorption. Gastroenterology *50:* 358 (1966).
21 Shimoda, S. S.; Saunders, D. R.; Rubin, C. E.: The Zollinger-Ellison syndrome with steatorrhea. Mechanism of fat and vitamin B_{12} malabsorption. Gastroenterology *55:* 705 (1968).
22 Corda, J. J.; Brooks, F. P.: Relationships between steatorrhea and an insufficiency of pancreatic secretion in the duodenum in patients with chronic pancreatitis. Am. J. med. Sci. *153:* 38 (1967).
23 Mansbach, C. M.; Newton, D.; Stevens, R. D.: Fat digestion in patients with bile acid malabsorption but minimal steatorrhea. Dig. Dis. Sci. *25:* 353 (1980).
24 Rosenberg, J. H.; Hardison, W. G.; Bull, D. M.: Abnormal bile salt patterns and intestinal bacterial overgrowth associated with malabsorption. New Engl. J. Med. *176:* 1391 (1967).
25 Falchuk, Z. M.: Update of gluten-sensitive enteropathy. Am. J. Med. *67:* 1085 (1979).
26 Sheehy, T. W.; Baggs, B.; Perez-Santiago, E.; Floch, M. H.: Prognosis of tropical sprue. A study of the effect of folic acid on the intestinal aspect of acute and chronic sprue. Ann. Intern. Med. *57:* 892 (1962).
27 Greenberger, N. J.; Isselbacher, K. J.: Malabsorption following irradiation injury to the gastrointestinal tract. Am. J. Med. *36:* 450 (1064).

28 Glickman, R. M.; Green, P. H. R.; Less, R. S.; et al.: Immunofluorescence studies of apolipoprotein in intestinal mucosa. Absence in abetalipoproteinaemia. Gastroenterology *76:* 288 (1979).
29 Theron, J. J.; Wittman, W.; Prinston, J. G.: The fine structure of the jejunum in kwashiorkor. Exp. molec. Path. *124:* 184 (1971).
30 Glickman, R. M.; Kirsch, K.: Lymph chylomicron formation during the inhibition of protein synthesis. J. clin. Invest. *52:* 2910 (1973).
31 Gross, J. B.; Wollaeger, E. E.; Sauer, W. G.; Huitzenga, K. A.; Dahlin, D. C.; Power, M. H.: Whipple's disease. Report of four cases including two in brothers, with observations on pathologic physiology, diagnosis, and treatment. Gastroenterology *39:* 65 (1959).
32 Heymsfield, S. B.; Bethel, R. A.; Ansley, J. D.; Nixon, D. W.; Rudman, D.: Enteral hyperalimentation: An alternative to central venous hyperalimentation. Ann. intern. Med. *90:* 63 (1979).
33 Mochizuki, H.; Trocki, O.; Dominioni, L.; Ray, M. B.; Alexander, J. W.: Optimal lipid content for enteral diets following thermal injury. J. parent. ent. Nutr. *8:* 638 (1984).
34 Mok, K. T.; Maiz, A.; Yamazaki, K.; Sobrado, J.; Babayan, V. K.; Moldawer, L. L.; Bistrian, B. R.; Blackburn, G. L.: Structures medium-chain and long-chain triglycerides emulsions are superior to physical mixtures in sparing body protein in the burned rat. Metabolism *33:* 901 (1984).
35 Maiz, A.; Yamazaki, K.; Sobrado, J.; Babayan, V. K.; Moldawer, L. L.; Bistrian, B. R.; Blackburn, G. L.: Protein metabolism during total parenteral nutrition (TPN) in injured rats using medium chain triglycerides. Metabolism *33:* 901 (1984).
36 Miller, B.; Strohmeyer, G.: Gastrale oder enterale Applikation? Z. Gastroenterologie (suppl.) *23:* 26 (1985).
37 Delany, H. M.; Carnevale, N. J.; Garvey, J. W.: Jejunostomy by a needle catheter technique. Surgery *73:* 786 (1973).

Wolfgang Stremmel, Medizinische Klinik D der Universität Düsseldorf, Moorenstr. 5, D-4000 Düsseldorf (FRG)

Dietze, Grünert, Kleinberger, Wolfram (eds.), Clinical Nutrition and Metabolic Research. Proc. 7th Congr. ESPEN, Munich 1985, pp. 119–132 (Karger, Basel 1986)

Optimal Nitrogen Source for Enteral Nutrition: Dipeptides versus Free Amino Acids

S. A. Adibi

Clinical Nutrition Unit and Dept. of Medicine, Montefiore Hospital and University of Pittsburgh School of Medicine, Pittsburgh, Pa., USA

An early observation which led to the discovery of large-scale oligopeptide absorption in intestine was that the rates of amino acid uptake are considerably greater from solutions containing dipeptides than from solutions containing a corresponding amino acid mixture [1]. This observation has been confirmed and extended by a number of studies [2–5]. Furthermore, it has been shown that competition for absorption is either greatly diminished or abolished by presenting the intestinal mucosa with a dipeptide rather than a corresponding amino acid mixture. An example of these studies is presented in figure 1. In this figure absorption rates of glycine and leucine during jejunal perfusion with test solutions containing glycyl-leucine or equimolar mixtures of free glycine and free leucine are compared. Two striking differences are apparent. First, over the range of concentration infused (20–100 mM), both glycine and leucine absorption rates are significantly greater from the dipeptide solutions than from the corresponding free amino acid solutions. Second, the difference between the absorption of glycine and leucine is much smaller from the dipeptide than from the corresponding amino acid solution. These differences in absorption can be explained by the fact that on a molar basis, glycyl-leucine is more rapidly absorbed than either glycine or leucine, and furthermore, an almost complete lack of hydrolysis prior to absorption largely prevents the neutral amino acid carrier system from exerting its preference for leucine over glycine.

The above observations on quantitative and qualitative differences in amino acid absorption from dipeptide and free amino acid solutions prompt the question of whether dipeptides or amino acids are the optimal nitrogen source for enteral nutrition. The answer to this question requires consideration of a number of factors including the following:

(1) tonicity
(2) solubility
(3) stability
(4) transport interaction
(5) intestinal disorders
(6) extraintestinal disorders
(7) malnutrition
(8) efficiency of absorption as a mixture.

Tonicity

Elemental diets with free amino acids as the nitrogen source are quite hypertonic. Exposure of the intestine to hypertonic solutions may have deleterious effects. For example, it has been shown that a single force-feeding of a hypertonic solution causes structural and functional damage to the rat jejunum [6]. The problems of hypertonicity can be greatly reduced or even eliminated by replacement of amino acids with dipeptides.

Solubility

Water solubility of some amino acids, particularly tyrosine, is limited. Water solubility of tyrosine can be greatly increased by the attachment of this amino acid to a water-soluble amino acid in dipeptide form. There is evidence that in certain situations synthesis of tyrosine from phenylalanine in the body is not sufficient to meet the substrate requirements for protein synthesis [7].

Stability

Some amino acids, such as cysteine and glutamine, are not stable in free form, but are highly stable as dipeptides. There are indications that in certain situations provision of cysteine and glutamine could be beneficial to protein nutrition [8, 9].

Transport Interaction

Enteral solutions besides nitrogen must contain adequate amounts of calories, vitamins, trace elements, minerals, and electrolytes. Therefore, the selection of the nitrogen source may require consideration of interaction between transport of amino acids and dipeptides with other nutrients. Such information is available as far as interactions with glucose, zinc, and sodium are concerned.

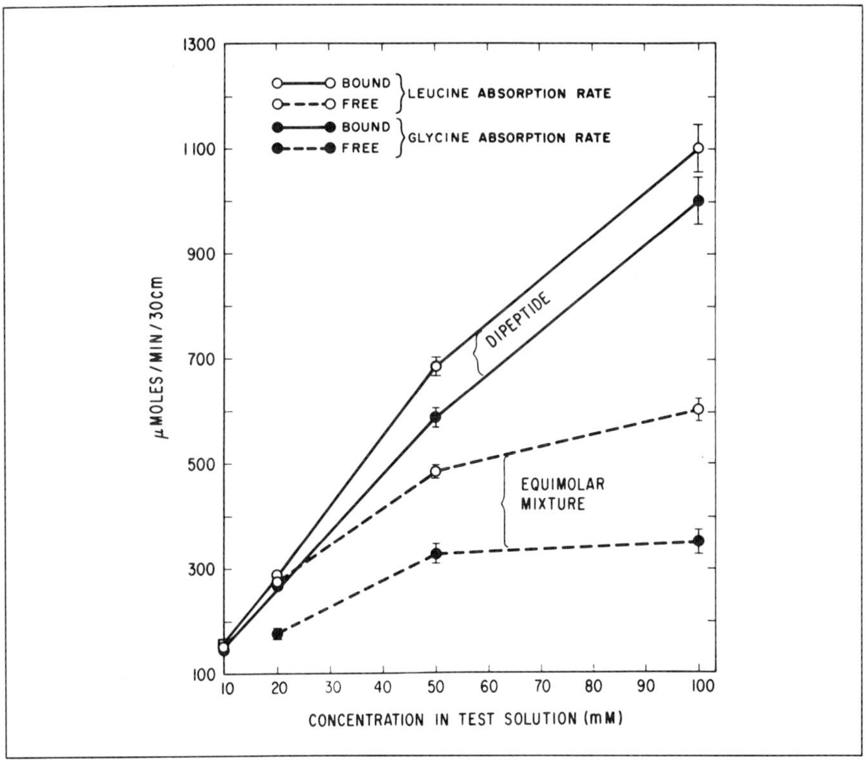

Fig. 1. Jejunal absorption rates of glycine and leucine (mean ± SEM) from test solutions containing either glycyl-L-leucine or an equimolar mixture of free glycine and free leucine in equivalent amounts. The studies were performed in 5 normal volunteers (reproduced from [2]).

Glucose

Glucose is usually the main source of calories in enteral solutions. Perfusion studies in human jejunum have shown that when 200 mM glucose is added to a test solution containing 100 mM glycine, the jejunal absorption rate of glycine is significantly reduced [10]. This interaction is diminished when dipeptides, instead of free amino acids, are used in the test solution. Jejunal absorption of glycine is reduced by 19% instead of 33% when 50 mM glycyl-glycine is substituted for 100 mM glycine [10]. Glycyl-glycine does not appear to have any significant effect on glucose absorption [10].

Zinc

Among trace elements, adequate zinc absorption appears to be most important. First, the requirement for zinc is far greater than for other trace elements. Second, growth and nitrogen balance are not maintained in patients with zinc depletions. Perfusion studies in human intestine have shown that zinc absorption is enhanced by dipeptides such as glycyl-leucine, but unaffected by a mixture of free glycine and leucine [11].

Sodium

The development of diarrhea during enteral nutrition is usually deleterious. Sodium absorption plays a key role in water absorption. Perfusion studies in human intestine have shown that amino acids stimulate sodium absorption and, consequently, water absorption [12–14]. Similar enhancements have also been found with dipeptides [13, 14]. However, it is not yet entirely clear that stimulation of sodium absorption with dipeptides is directly related to dipeptide transport or related to transport of amino acids released from peptide hydrolysis on the cell surface.

Intestinal Disorders

Enteral nutrition may be used in patients with intestinal disorders which reduce absorption. The selection of proper nitrogen source for enteral nutrition in these patients requires studies of amino acid and peptide absorption in malabsorptive states. Such studies have been performed in the intestine of patients with celiac sprue, cystic fibrosis, and jejunoileal bypass.

Celiac Sprue

Patients with celiac sprue often have protein malnutrition. There is evidence that amino acid absorption is significantly reduced in the jejunum of these patients [15]. Three groups of investigators have examined amino acid and dipeptide absorption in the intestine of patients with celiac sprue. Adibi and coworkers [16] found intestinal absorption of glycyl-glycine and glycyl-leucine to be significantly reduced. However, they found a striking difference between amino acid and dipeptide absorption when they compared the rate of glycine absorption from test solutions containing 50 mM glycyl-glycine or an equivalent amount of free glycine (100 mM) infused into the intestine of the same patient. The results of this study are shown in figure 2. Normally, there is less than a 2-fold difference in the rate of glycine uptake from 100 mmol glycine and 50 mM glycyl-glycine test solutions [16]. In patients with celiac sprue, the difference in rates of glycine uptake from these infusion solutions is increased 3- to 6-fold (fig. 2). In fact, in one patient (E.K.) there was an actual secretion of glycine into the lumen when the free glycine solution was infused. In contrast, there was glycine absorption when the jejunum of this patient was infused with glycyl-glycine test solution. These data indicate that in some patients the jejunal absorption rates of dipeptides are less severely affected than those of free amino acids. This unequal impairment allows a greater amino acid transport through the dipeptide than through the free amino acid carrier system.

Silk et al. [17] found that patients with adult celiac disease may have no significant reduction in their intestinal uptake of alanine and glycine from a test solution containing glycyl-alanine, but have impaired absorption of these amino acids from a test solution containing a corresponding free amino acid mixture. Nutzenadel et al. [18] found a reduction in intestinal absorption of glycine and phenylalanine from test solutions containing either glycyl-phenylalanine or the corresponding free amino acid mixture. However, these investigators observed the advantage of amino acid absorption from dipeptides to be maintained in these patients.

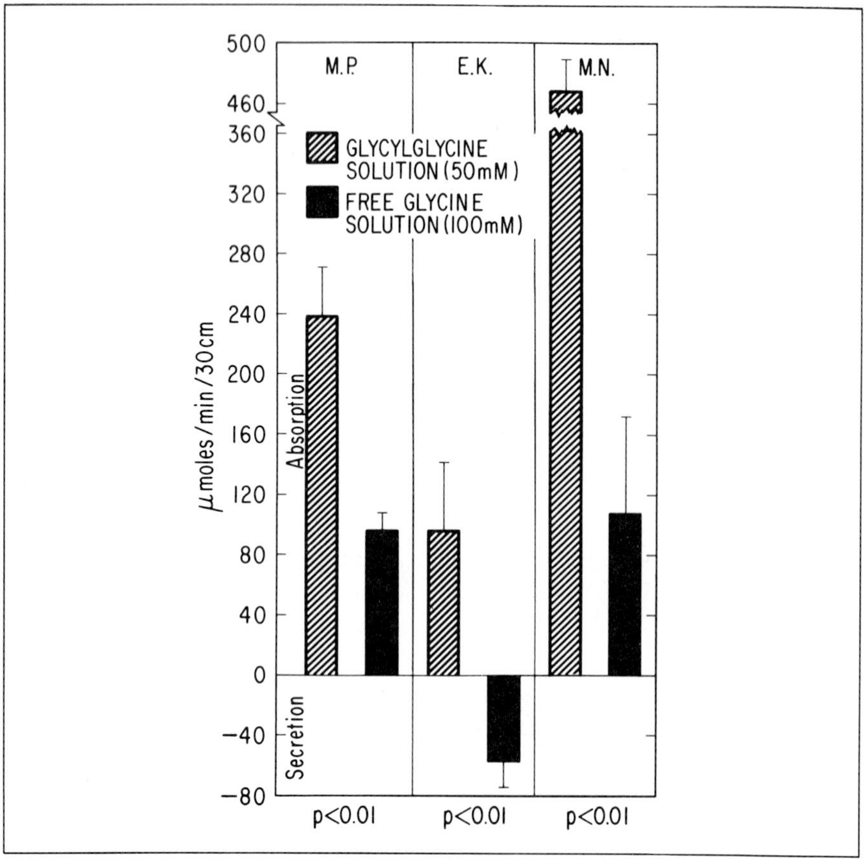

Fig. 2. Jejunal absorption rates (mean ± SEM) of glycine from test solutions containing equal amounts of glycine in free and dipeptide forms in 3 untreated celiac-sprue patients (reproduced from [16]).

Cystic Fibrosis

There is evidence that patients with cystic fibrosis have amino acid malabsorption. Milla et al. [19] investigated jejunal absorption rates of glycine and phenylalanine from test solutions containing glycyl-phenylalanine and a mixture of free glycine and phenylalanine in these patients. They found that while absorption rates of glycine and phenylalanine from the amino acid solution were significantly reduced, the absorption of glycine and phenylalanine from the dipeptide solution was either normal or increased in cystic fibrosis.

Jejunoileal Bypass

During the last two decades, jejunoileal bypass was extensively used for treatment of morbid obesity [20]. Fogel and coworkers [21] investigated rates of amino acid and peptide absorption in the jejunum of a group of obese patients before and after jejunoileal bypass. They found a significant reduction in the rate of amino acid absorption, but none in the rate of dipeptide absorption after the surgery. The data seem to suggest that in an altered nutritional state the dipeptide transport system is more resistant to change than the amino acid transport system.

Extraintestinal Disorders

Renal failure in experimental animals has been shown to be associated with a decrease in intestinal absorption of amino acids. Sterner et al. [22] investigated plasma α-amino nitrogen levels after oral loads of glycine and glycyl-glycine in a group of patients with chronic renal insufficiency. They found that uremic patients had significantly lower levels of plasma α-amino nitrogen after glycine than after glycyl-glycine. From these results, Sterner et al. concluded that even in uremic patients dipeptide absorption is more efficient than amino acid absorption.

Malnutrition

Patients who require support with enteral nutrition are often malnourished. Malnutrition has profound effects on the intestine. For example, studies in the intestine of human volunteers have shown that starvation and protein deprivation for a period of 2 weeks reduces the jejunal absorption rates of amino acids [23]. These reductions occurred without any apparent change in intestinal morphology as examined by light and electron microscopy [23]. To investigate the effect of malnutrition on intestinal absorption rates of amino acids in free and peptide form, Vazquez and colleagues [24] have studied the jejunal absorption rates of glycine from triglycine and glycine test solutions before and after 2 weeks of starvation in a group of obese patients. The concentration of glycine in free and peptide form was similar. They found that before starvation glycine absorption was significantly greater from the triglycine than from the glycine test solution. Although starvation significantly decreased glycine absorption from both solutions, the greater amino acid absorption from the triglycine than from the glycine test solution was maintained.

Efficiency of Absorption as a Mixture

The use of dipeptides as the nitrogen source requires design of molecular structures which are best suited for enteral nutrition. Among many various possibilities, Steinhardt and Adibi [25] have proposed that dipeptides should commonly have glycine as the N-terminal amino acid residue, and an essential or nonessential amino acid in the C-terminus. Dipeptides with glycine as the N-terminal amino acid residue have the following properties:

Solubility

Glycine is the most water-soluble amino acid. This property is of value for increasing the water solubility of other amino acids. For example, unlike tyrosine, glycyl-tyrosine is quite water-soluble.

Utilization

An objective of enteral nutrition is the delivery of an adequate amount of nitrogen. Glycine is an excellent source of nitrogen. In fact, studies in subhuman primates have shown efficient utilization of a large load of glycine, and maintenance of nitrogen equilibrium with a dipeptide mixture composed exclusively of glycyl-dipeptides [26].

Hydrolysis

For dipeptides to be suitable substrates for enteral nutrition, they must have minimal hydrolysis in the gut lumen. Otherwise, they would behave like free amino acids. As far as dipeptide hydrolysis is concerned, the amino acid in the N-terminus is more important than the amino acid in the C-terminus, since the activity of peptidases are generally directed toward the N-terminal of peptides. Studies of dipeptide hydrolysis by a brush-border membrane preparation of intestinal mucosa of man (Adibi and Morse, unpublished observation) have shown that dipeptides with glycine as the N-terminal amino acid residue generally have a slower rate of hydrolysis than dipeptides with the other amino acids in this position.

Transport

Another important requirement for nutritional use of dipeptides is that they be substrates for the peptide transport system. Studies of mechanisms of assimilation of dipeptides in human jejunum have shown that the luminal disappearance of glycyl-dipeptides occurs largely as intact peptides rather than as free amino acids [2, 27].

The use of glycyl-dipeptides as the nitrogen source for enteral nutrition requires their provision as a dipeptide mixture. The suggestion for the use of such a mixture may prompt the following question. Is there any advantage in efficiency of absorption if the intestinal mucosa is presented with a mixture of dipeptides containing all essential amino acids and a variety of non-essential amino acids instead of a mixture of free amino acids? The evidence that the rates of amino acid uptake from a test solution containing a single glycyl-dipeptide are significantly greater than from a corresponding amino acid solution cannot be extrapolated to the rate of amino acid absorption from a dipeptide mixture. Intestinal perfusion studies in man have shown that the kinetics of amino acid absorption is vastly different when an amino acid is presented to the intestine singly or together with other amino acids [28–30].

As a first step toward development of a glycyl-dipeptide mixture for enteral nutrition, Steinhardt and Adibi [25] have investigated kinetics and characteristics of jejunal absorption of individual dipeptides from an equimolar mixture of 12 dipeptides. All dipeptides contained glycine in the N-terminal position and all 8 essential amino acids (methionine, isoleucine, leucine, valine, phenylalanine, lysine, threonine, and tryptophan) and 4 nonessential amino acids (arginine, proline, histidine, and alanine) in the carboxyl position. Furthermore, these investigators compared absorption rates of amino acids from this dipeptide mixture with those from a corresponding free amino acid mixture. The results of these studies, which were performed in the jejunum of healthy human volunteers, are summarized in figures 3 and 4. The rate of absorption from the free amino acid solution was characterized by the following pattern: methionine, isoleucine, and leucine had the fastest rates, and histidine and tryptophan had the lowest rates of absorption (fig. 3). Between these two extremes, in decreasing order were the absorption rates of valine, arginine, alanine, phenylalanine, proline, lysine, and threonine. This pattern of selective absorption was not observed when the dipeptide mixture was infused, due mainly to large increases in the absorption rates of amino acids which were slowly absorbed from the free amino acid mixture (fig. 3). For example, histidine, which was not absorbed at a measurable rate from the free amino acid mixture, had a substantial rate of absorption from the dipeptide mixture. In another example, the absorption rate of threonine was over 3-fold greater from the dipeptide than from the free amino acid mixture. Except for arginine, the rates of absorption were generally greater from the dipeptide than from the free amino acid mixture. For these studies, the concentration of each dipeptide or amino acid in the test solutions was either 6 or 2 mM. These concentrations were

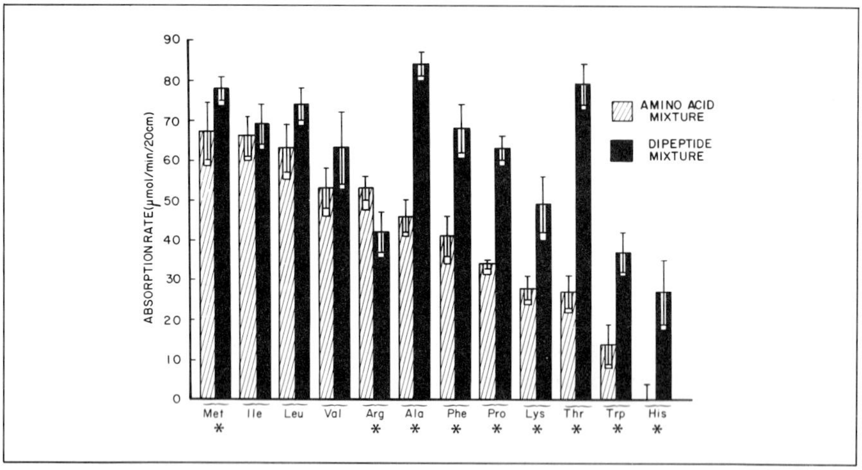

Fig. 3. Amino acid absorption rates (mean ± SEM) from a mixture of 12 glycyl-dipeptides and a mixture of corresponding amino acids. The concentration of each dipeptide and corresponding amino acid in the test solution was 6 mM. The studies were performed in the intestine of 5 normal volunteers. The asterisk indicates that the difference was statistically significant (reproduced from [25]).

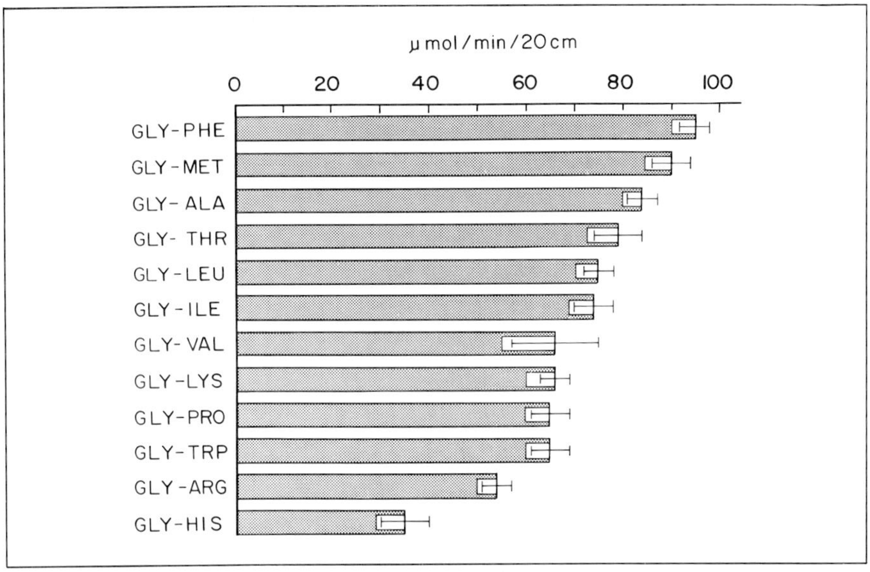

Fig. 4. Dipeptide absorption rates (mean ± SEM) from the 6 mM equimolar mixture of 12 glycyl-dipeptides. The studies were performed in the intestine of 5 normal volunteers (reproduced from [25]).

within the range of concentrations found in the gut lumen after a protein meal [31]. At the 2 mM infusion concentration, in contrast to rates of amino acid absorption, the absorption rates of all 12 dipeptides were approximately similar [25]. In contrast, at 6 mM infusion concentration, there was some selectivity in absorption rates of dipeptides (fig. 4). Absorption rates were fastest for glycyl-phenylalanine and glycyl-methionine, and slowest for glycyl-histidine and glycyl-arginine. However, between the two ends of this spectrum, the absorption of other dipeptides differed only modestly from each other.

Conclusion

In healthy or in diseased states, dipeptide absorption is more efficient than amino acid absorption. This efficiency persists even when a mixture of 12 glycyl-dipeptides containing all essential amino acids and several nonessential amino acids are presented to the intestinal mucosa. The mechanism of this efficiency in absorption appears to be the result of uptake by a system which has a greater transport capacity than amino acid carrier systems, thus minimizing competition among its substrates. In addition to efficiency of absorption, use of dipeptides instead of free amino acids as the nitrogen source for enteral nutrition allows reduction in hypertonicity, and provision of amino acids which are either poorly soluble in water (e.g., tyrosine) or unstable in free form (e.g., glutamine and cysteine).

Finally, all the studies performed thus far must be considered as preliminary evidence for establishing the superiority of dipeptides over amino acids as substrates for enteral nutrition. The definitive study which has yet to be performed will have to show the maintenance of a better protein nutrition with dipeptides than amino acids as the nitrogen source in patients requiring enteral nutrition.

References

1 Matthews, D. M.; Adibi, S. A.: Peptide absorption. Gastroenterology *71:* 151–161 (1976).

2 Adibi, S. A.: Intestinal transport of dipeptides in man: Relative importance of hydrolysis and intact absorption. J. clin. Invest. *50:* 2266–2275 (1971).

3 Hellier, M. D.; Holdsworth, C. D.; McColl, I.; Perrett, D.: Dipeptide absorption in man. Gut *13:* 965–969 (1972).

4 Silk, D. B. A.; Perrett, D.; Clark, M. L.: Intestinal transport of two dipeptides containing the same two neutral amino acids in man. Clin. Sci. mol. Med. *45:* 291–299 (1973).

5 Cook, G. C.: Independent jejunal mechanisms for glycine and glycyl-glycine transfer in man in vivo. Br. J. Nutr. *30:* 13–19 (1973).

6 Teichberg, S.; Lifshitz, F.; Pergalizzi, R.; Wapnir, R. A.: Response of rat intestine to a hypertonic feeding. Pediat. Res. *12:* 720–725 (1978).

7 Daabees, T. T.; Stegink, L. D.: L-alanyl-L-tyrosine as a tyrosine source during total parenteral nutrition. Infusion at 0.5 and 2 mmoles/kg/day in adult rats. Pediat. Res. *13:* 894–899 (1979).

8 Rudman, D.; Kutner, M.; Ansley, J.; Jansen, R.; Chipponi, J.; Bain, R. P.: Hypotyrosinemia, hypocystinemia, and failure to retain nitrogen during total parenteral nutrition of cirrhotic patients. Gastroenterology *81:* 1025–1035 (1981).

9 Amberger, I.; Fürst, P.; Godel, H.; Graser, T.; Stehle, P.; Pfaender, P.: The potential parenteral application of the peptide L-alanyl-L-glutamine as a nitrogen source in severe catabolic states. Hoppe-Seyler's Z. physiol. Chem. *364:* 1253–1254 (1983).

10 Cook, G. C.: Comparison of intestinal absorption rates of glycine and glycyl-glycine in man and the effect of glucose in the perfusing fluid. Clin. Sci. *43:* 443–453 (1972).

11 Steinhardt, H. J.; Adibi, S. A.: Interaction between transport of zinc and other solutes in human intestine. Am. J. Physiol. *247:* G176–G182 (1984).

12 Adibi, S. A.: Leucine absorption rate and net movements of sodium and water in human jejunum. J. appl. Physiol. *28:* 753–757 (1970).
13 Hellier, M. D.; Thirumalai, C.; Holdsworth, C. D.: The effect of amino acids and dipeptides on sodium and water absorption in man. Gut *14:* 41–45 (1973).
14 Silk, D. B. A.; Fairclough, P. D.; Park, N. J.; Lane, A. E.; Webb, J. P. W.; Clark, M. L.; Dawson, A. M.: A study of relations between the absorption of amino acids, dipeptides, water and electrolytes in the normal human jejunum. Clin. Sci. mol. Med. *49:* 401–408 (1975).
15 Schedl, H. P.; Pierce, C. E.; Rider, A.; Clifton, J. A.: Absorption of L-methionine from the human small intestine. J. clin. Invest. *47:* 417–425 (1968).
16 Adibi, S. A.; Fogel, M. R.; Agrawal, R. M.: Comparison of free amino acid and dipeptide absorption in the jejunum of sprue patients. Gastroenterology *67:* 586–591 (1974).
17 Silk, D. B. A.; Kumar, P. J.; Perrett, D.; Clark, M. L.; Dawson, A. M.: Amino acid and peptide absorption in patients with coeliac disease and dermatitis herpetiformis. Gut *15:* 1–8 (1974).
18 Nutzenadel, W.; Fahr, K.; Lutz, P.: Absorption of free and peptide-linked glycine and phenylalanine in children with active celiac disease. Pediat. Res. *15:* 309–312 (1981).
19 Milla, P. J.; Kilby, A.; Rassam, U. B.; Ersser, R.; Harries, J. T.: Small intestinal absorption of amino acids and a dipeptide in pancreatic insufficiency. Gut *24:* 818–824 (1983).
20 Adibi, S. A.; Stanko, R. T.: Perspectives on gastrointestinal surgery for treatment of morbid obesity: The lesson learned. Gastroenterology *87:* 1381–1391 (1984).
21 Fogel, M. R.; Ravitch, M. M.; Adibi, S. A.: Absorptive and digestive function of the jejunum after jejunoileal bypass for treatment of human obesity. Gastroenterology *71:* 729–733 (1976).
22 Sterner, G.; Lindberg, T.; Denneberg, T.: Small intestinal absorption of glycine and glycyl-glycine in patients with chronic renal failure. Acta med. scand. *213:* 375–379 (1983).
23 Adibi, S. A.; Allen, E. R.: Impaired jejunal absorption rates of essential amino acids induced by either dietary caloric or protein deprivation in man. Gastroenterology *69:* 404–413 (1970).
24 Vazquez, J. A.; Morse, E. L.; Adibi, S. A.: Effect of starvation on amino acid transport and peptide hydrolysis in man. Am. J. Physiol. *249:* G563–G566 (1985).
25 Steinhardt, H. J.; Adibi, S. A.: Kinetics and characteristics of absorption from an equimolar mixture of twelve glycyl-dipeptides in human jejunum. Gastroenterology (in press).
26 Steinhardt, H. J.; Paleos, G. A.; Brandl, M.; Fekl, W. L.; Adibi, S. A.: Efficacy of a synthetic dipeptide mixture as the source of amino acids for total parenteral nutrition in a subhuman primate (baboon): Plasma concentration, metabolic clearance, and urinary excretion of a series of dipeptides. Gastroenterology *86:* 1562–1569 (1984).
27 Adibi, S. A.; Soleimanpour, M. R.: Functional characterization of dipeptide transport system in human jejunum. J. clin. Invest. *53:* 1368–1374 (1974).
28 Adibi, S. A.; Gray, S. J.: Intestinal absorption of essential amino acids in man. Gastroenterology *52:* 837–845 (1967).
29 Adibi, S. A.; Gray, S. J.; Menden, E.: The kinetics of amino acid absorption and

alteration of plasma composition of free amino acids after intestinal perfusion of amino acid mixtures. Am. J. clin. Nutr. *20:* 24–33 (1967).

30 Adibi, S. A.: The influence of molecular structure of neutral amino acids on their absorption kinetics in the jejunum and ileum of human intestine in vivo. Gastroenterology *56:* 903–913 (1969).

31 Adibi, S. A.; Mercer, D. W.: Protein digestion in human intestine as reflected in luminal, mucosal, and plasma amino acid concentrations after meals. J. clin. Invest. *52:* 1586–1594 (1973).

Siamak A. Adibi, M.D., Ph.D., Montefiore Hospital, 3459 Fifth Avenue, Pittsburgh, PA 15213 (USA)

Dietze, Grünert, Kleinberger, Wolfram (eds.), Clinical Nutrition and Metabolic Research. Proc. 7th Congr. ESPEN, Munich 1985, pp. 133–142 (Karger, Basel 1986)

Carbohydrate Absorption and Related Sodium and Water Absorption in the Critically Ill

B. J. M. Jones

The London Hospital, Whitechapel, London, UK

Introduction

Carbohydrate absorption depends upon intake, gastric emptying, luminal hydrolysis, brush border hydrolysis and finally translocation of substituent monosaccharides across the enterocytes to the portal venous system via specific carrier systems [1]. In the critically ill patient, carbohydrate absorption may be impaired at any of the above stages. Three topics can be identified for discussion:

(i) General factors arising from the effect of a non-alimentary illness on the alimentary tract;

(ii) specific problems arising from primary alimentary tract disease;

(iii) achievement of energy balance by optimisation of the carbohydrate content of enteral diets for use in the critically ill.

It should be noted that the very nature of a critical illness in man complicates investigation of nutrient absorption, a situation compounded by a tendency to opt, often unnecessarily, for parenteral rather than enteral nutrition in such patients. Much work has therefore been done in animals.

General Factors Affecting Carbohydrate Absorption

Gastric Emptying

Gastric emptying is often markedly impaired in injured patients so that carbohydrate absorption cannot be assessed by standard tolerance tests. When gastric function is unaffected, emptying is determined by volume, temperature, particulate profile, energy density and osmolality [2]. In conventional polymeric enteral diets, most of the osmolality is due to the carbohydrate and ionic moieties. Hitherto, energy density was held to determine emptying [3] but recently, osmolality has been considered more important [4]. Thus maltodextrins (glucose polymer mixtures with median chain length of about 10 glucose residues) empty faster than isocaloric free glucose solution [5]. The negative feedback loop depends also upon vagal and pyloric integrity as well as duodenal osmoreceptor detection of osmotically active carbohydrate so that both hypolactasia and pancreatic insufficiency lead to rapid gastric emptying [6]. All these considerations are rendered irrelevant by the introduction of continuous nasogastric nutrient infusion at rates well below the maximal gastric emptying rate.

Small Bowel Motility

Until recently, postoperative ileus meant no enteral feeding. The realisation that jejunoileal motility and function return well before that of the stomach or colon has led to early postoperative nasoenteric or enterostomy feeding. Normal glucose and sodium absorption have been demonstrated in the early postoperative period in man [7] but in rats subjected to 40% burns, 3-0-methylglucose, calcium and cycloleucine absorption were markedly reduced 18 h post burn [8]. This suggested that severe trauma may have a specific effect on nutrient absorption independent of its effect on motility. Decreased motility and luminal flow directly affect absorption by increasing the depth of the unstirred water layer adjacent to the brush border, thus hindering access of sugars, particularly complex ones, to the brush border hydrolysis sites [9].

Brush Border Function

Starvation and Bowel Rest

The most profound effects on small bowel mucosal structure and function in the critically ill are the result of starvation. Lack of luminal nutrients plays a crucial role not reversed by total parenteral nutrition

[10]. Loss of villous height, thinning of the mucosa and decreased protein synthesis lead to reduced carbohydrate activity, particularly of lactase but sucrase and maltase are also affected [11]. Pancreatic enzyme secretion is also reduced but this is of minor significance (see below). Since lactose hydrolysis is normally rate limiting for absorption, lactose intolerance is the most common form of carbohydrate intolerance and may lead to secondary malabsorption of other sugars as a result of small bowel bacterial overgrowth [11]. Whether malabsorption of starch, glucose polymers, maltose or sucrose is ever of clinical significance when lactose free enteral diets are used in starvation is doubtful. When significant carbohydrate malabsorption does occur diarrhoea results from the osmotic effects of unchanged sugars and their organic acid bacterial degradation products within the colon [11]. Exchange of bicarbonate for hydrions may lead to acidosis, particularly in children [11].

Glucose monomer absorption is also reduced by lack of luminal glucose so that the normal gradient for glucose absorption from jejunum to ileum is abolished without structural abnormality [12]. This work suggests that glucose carrier sites can be induced by luminal glucose.

It is important to emphasise that impairment of carbohydrate absorption may not be reflected by clinically significant carbohydrate intolerance, particularly when continuous rather than bolus infusion techniques are used. It is also vital to recognize that other factors such as concurrent antibiotic therapy are more probable explanations of diarrhoea occurring during reintroduction of enteral nutrition in starved patients [13, 14].

Miscellaneous Factors Affecting Brush Border Function

Injured and septic patients often demonstrate insulin resistant hyperglycaemia. There is no evidence that a reduction in luminal-serosal glucose gradients reduces glucose absorption although recent evidence suggests a role for insulin in mucosal glucose translocation [15]. Sucrose activity [16] and glucose absorption [17] are enhanced in diabetes mellitus. Glucocorticoids enhance carbohydrase activity and adaptive ileal hyperplasia [18]. Alcohol reduces disaccharidase activity [19], glucose and water absorption but not sodium absorption [20]. Folic acid deficiency may be important in these patients [19].

Small bowel ischaemia up to the point of irreversible mucosal damage produces remarkably little disturbance of carbohydrate absorption [21]. In most cases of chronic ischaemia, reduced intake explains loss of weight [21].

Further studies are required to establish the incidence and relevance of intestinal hypoalbuminaemic oedema. Modulation of the serosal glucose carrier sites by substances such as ATP may also prove interesting [22].

Carbohydrate Absorption and Primary Alimentary Tract Disorders

Basic Concepts

Although colonic spillage of malabsorbed carbohydrate may be physiological on a normal diet [23], the carbohydrate moieties of liquid enteral diets are almost entirely absorbed by the duodenum and proximal jejunum [4]. Since carbohydrate absorption falls off distally to the ileum, disease or resection of the jejunum has a more profound effect than that of the ileum. However, the ileum is capable of marked adaptation so that clinical carbohydrate intolerance does not invariably follow upon loss of jejunal absorption. This is best illustrated by coeliac disease [24].

With the exception of lactose, hydrolysis of disaccharides and glucose polymers is not rate limiting for absorption [1]. However, some sugars are absorbed faster than others, a phenomenon known as 'kinetic advantage'. Evidence from in vivo human jejunal segmental perfusion studies has shown that maltose, maltotriose, glucose oligomers and amylase hydrolysates of starch are all absorbed significantly faster than isocaloric free glucose [25–29]. This kinetic advantage phenomenon holds true over a wide concentration range (e.g., 5.7 −111 mM maltose [27, 28]) unlike the kinetic advantage of oligopeptides [30].

The jejunum is a 'leaky' epithelium so that the luminal contents remain isotonic despite luminal and brush border hydrolysis. Water is passively absorbed or secreted according to the net loss or gain of osmotically active particles within the lumen. Stool water content is determined by the less leaky ileal and colonic epithelia which are also able to absorb sodium against a greater concentration gradient than the jejunum where active uphill sodium absorption must first overcome passive sodium secretion [31]. Sugars, amino acids, glycerides and bicarbonate are the principal stimulants of sodium absorption [31].

Gastroenteritis

In both enterotoxogenic bacterial diarrhoea (e.g., cholera) and cytopathic viral diarrhoea (e.g., rotavirus, Norwalk agents), glucose stimulated sodium absorption remains intact so that glucose-electrolyte solutions are now advocated for rehydration in these conditions [32]. More recently, alternative carbohydrate substrates such as sucrose or rice water [33, 34] have also been found to promote rehydration even in viral gastroenteritis in which a marked reduction in brush border carbohydrase activity occurs [33]. The correct sodium content of such solutions to avoid hypernatraemia remains controversial, particularly in temperate climates and viral enteritis in which stool sodium content is low.

Coeliac Disease

Jejunal carbohydrase activity and monosaccharide absorption are usually markedly reduced but the proximal nature of this disease allows the unaffected ileum to adapt so that clinical carbohydrate intolerance is a late manifestation of severe coeliac disease unless small bowel bacterial overgrowth supervenes. The kinetic advantage of oligopeptides compared to free amino acids is preserved even with severe villous atrophy [24] whereas the kinetic advantage of maltose and complete amylase hydrolysates of starch is less clearly preserved [Jones, unpublished data]. The reduction in carbohydrase activity and absorptive surface area is partially offset by a reduction in the thickness of the unstirred water layer [35].

Pancreatic Exocrine Insufficiency

Gastric emptying of starch and maltodextrins is enhanced in physiological and pathological pancreatic exocrine insufficiency (PI) [6, 36]. In neonates up to 6 months of age this leads to starch loss in the stools but maltodextrins such as Caloreen still confer nutritional benefit in low birth weight infants [37]. In adults, amylase secretion greatly exceeds requirements but even a 90% reduction in luminal amylase concentration leads only to a small increase in mean chain length of starch hydrolysis products from 3 to 4.5 glucose units at the duodenojejunal junction [38]. Brush border enzymes, particularly glucoamylase, are capable of hydrolysing starch in the absence of amylase [39]. This is well demonstrated in rat Thiry-Vella loops in which maltodextrins (Polycose) were absorbed almost as fast as free glucose [40]. In man, maltodextrins (Caloreen) were absorbed as fast as free glucose [28] but high molecular weight glucose polymers were absorbed more slowly [28] during perfusion of 25 cm jejunal segments. This is unlikely to lead to carbohydrate intolerance provided the small bowel is anatomically and functionally normal so that maltodextrins can be used as supplements in pancreatic insufficiency [41].

Crohn's Disease and the Short Bowel Syndrome (SBS)

Carbohydrate intolerance in Crohn's disease usually reflects lactose intolerance or small bowel bacterial overgrowth. Malabsorption of glucose polymers, disaccharides or glucose is so uncommon that current interest in Crohn's disease centres around the remarkable improvements associated with enteral diets which contain large quantities of maltodextrins [42]. However, in a few patients multiple resections of small and large bowel lead to the SBS. Originally it was thought that glucose monomer would provide optimal carbohydrate uptake in SBS but maltodextrins have now completely replaced free glucose. Simulation of SBS in perfusion studies of short segments of normal human jejunum has demonstrated that maltose, glucose oligomers and complete amylase hydrolysates of Caloreen and high molecular weight glucose polymers are all absorbed faster than isocaloric free glucose [25–29, 43]. Caloreen and potato starch solutions are absorbed as well as free glucose in SBS patients with as little as 25 cm jejunum [44]. Provided pancreatic function is intact, maltodextrins or high molecular weight glucose polymers can provide increased energy supply at no osmotic cost.

In many SBS patients, it is not malnutrition but loss of water and electrolytes which provides the greatest problems. It is now clear that the sodium content of enteral rehydration solutions is crucial to the establishment of net sodium and water absorption in SBS. Low Na^+ drinks, e.g., water or tea, cause sodium wastage [45]. Perfusion data with sugar saline solutions or isotonic enteral diets (Vivonex and Ensure) clearly shows that net sodium absorption from the jejunum depends upon the initial Na^+ concentration which must exceed 70–90 mmol/l in the presence of carbohydrate [46, 47]. Isotonicity of rehydration solutions and complete enteral diets is essential to avoid excessive water losses in SBS. However, perfusion of isotonic Vivonex was also associated with marked water secretion from a 25 cm jejunal segment [47]. Scrutiny of available data in patients with SBS confirms the crucial role of sodium concentration in rehydration solutions [44, 45]. The longer the residual bowel, the less important this becomes. The ideal carbohydrate substrate for enteral sugar-electrolyte 'rehydration' solutions is controversial. Some favour free glucose [45], other maltodextrins [48]. Personal data would suggest that a glucose oligomer mixture requiring minimal luminal hydrolysis might prove ideal.

Water absorption from 25 cm jejunal segments perfused with a variety of monomeric and polymeric sugar-saline solutions was similar. Available evidence suggests that glucose polymers contribute little to water absorption except by stimulation of active Na^+ absorption. It is the electrolyte content of glucose polymer-saline solutions which determines water absorption. So once again, an adequate electrolyte content is essential for rehydration in SBS [49].

Optimisation of Carbohydrate Absorption – The Role of Energy Dense Formulations and Sucrose

The increased demands for energy associated with injury and sepsis can be satisfied by increasing the administered volume of standard 1 kcal/ml enteral feed or increasing its energy density. Such patients are often 'volume intolerant'. Formulations of 1.5–2.0 kcal/ml are now available and well tolerated in patients with extensive burns despite the obligatory rise in diet osmolality [50]. When severe volume restriction is indicated as in cardiac, respiratory or renal failure and after head injury or neurosurgery, presently available energy dense diets may not enable achievement of energy balance. High molecular weight glucose polymers with negligible osmotic effect are absorbed as efficiently as free glucose when luminal amylase is present and would provide adequate energy at minimal osmotic cost [43].

Sucrose is also a valuable addition to enteral diets since total monosaccharide absorption from sucrose during perfusion studies exceeds that from isocaloric glucose [51]. Furthermore, the alternative pathway used for fructose transport allows saturated glucose transport to be supplemented with enteral diets such as Ensure [52].

References

1 Gray, G.: Carbohydrate absorption and malabsorption; in Johnson, Physiology of the gastrointestinal tract, pp. 1063–1072 (Raven Press, New York 1981).

2 Minami, H.; McCallum, R.: The physiology and patho-physiology of gastric emptying in humans. Gastroenterology *86:* 1592–1610 (1984).

3 Hunt, J.; Stubbs, D.: The volume and energy density of meals as determinants of gastric emptying. J. Physiol. *245:* 209–225 (1975).

4 Ruppin, H.; Bar-Meir, S.; Soergel, K.; Wood, C.: Effects of liquid formula diets on proximal gastrointestinal function. Dig. Dis. Sci. *26:* 202–207 (1981).

5 Foster, C.; Costill, D.; Fink, W.: Gastric emptying characteristics of glucose and glucose polymer solutions. Res. Q. Exerc. Sport. *51:* 299–315 (1980).

6 Mallinson, C.: Effect of pancreatic insufficiency and intestinal lactase deficiency on the gastric emptying of starch and lactose. Gut *9:* 737 (1968).

7 Glucksman, D.; Kalser, M.; Warren, D.: Small intestinal absorption in the immediate postoperative period. Surgery *60:* 1020–1025 (1966).

8 Molnar, J.; Bell, S.; Goodenough, R.; Burke, J.: Enteral nutrition in patients with burns or trauma; in Rombeau, Caldwell, Clinical nutrition, vol. 1, Enteral and tube feeding, pp. 412–433 (Saunders, Philadelphia 1984).

9 Rey, F.; Drillet, F.; Schmitz, J.; Rey, J.: Influence of flow rate on the kinetics of the intestinal absorption of glucose and lysine in children. Gastroenterology *66:* 79–85 (1974).

10 Dowling, R.: Small bowel adaptation and its regulation. Scand. J. Gastroent. *17:* suppl. 74, pp. 53–74 (1982).

11 Harries, J.; Muller, D.: Basic causes of carbohydrate malabsorption; in Burman, Holton, Pennock, Inherited disorders of carbohydrate metabolism, pp. 21–37 (MTP Press, Lancaster 1980).

12 Diamond, J.; Karasov, W.: Effect of dietary carbohydrate on monosaccharide uptake by mouse small intestine in vitro. J. Physiol. (Lond) *359:* 419–440 (1984).

13 Jones, B.; Lees, R.; Andrews, J.; Frost, P.; Silk, D.: Comparison of an elemental and polymeric enteral diet in patients with normal gastrointestinal function. Gut *24:* 78–84 (1983).

14 Keohane, P.; Attrill, H.; Jones, B.; Brown, I.; Frost, P.; Silk, D.: The roles of lactose and clostridium difficile in the pathogenesis of enteral feeding associated diarrhoea. Clin. Nutr. *1:* 259–264 (1983).

15 Lucas, M.: Physiology of the small intestine. Curr. Opinion Gastroenterol. *1:* 203–211 (1985).

16 Olsen, W.; Korsmo, H.: The intestinal brush border membrane in diabetes. Studies of sucrase-isomaltase metabolism in rats with streptozotocin diabetes. J. clin. Invest. *60:* 181–188 (1977).

17 Vinnick, I.; Kern, F.; Sussman, K.: The effect of diabetes mellitus and insulin on glucose absorption by the small intestine in man. J. Lab. clin. Med. *66:* 131–136 (1965).

18 Batt, R.; Scott, G.: Response of the small intestinal mucosa to oral glucocorticoids. Scand. J. Gastroent. *17:* suppl. 74, pp. 75–88 (1982).

19 Perlow, W.; Baraona, G.; Lieber, C.: Symptomatic intestinal disaccharidase deficiency in alcoholism. Gastroenterology *72:* 680–684 (1977).
20 Russell, R.: Alcohol and the small intestine. Curr. Opinion Gastroenterol. *1:* 232–234 (1985).
21 Marston, A.; Clarke, M.; Garcia, J.; Miller, A.: Intestinal function and intestinal blood supply. Gut *26:* 656–666 (1985).
22 Kimmich, G.: Intestinal absorption of sugar; in Johnson, Physiology of the gastrointestinal tract, pp. 1053–1062 (Raven Press, New York 1981).
23 Levitt, M.: Malabsorption of starch: A normal phenomenon. Gastroenterology *85:* 769–770 (1983).
24 Silk, D.; Kumar, P.; Webb, J.; Lane, A.; Clark, M.; Dawson, A.: Ileal function in patients with untreated coeliac disease. Gut *16:* 261–267 (1975).
25 Cook, G.: Comparison of absorption rates of glucose and maltose in man in vivo. Clin. Sci. mol. Med. *44:* 425–428 (1973).
26 Fairclough, P.; Silk, D.; Webb, J.; Clark, M.; Dawson, A.: A reappraisal of osmotic evidence for intact peptide absorption. Clin. Sci. mol. Med. *53:* 241–248 (1977).
27 Sandle, G.; Lobley, R.; Holmes, R.: Maltose hydrolysis and absorption in the human jejunum. Digestion *24:* 137–145 (1982).
28 Jones, B.; Brown, B.; Loran, J.; Edgerton, D.; Kennedy, J.; Stead, J.; Silk, D.: Glucose absorption from starch hydrolysates in the human jejunum. Gut *24:* 1152–1160 (1983).
29 Jones, B.; Brown, B.; Silk, D.: Intestinal absorption of maltotriose and maltopentaose-hexaose mixture in man. Gut *22:* A 969 (1981).
30 Hegarty, J.; Fairclough, P.; Moriarty, K.; Kelly, M.; Clark, M.: Effects of concentration on in vivo absorption of a peptide containing hydrolysate. Gut *23:* 304–309 (1982).
31 Schultz, S.: Salt and water absorption by mammalian small intestinel, in Johnson, Physiology of the gastrointestinal tract, pp. 983–989 (Raven Press, New York 1981).
32 Hirschorn, N.: The treatment of acute diarrhoea in children. An historical and physiological perspective. Am. J. clin. Nutr. *33:* 637–663 (1980).
33 Sack, D.; Chowdhury, A.; Eusof, A.; Ali, A.; Merson, M.; Islam, S.; Black, S.; Brown, K.: Oral rehydration in rotavirus diarrhoea: A double blind comparison of sucrose with glucose electrolyte solution. Lancet *ii:* 280–283 (1978).
34 Molla, A.; Parker, S.; Hossain, M.; Molla, A.; Greenough, W.: Rice powder electrolyte solution as oral therapy in diarrhoea due to vibrio cholerae and escherichia coli. Lancet *i:* 1317–1319 (1982).
35 Read, N.; Barber, D.; Levin, R.; Holdsworth, C.: Unstirred layer and kinetics of electrogenic glucose absorption in the human jejunum in situ. Gut *18:* 865–876 (1977).
36 Husband, J.; Husband, P.; Mallinson, C.: Gastric emptying of starch meals in the newborn. Lancet *ii:* 290–292 (1970).
37 Raffles, A.; Schiller, G.; Erhardt, P.; Silverman, M.: Glucose polymer supplementation of feeds for very low birth weight infants. Brit. med. J. *286:* 935–936 (1983).
38 Fogel, M.; Gray, G.: Starch hydrolysis in man: An intraluminal process not requiring membrane digestion. J. appl. Physiol. *35:* 263–267 (1973).
39 Kelly, J.; Alpers, D.: Properties of human intestinal glucoamylase. Biochim. biophys. Acta. *315:* 113–120 (1973).

40 Kerzner, B.; Sloan, Y.; Haase, G.; McGlung, K.; Ailabouni, A.: The jejunal absorption of glucose oligomers in the absence of pancreatic enzymes. Pediat. Res. *15:* 250–253 (1981).
41 Berry, H.; Kellog, F.; Hunt, M.; Ingberg, R.; Richter, L.; Gutjahr, C.: Dietary supplement and nutrition in children with cystic fibrosis. Am. J. Dis. Child. *129:* 165–171 (1975).
42 O'Moráin, C.; Segal, A.; Levi, A.: Elemental diet as primary treatment of acute Crohn's disease: A controlled trial. Br. med. J. (Clin. Res.) *288:* 1859–1862 (1984).
43 Jones, B.; Brown, B.; Grimble, G.; Silk, D.: The formulation of energy dense enteral diets – the use of high molecular weight glucose polymers. J. parent. ent. Nutr. *5:* 359 (1981).
44 Griffin, G.; Fagan, E.; Hodgson, H.; Chadwick, V.: Enteral therapy in the management of massive gut resection complicated by chronic fluid and electrolyte depletion. Dig. Dis. Sci. *27:* 902–908 (1982).
45 Newton, C.; Gonvers, J.; McIntyre, P.; Preston, D.; Lennard-Jones, J.: Effect of different drinks on fluid and electrolyte losses from a jejunostomy. J. R. Soc. Med. *78:* 27–34 (1985).
46 Jones, B.; Higgins, B.; Silk, D.: Jejunal Na^+ absorption is concentration dependent. Gut *25:* A 1163 (1984).
47 Spiller, R.; Jones, B.; Brown, B.; Silk, D.: Influence of Na^+ content of enteric diets on water absorption from the human jejunum. J. parent. ent. Nutr. *6:* 342 (1982).
48 Saunders, D.; Sillery, J.: Absorption of carbohydrate-electrolyte solutions in rat duodenojejunum: Implications for the composition of oral electrolyte solutions in man. Dig. Dis. Sci. *30:* 154–160 (1985).
49 Jones, B.; Silk, D.: Glucose polymers and jejunal water absorption. Gut *26:* A 550 (1985).
50 Desai, M.; Teres, D.: New high caloric density supplement for enteral nutrition in burned patients. Nutr. Support. Services *2:* 20–22 (1982).
51 Jones, B.; Higgins, B.; Silk, D.: Glucose absorption from maltotriose, glucose oligomers and sucrose in the human jejunum: The kinetic advantage of (1–4) linked oligomers (submitted for publication).
52 Spiller, R.; Jones, B.; Brown, B.; Silk, D.: Enhancement of carbohydrate absorption by the addition of sucrose to enteric diets. J. parent. ent. Nutr. *6:* 321 (1982).

B. J. M. Jones, B.Sc., M.D., M.R.C.P., Senior Medical Registrar, Dept. of Gastroenterology, The London Hospital (Whitechapel), GB-London E1 1BB (UK)

Dietze, Grünert, Kleinberger, Wolfram (eds.), Clinical Nutrition and Metabolic Research. Proc. 7th Congr. ESPEN, Munich 1985, pp. 143–155 (Karger, Basel 1986)

Intestinal Absorption of Water-Soluble Vitamins and Essential Trace Elements

A. Shenkin, R. Richardson, O. J. Garden

Royal Infirmary, Glasgow, Scotland, UK

Introduction

Provision of micronutrients in a modern tube feed should, in theory, be more accurately defined than similar provision in the oral diet. The micronutrients in a normal mixed diet are present in a variety of chemical forms, which may vary considerably in the proportion of the active substance absorbed into the portal vein. Thus iron in haem is better absorbed than inorganic iron [1], but in tube feeds, all iron present will be inorganic. Similarly, certain water-soluble vitamins such as riboflavin, nicotinic acid, or folic acid may be unavailable to a variable extent because of the need to digest, from a complex matrix, the naturally occurring coenzyme forms, such as flavine and nicotinamide nucleotides [2, 3], or folic acid polyglutamates [4]. In tube feeds, all vitamins and minerals are added in the 'pure' chemical form so that the amount of each absorbed should be predictable. There are, however, still a number of factors which can alter the efficiency of absorption.

In this discussion, some of the factors of importance in absorption of water-soluble micronutrients from a 'chemically defined' tube feed will be considered. For many of the nutrients, the detailed mechanism of absorption is not clear.

Factors Affecting Absorption of Micronutrients

The Amount of Individual Nutrients

It is not surprising that, in general, the more of a nutrient present, the more is absorbed. This is the case not only for substances usually absorbed by passive diffusion, such as ascorbic acid, folic acid [5] or thiamine [6], but also for certain substances such as iron where a specific transport mechanism is involved [1]. When provision of these substances is limited, other mechanisms may be used including an active transport system for the vitamins, or increased transfer of iron across the mucosal cell, thus ensuring more efficient absorption.

Complex Formation between Nutrients and Other Substances

Although chemical analysis may indicate the total amount of a nutrient present, many factors can affect the biological availability, especially of minerals [7]. Micronutrients are likely to form complexes with a variety of substances in the diet. Iron absorption is inhibited by complexing tannins of polyphenols (e.g., from tea) [1], zinc absorption is reduced by phytate [8] and dietary fibre may reduce absorption of a number of minerals, including copper, zinc and magnesium [9]. Such effects may occur to a variable extent in tube-fed patients, since many are able to take oral fluids or diet, and some tube feeds are now available which contain significant amounts of fibre. The significance of these interactions in the seriously ill patient remains to be established.

Certain types of complexes may improve absorption of micronutrients. The binding of zinc to low molecular ligand such as picolinic acid [10] or citric acid [11] may improve zinc absorption from human milk. Complexing with amino acids, e.g., copper – histidine, may also improve absorption [12] and vitamin B_{12} requires to form a complex with intrinsic factor for absorption in the terminal ileum.

Other Types of Interaction between Micronutrients

Interaction of vitamin C with iron is valuable in reducing ferric iron to ferrous, and thus increasing the proportion absorbed [1]. Indeed, ascorbic acid is often present in excess in tube feeds, to protect nutrients from oxidative change. By contrast, folic acid supplements may reduce zinc absorption, possibly by formation of insoluble chelates, but does not alter iron or copper absorption [13].

The proportion absorbed may also depend upon interactions of other elements which have similar absorption pathways. Zinc absorption can be inhibited by inorganic iron or tin [14], whereas zinc supplements may reduce copper status [15]. We have recently observed severe zinc deficiency in a patient receiving supplementary home intravenous nutrition, the onset being associated with the introduction of oral copper supplements (fig. 1) [16]. The use of individual element supplements must, therefore, be carefully monitored to prevent unbalanced provision and absorption of micronutrients.

Length and Integrity of Small Intestine

Patients who require enteral nutrition are likely to have diseases which may directly, or as a result of surgery, have altered the digestive

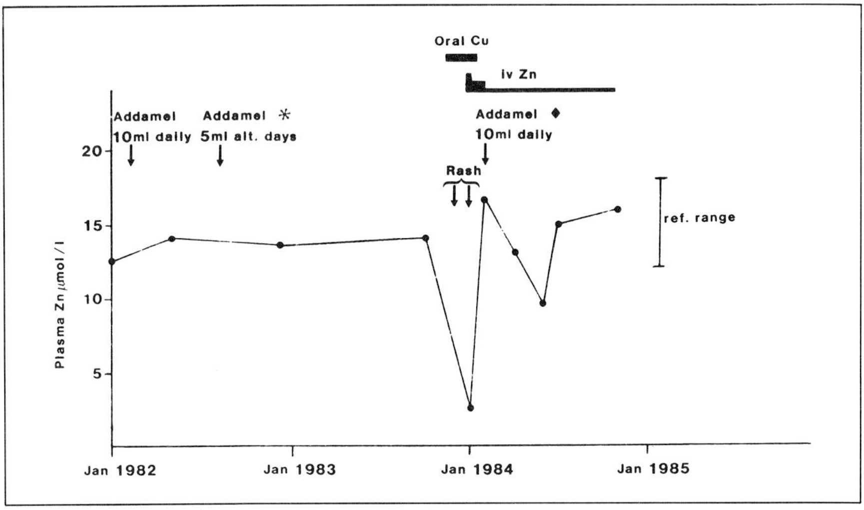

Fig. 1. Plasma zinc in a patient receiving home IVN. Oral copper supplements (1 mg/day) were commenced because of a low serum copper concentration. Zinc intake at that time was on average 5 µmol/day plus an unknown amount from oral diet.

area or mechanism of absorption for particular nutrients. It is axiomatic that an adequate length of gut is necessary to permit adequate absorption. The minimum length necessary for absorption of micronutrients is not established, but a study of 7 patients with short bowel remnants of 40–110 cms demonstrated normal iron, zinc and copper balance [17]. The type of healthy small bowel is important – iron is better absorbed in duodenum than ileum, partly as a result of the more acid pH, but also because duodenal mucous membrane is specially adapted for the purpose [1]. Similarly, the vitamin-B_{12}-intrinsic factor complex is only absorbed by the specialised cells of the terminal ileum. Hence, loss of a segment of small bowel may have a variable effect on the different micronutrients.

Alterations within the Enterocyte

After absorption from the lumen of the gut, micronutrients may be modified in a number of ways. Metals, such as zinc and copper, may bind extensively to metallothionein within the mucosal cell [18], and are then released into the portal blood. Similarly, iron may be bound to a transferrin-like protein for transfer across the mucosal cell to the circulation, or excess iron may be stored as ferritin. The ratio of these two proteins alters depending on whether more iron is to be transferred or excluded [19]. Metabolic changes may also occur to produce the active form of the micronutrient – for example, mucosal cells can reduce and methylate oxidized folate to produce methyltetrahydrofolate monoglutamate, the main active form of folate in man [20].

Summary of Factors Affecting Absorption

From the above brief review, it is apparent that the amount of individual micronutrients finally delivered to the tissues of the body is the net result of a number of interacting mechanisms. Apart from those mechanisms acting within the gut lumen, the physiological state of the patient in terms of deficiency or excess of a nutrient may alter the efficiency of uptake and transfer across the mucosa. Although this is an important control mechanism, it is not readily manipulated. Thus the absolute content of the enteral feed and the relative amounts of the various nutrients is of paramount importance in provision of an adequate tube feed.

Table I. Assessment of patients on referral for nutritional support (results are mean ± SD)

	Albumin g/l	Transferrin g/l	Vit A μmol/l	Vit B_1 (% activation*)	P mmol/l	Mg mmol/l	Zn μmol/l	Cu μmol/l
Died (88)	27.6 ± 5.6	1.57 ± 0.53	1.10 ± 0.65	18.3 ± 13.3	0.87 ± 0.31	0.71 ± 0.13	10.8 ± 3.1	18.2 ± 5.2
Discharged (304)	30.1 ± 5.8	1.84 ± 0.68	1.27 ± 0.79	14.0 ± 10.2	1.00 ± 0.32	0.77 ± 0.23	11.9 ± 3.7	19.8 ± 5.1
p <	0.001	0.001	0.05	0.02	0.001	0.01	0.01	0.01
Lab reference ranges	33–35	2.0–4.0	1.0–3.5	< 25	0.7–1.4	0.7–1.0	12–18	10–22

* Vitamin B_1 status was assessed by rbc transketolase activation. High activations are associated with vitamin B_1 deficiency.

Dietary Requirements for Micronutrients

By definition, an inadequate intake of the essential inorganic micronutrients (trace elements) or organic micronutrients (vitamins) leads to development of a clinical deficiency syndrome, which can be reversed by provision of the relevant substances. For many of these micronutrients, recommendations for dietary intake have been made by the Food and Nutrition Board, National Research Council in the United States [21], and by the Department of Health in the United Kingdom [22]. The United States recommendations are considered to be 'adequate to meet the known nutrition needs of practically all healthy persons', whereas the United Kingdom figures should be 'the average intake of individuals in a group'. Where data is insufficient to make a firm recommendation, 'safe and adequate daily dietary intakes' have been proposed [21]. The problem with these recommendations is that they are not necessarily applicable to patients with a variety of disease states.

It is probable that vitamin and trace element requirements are greater in disease, especially during the anabolic phase of tissue repair and regeneration. In a recent retrospective study of 392 patients with a variety of surgical complications, managed by our Nutrition Group, a biochemical assessment of several trace elements and vitamins was performed at the time of referral. Apart from frequent individual abnormalities, it was found that the 88 patients who subsequently died had, in general, a poorer status of magnesium, zinc, copper, and vitamin B_1, than the 304 patients who survived (table I). Such abnormalities are therefore associated with more severe illness. Although the clinical benefit of correcting such abnormalities has not been established, it would seem logical to attempt to provide, by the enteral route, a slight excess of such nutrients. The control of absorption at gut level, and subsequent immediate transfer to the liver of most micronutrients, makes it unlikely that significant over-provision would occur.

Provision of Micronutrients from Chemically Defined Diets

Most commercial preparations take account of the increased requirements in disease, by providing amounts of essential micronutrients in excess of the recommended dietary allowances (table II). Moreover, to allow for some chemical degradation, additional amounts of vitamins

Table II. Commercial preparations provide amounts of essential micronutrients in excess of the recommended dietary allowances

Composition/ 2000 mls	Clinifeed (1)		Ensure (2)		Triosorbon (3)		Reabilan (4)	Fortison (5)	Vivonex (6)	Nutrauxil (7)	RDI*
	ISO	favour	new	old+	new	old+					
Kcal	2000	2000	2100	2060	2000	2000	2000	2000	2000	2000	
Protein (g)	56	75	74	72	81	81	63	80	41	76	
Fat (g)	82	66	74	72	81	81 (MCT 64.5)	78	80	3	68	
Carbohydrate (g)	261	280	290	282	238	238	263	240	460	276	
Vitamin A (µg/IU)	901 µg/3000 IU	1802 µg/6000 IU	1580 µg/5264 IU	1606 µg/5300 IU	1000 µg/3330 IU	1595 µg/5315 IU	1600 µg/5320 IU	1261 µg/4200 IU	1665 µg/5544 IU	1200 µg/3996 IU	F 1000 µg M 800 µg
Vitamin D_3 (µg/IU)	8.5 µg/340 IU	9.1 µg/360 IU	10 µg/400 IU	10 µg/400 IU	10 µg/400 IU	10 µg/400 IU	10 µg/400 IU	10 µg/400 IU	11 µg/440 IU	10 µg/400 IU	5 µg
Vitamin E (mg/IU)	20.2 mg/20 IU	80 mg/80 IU	48 mg/48 IU	64 mg/64 IU	10 mg/10 IU	16 mg/16 IU	30 mg/30 IU	70 mg/70 IU	33 mg/33 IU	30 mg/30 IU	F 10 mg M 8 mg
Vitamin K_1 (µg)	–	–	76	–	105	105	100	–	74	220	
Vitamin C (mg)	80	80	320	320	90	66	200	100	67	100	60 mg
Folic acid (mg)	277	501	422	420	400	199	500	500	466	400	400 mg
Vitamin B_1 (mg)	2.0	2.0	7.6	3.2	1.4	1.6	3.0	1.4	1.6	2.2	1.2–1.5 mg
Vitamin B_2 (mg)	2.4	2.0	3.6	3.6	1.6	1.9	3.0	2.0	1.8	2.6	1.2–1.7 mg
Vitamin B_6 (mg)	3.0	2.4	4.0	4.2	2.2	2.2	4.0	2.0	2.2	2.4	1.6–2.2 mg
Vitamin B_{12} (µg)	5.0	5.0	12.6	12.6	3.0	3.2	4.0	4.0	6.6	6.0	3.0 µg
Niacin (mg)	24.0	24.0	42.0	42.2	18.0	21.2	40.0	20.0	22.2	18.0	13–19 mg
Biotin (µg)	91	160	320	400	150	450	200	300	333	240	(Av. intake 100–300 µg)
Choline (g)	–	–	1.1	1.4	–	–	0.4	0.9	1	0.6	(Av. intake 0.4–0.9 g)
Pantothenic acid (mg)	Ca Panto.	Ca Pantothenate									
	18.1	12.0	10.5	10.5	5.5	8.5	10.0	10.0	11.1	13.8	
Sodium (mmols)	30	61	74	64	85	85	61	70	75	66	
Potassium (mmols)	77	56	80	65	85	85	64	77	60	64	
Chloride (mmols)	59	65	81	60	105	106	65	45	104	66	
Calcium (mmols)	30	23	27	26	26	26	25	25	28	25	20
Phosphorus (mmols)	29	22	35	34	38	38	32	25	36	39	26
Magnesium (mmols)	9.8	16.4	17.4	17.3	15	14.9	20.5	12.5	18.2	10.7	F 14 mmols M 12 mmols
Manganese (µmols)	77	70	76	76	45	–	73	146	57	55	46–91 µmols
Iodine (µmols)	–	–	1.3	–		–	1.2	0.9	1.3	1.2	1.2 µmols
Copper (µmols)	32	34	33	35	31	2.4**	31	31	35	31	32–48 µmols
Iron (µmols)	240	286	339	339	321	285	357	357	357	357	F 178 M 321
Zinc (µmols)	277	244	484	480	229	38**	305	214	254	229	229
Selenium (µmols)	–	–	–	–	–	–	1.3	–	–	–	0.6–2.5

* RDI – recommended dietary intake [21]
** GRI analysis
\+ Old formulations were used for the studies quoted in figs. 2–7. They have now been replaced by the new formulations.

(1) Clinifeed: Roussel Laboratories Ltd, Uxbridge, Middlesex
(2) Ensure: Abbott Laboratories Ltd, Queensborough, Kent
(3) Triosorbon: E. Merk Ltd, Alton, Hampshire
(4) Reabilan: Roussel Laboratories Ltd, Uxbridge, Middlesex
(5) Fortison: Cow & Gate Ltd, Trowbridge, Wiltshire
(6) Vivonex: Norwich Eaton Ltd, Woking, Surrey
(7) Nutrauxil: Kabi Vitrum Ltd, Uxbridge, Middlesex

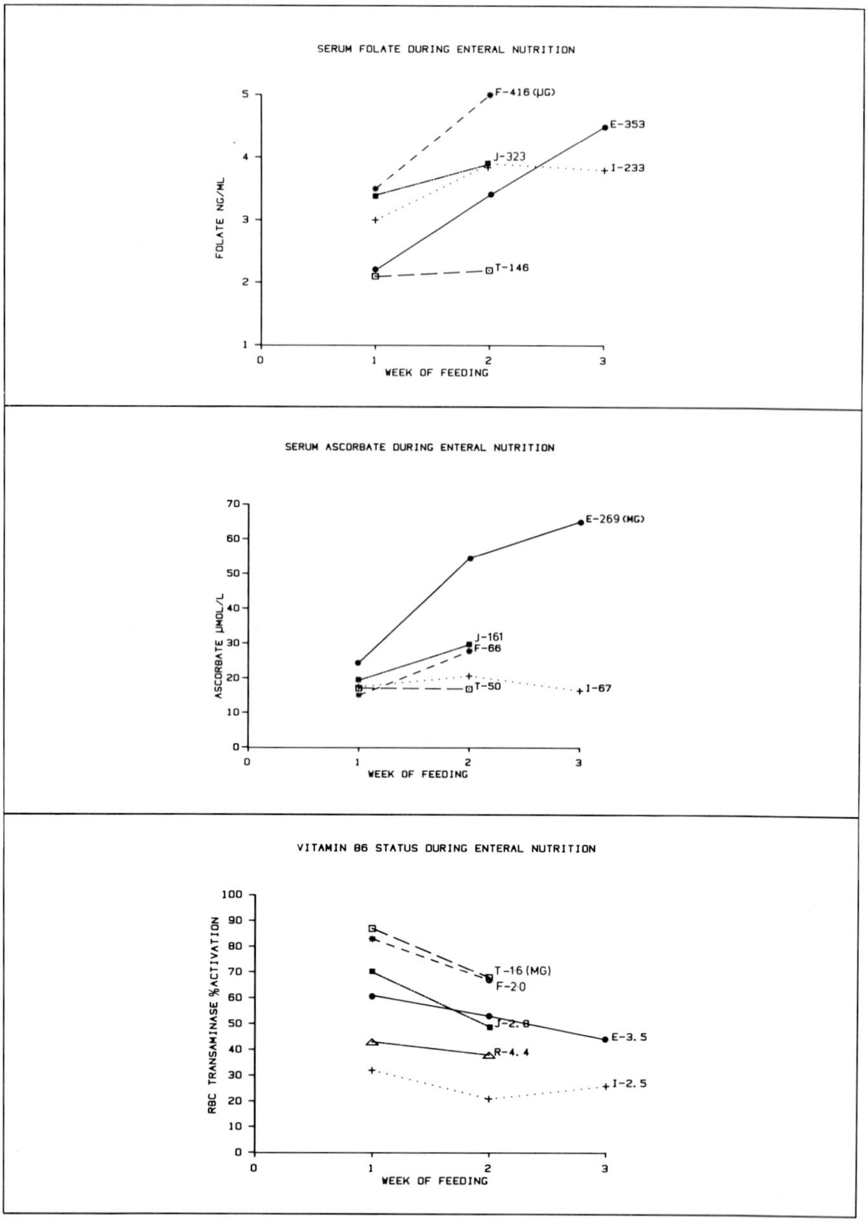

2

3

4

Fig. 2–7. Changes in micronutrients during enteral feeding. E = Ensure, F = Clinifeed Favour, I = Clinifeed ISO, J = Jejunostomy feeding, R = Reabilan, T = Triosorbon. Amounts are the mean daily input of the micronutrient from the feed under study.

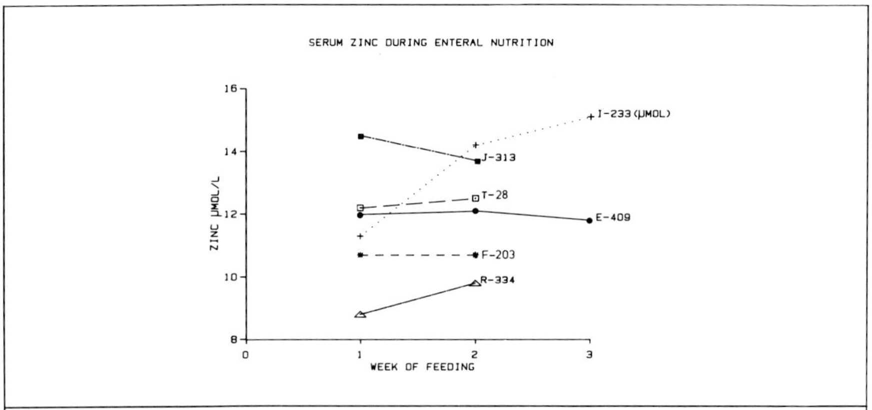
SERUM ZINC DURING ENTERAL NUTRITION
ZINC µMOL/L
16
14
12
10
8
0
1
2
3
WEEK OF FEEDING
I-233 (µMOL)
J-313
T-28
E-409
F-203
R-334

5

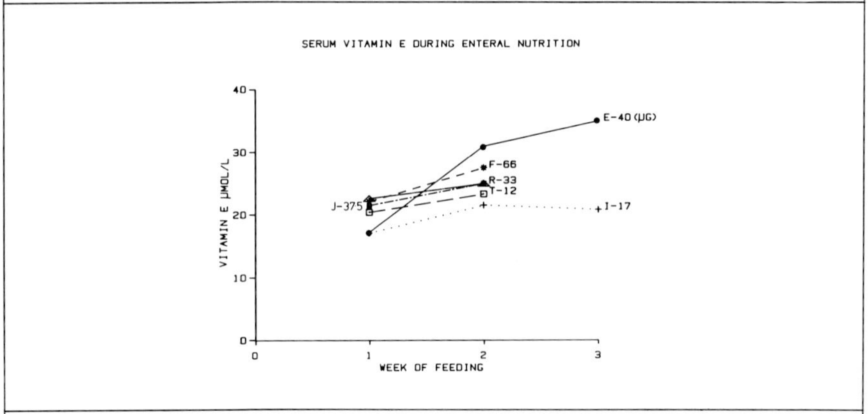
SERUM VITAMIN E DURING ENTERAL NUTRITION
VITAMIN E µMOL/L
40
30
20
10
0
0
1
2
3
WEEK OF FEEDING
E-40 (µG)
F-66
R-33
T-12
J-375
I-17

6

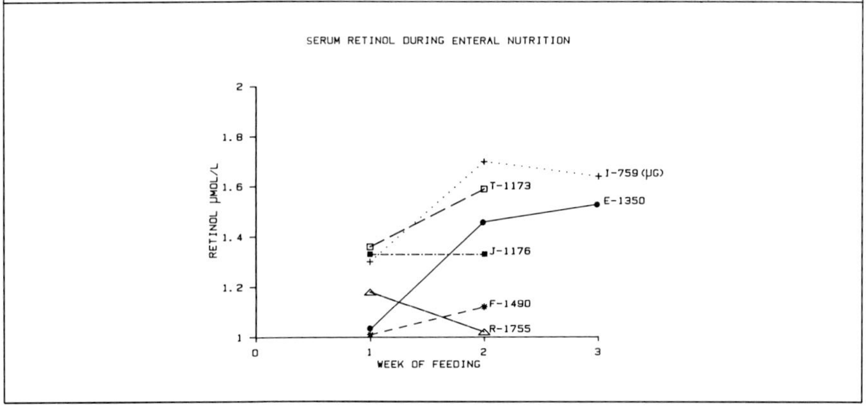
SERUM RETINOL DURING ENTERAL NUTRITION
RETINOL µMOL/L
2
1.8
1.6
1.4
1.2
1
0
1
2
3
WEEK OF FEEDING
I-759 (µG)
T-1173
E-1350
J-1176
F-1490
R-1755

7

('overage') are usually also included. In many cases, particularly for the essential trace elements [23], the amount actually present on analysis has differed substantially from the theoretical specification. Since large variations in micronutrient provision exist in different preparations, we have compared changes in micronutrient status at different levels of supply.

Five tube feed preparations were supplied by the nasogastric route and, in addition, several patients were fed by jejunostomy. Table III summarises the patient details and nutritional input. Only patients fed for a minimum period of 7 days were included, although the majority received 14–21 days nutritional support. Assessments of protein energy, vitamin and trace element status were performed by standard methods [24] at weekly intervals. For most micronutrients, no substantial changes were observed during the feeding periods. Those measurements which showed most variation with time are shown in the figures 2–7, with a note of the mean intake of each nutrient from the feed under study. The conclusions which can be reached from the study are:

(1) In a short-term study, with intakes ranging from about 1,500–2,200 kcal/day in this heterogenous population, no significant deterioration in micronutrient status was observed despite substantial differences in intake of vitamins and essential elements from the different preparations.

(2) Serum concentrations of certain micronutrients, especially folate, ascorbate, and vitamin E, as well as vitamin B_6 status, showed a substantial improvement even in a 2-week period, and the extent of this change was usually related to the level of supply.

(3) Serum zinc concentration was maintained in patients receiving the 2 preparations which contain soya-based protein, and hence also phytate. Interpretation of the zinc results is difficult, since serum zinc is unlikely to reflect body zinc status in the type of patient under study.

(4) The results from jejunostomy feeding were similar to those obtained from nasogastric feeding. Absorption of micronutrients from jejunal supply is, therefore, adequate for most patients.

Conclusions

Commercial chemically defined preparations which are designed for nasogastric or jejunal feeding in general contain adequate amounts of essential elements and vitamins. The optimal levels of supply in illness are,

Table III. Details of tube feed study

	Ensure* (E)	Clinifeed ISO (I)	Clinifeed Favour (F)	Triosorbon* (T)	Reabilan (R)	Jejunostomy feed (J)
No. of patients	18	16	7	12	5	8
Mean age	60	63	55	57	63	55
(range)	(30–77)	(40–76)	(45–61)	(16–79)	(52–69)	(15–75)
Post-op : pre-op	12 : 6	12 : 4	7 : 0	11 : 1	4 : 1	8 : 0
Average input						
kcal/day	1732	1685	1663	1450	2145	1648
nitrogen (g)	9.7	7.6	10.0	8.8	11.0	8.9
Protein source	casein + soy protein	casein/ whey	casein + soy protein	casein/ whey	peptides of whey/casein	4 ensure 2 C. ISO 2 C. favour

* The ensure and triosorbon used were both old formulations, which have subsequently been modified (table II).

however, poorly defined. Because enteral feeds usually contain synthetic 'pure' micronutrients, problems of bioavailability are reduced. However, interactions within the feed may occur, especially if supplements of individual nutrients are added to correct specific depletion or deficiency states. In such situations, careful monitoring of relevant vitamin or essential element status is indicated.

Acknowledgements

We are grateful to Roussel Laboratories, Middlesex, and to Abbott Laboratories, Kent, for financial support during this study.

References

1 Charlton, R. W.; Bothwell, T. H.: Iron Absorption. Annu. Rev. Med. *39:* 55–68 (1983).
2 Baum, C. L.; Selhub, J.; Rosenberg, I. H.: The hydrolysis of nicotinamide adenine dinucleotide by brush border membranes of rat intestine. Biochem. J. *204:* 203–207 (1982).
3 Akiyama, T.; Selhub, J.; Rosenberg, I. H.: FMN phosphatase and FAD pyrophosphatase in rat intestinal brush borders. Role in intestinal absorption of dietary riboflavin. J. Nutr. *112:* 263–268 (1982).
4 Lavoie, A.; Tripp, E.; Hoffbrand, A. V.: Sephadex-gel filtration and heat stability of human jejunal and serum pteroylglutamic hydrolase (folate conjugase). Evidence for two different forms. Biochem. Med. *13:* 1–6 (1975).
5 Selhub, J.; Dhar, G. J.; Rosenberg, I. H.: Gastrointestinal absorption of folates and antifolates. Pharmacol. Ther. *20:* 397–418 (1983).
6 Thomson, A. D.; Leevy, C. M.: Observations on the mechanism of thiamine hydrochloride absorption in man. Clin. Sci. *43:* 153–163 (1972).
7 Rosenberg, I. H.; Solomons, N. W.: Biological availability of minerals and trace elements: A nutritional overview. Am. J. clin. Nutr. *35:* 781–782 (1982).
8 Lonnerdal, B.; Cederblad, A.; Davidsson, L.; Sandstrom, B.: The effect of individual components of soy formula and cows' milk formula on zinc bioavailability. Am. J. clin. Nutr. *40:* 1064–1070 (1984).
9 Drews, L. M.; Kies, H. M.: Effect of dietary fibre on copper, zinc and magnesium utilisation by adolescent boys. Am. J. clin. Nutr. *32:* 1893–1897 (1979).
10 Evans, G. W.; Johnson, P. E.: Purification and quantification of a zinc binding ligand in human milk. Pediat. Res. *14:* 876–880 (1980).
11 Hurley, L. S.; Lonnerdal, B.; Stanislowski, A. G.: Zinc citrate, human milk and acrodermatitis enteropathica. Lancet *i:* 677–678 (1979).
12 Evans, G. W.: Copper homeostasis in the mammalian system. Physiol. Rev. *53:* 535–570 (1973).

13 Milne, D. B.; Canfield, W. K.; Mahalko, J. R.; Sandstead, H. H.: Effects of oral folic acid supplements on zinc, copper and iron absorption and excretion. Am. J. clin. Nutr. *39:* 535–539 (1984).
14 Valberg, L. S.; Flanagan, P. R.; Chamberlain, M. J.: Effects of iron, tin and copper on zinc absorption in humans. Am. J. clin. Nutr. *40:* 536–541 (1984).
15 Fischer, P. W. F.; Giroux, A.; Abbe, M. R. L.: Effect of zinc supplementation on copper status in adult man. Am. J. clin. Nutr. *40:* 743–746 (1984).
16 De Caestecker, J. S.; Shenkin, A.; Fell, G. S.; Heading, R. C.: Hazards and benefits in a patient on long-term total parenteral nutrition. Proc. Nutr. Soc. (in press).
17 Engels, L. G. J.; van der Hamer, C. J. A.; van Tongeren, J. H. M.: Iron, zinc and copper balance in short bowel patients on oral nutrition. Am. J. clin. Nutr. *40:* 1038–1041 (1984).
18 Cherian, M. G.; Goer, R. A.: Metallothioneins and their role in the metabolism and toxicity of metals. Life Sci. *23:* 1–10 (1978).
19 Savin, M. A.; Cook, J. D.: Mucosal iron transport by rat intestine. Blood *56:* 1029–1035 (1980).
20 Strum, W.; Nixon, P. F.; Bertino, J. B.; Binder, H. J.: Intestinal folate absorption 1. 5-methyltetrahydrofolic acid. J. clin. Invest. *50:* 1910–1916 (1971).
21 Food and Nutrition Board. Recommended dietary allowances; 9th ed (National Acad. Sci., Washington DC 1980).
22 Committee on medical aspects of food policy. Recommended daily amounts of food energy and nutrients for groups of people in the United Kingdom (DHSS., London 1979).
23 Bunker, V. W.; Clayton, B. E.: Trace element content of commercial enteral feeds. Lancet *ii:* 426–428 (1983).
24 Shenkin, A.: Assessment and monitoring of nutritional status; in Russell, Elemental Diets, pp. 27–45 (CRC Press, Boca Raton 1981).

Dr. A. Shenkin, Department of Biochemistry, Royal Infirmary, GB-Glasgow, G4 OSF (UK)

Dietze, Grünert, Kleinberger, Wolfram (eds.), Clinical Nutrition and Metabolic Research. Proc. 7th Congr. ESPEN, Munich 1985, pp. 156–168 (Karger, Basel 1986)

Variations of the Natural Isotope Abundance in Diet – Causes of Artifacts or the Base of New Possibilities in Stable Isotope Tracer Work?

H.-L. Schmidt, C. Metges

Dept. of General Chemistry and Biochemistry, Technical University of Munich, Freising-Weihenstephan, FRG

Natural Abundance of Stable Isotopes and Causes for Their Variations

The bioelements hydrogen, carbon, nitrogen, oxygen, and sulfur occur in nature as mixtures of stable isotopes, in which the light isotopes are by far in excess. The relative natural abundance of the main heavy isotopes (^{2}H, ^{13}C, ^{15}N, ^{18}O, ^{34}S, table I) is generally regarded as constant, however, in practice it varies within certain limits depending on origin, pretreatment, and pool of the compound in question.

The different number and symmetry of the neutrons within the nuclei of the isotopes of an element have consequently differences in their mass, polarization, and nuclear spin, which on their part – depending on their position within a molecule – influence mass, polarity, and binding energies within and between the molecules in which they occur. Any organic substance thus consists of a mixture of isotopomer molecules, in which – according to the mean abundance of a given stable isotope – any position can be statistically labeled with the isotope nucleus.

Due to the small differences in total energy content, binding energy, and intermolecular interdependence, isotopomers have slightly different physical properties, e.g. phase equilibrium constants, and show differences in the velocities of chemical or biochemical reactions, especially when binding with the isotope substitution is involved. Phenomena directly or indirectly caused by these different behaviors are called thermodynamic, kinetic, or nuclear spin isotope effects [2].

Isotope effects of vapour pressure or diffusion velocity of small molecules are used in multiple step processes for the separation of stable isotopes, leading to an enrichment of the heavy isotope up to 99% and more. Enriched molecules like $^{13}CO_2$ and $^{15}NH_3$ are the starting materials for the preparation of labeled organic compounds by means of chemical or biochemical synthesis. The heavy isotope may be uniformly distributed over the molecules or located in defined positions. Labeled molecules – with the exception of highly deuterated compounds, especially when bearing ^2H in certain positions – are absolutely physiologically equivalent to the corresponding normal molecules and thus can serve as tracers in the life sciences. The interference of natural variations with corresponding tracer work is subject of this paper.

Isotope effects are also implied in natural processes and are – especially in the biosphere – the cause for small but perceptible separations of isotopomers in the cycles of hydrogen, carbon, nitrogen, oxygen, and sulfur [2]. As the resulting variations of the natural abundance are very small, they are expressed as δ-values, abundance relative to those of international standards (table I).

One of the main reasons for isotopic shifts of the hydrogen and oxygen isotope abundance is isotope effects of water evaporation and conden-

Table I. Concentration scales and standards of stable isotopes [1]

Element and main heavy isotope	Mean natural abundance [atom-%]	Name*	Standard abundance [atom-%]	Isotope ratio
Hydrogen (^2H)	0.0145	SMOW	0.0158	0.00015576
Carbon (^{13}C)	1.108	PDB	1.111	0.0112372
Nitrogen (^{15}N)	0.3663	atmosph.N_2	0.3663	0.0036765
Oxygen (^{18}O)	0.2039	SMOW	0.2000	0.0020052
Sulfur (^{34}S)	4.215	CDT	4.275	0.0450045

Isotope abundance: $\frac{c_{isotope}}{\Sigma c_{isotopes}} \times 100$ (atom-%)

Isotope ratio R: $\frac{c_{isotope}}{c_{main\ isotope}}$

δ-value: $\frac{R_{sample}-R_{standard}}{R_{standard}} \times 1000$ (‰)

* SMOW = Standard Mean Ocean Water; PDB = PeeDeeBee-Belemnite (carbonate); CDT = Canyon Diablo Troilite (FeS); c = concentration; R = isotope ratio of heavy and light isotopes

sation. The water molecules with the light hydrogen and oxygen isotopes become enriched in the vapour phase, while those with heavy isotopes are concentrated in the condensate. Correspondingly, due to isotope effects of evaporation, the leaf water in plants is enriched in ^{2}H and ^{18}O relative to the ground water. Isotope effects of the biosynthesis of organic substances have consequently further isotope separations between different hydrogen and oxygen pools and, in the case of oxygen, isotope effects of oxygenation reactions are of great importance.

The main pool for nitrogen is atmospheric N_2. As nitrogen assimilation (nitrogenase reaction) proceeds without isotope discrimination, the δ-value of the organic nitrogen in legumes is not far from that of N_2. On the other hand, different reactions and processes in the nitrogen cycle proceed with isotope discrimination. However, as the interdependence between the different pools and oxidation states of nitrogen is very complicated, no generally valuable correlation between origin and δ-value of nitrogen-containing compounds can be stated. One can observe that an enrichment of the heavy nitrogen isotope ^{15}N occurs in the biomass in the course of food chains, e.g. from plants to animals.

In the case of carbon, isotope discriminations in nature are well investigated and understood. Two different primary reactions of the photosynthetic CO_2-fixation occur in the vegetable kingdom, leading either to 3-phosphoroglycerate, a C_3-product (ribulosebisphosphate carboxylase-reaction), respectively to oxaloacetate, a C_4-product (phosphoenolpyruvate carboxylase-reaction). These reactions proceed with different kinetic isotope effects, consequently the $\delta^{13}C$-values of the organic material in 'C_3-plants' are between −32 to −24‰, while those in 'C_4-plants' range from −15 to −9‰ [3]. In addition, due to a thermodynamic isotope effect between the carbon sources in the atmosphere (CO_2, $\delta^{13}C = -7‰$) and in the hydrosphere (HCO_3^-, $\delta^{13}C = 0‰$), the products of C_3-plants in water are 'heavier' by about 7‰. Finally, isotope effects in the secondary metabolism, mainly of the pyruvate dehydrogenase reaction [4, 5], are responsible for the depletion of lipids in each group of plants by about −5 to −7‰, while the proteins have $\delta^{13}C$-values similar to that of the carbohydrates. Differences between distinct amino acids originate from carbon isotope discriminations in the Krebs cycle [1]. The most important C_4-culture plants are corn and sugar cane, while ordinary cereals, sugar beet, and vegetables belong to the group of the C_3-plants.

The products of these processes are or belong to our food, hence our proper biomass originates from them. The δ-value of any biological compound is determined by that of its starting material and isotope effects during its biosynthesis and metabolism; it is thus typical for the origin of the material. On the other hand variations of the natural isotope abundance in food can interfere with tracer experiments performed with labeled molecules.

Analytical Methods for the Determination of Stable Isotopes in Organic Material

Any result of a quantitative analysis of stable isotopes – and this is quite different from the situation with radioactive tracers – is dependent on the amount of isotopes introduced into the sample by carrier molecules or matrix. As any organic material contains the stable isotopes in their natural abundance, the precision of a tracer experiment depends on the amount and actual isotope content of the background and, therefore, in many cases it is indispensable to isolate the compound in question in a pure state before isotope analysis.

Apart from special methods for isotope analysis [6], the main procedures used are isotope ratio mass spectrometry (IRMS), which implies an elemental analytical preparation procedure, and gas chromatography/mass spectrometry with selected ion monitoring (SIM-GCMS) [7]. While the latter method can be exclusively used for the identification and the semiquantitative determination of labeled molecules, the former is a real quantitative method, but in general only yields mean global values of the isotope content of a complete molecule.

For IRMS relatively high amounts (~ 1 mg = a few μmol) of an organic substance are combusted in a vacuum system or in sealed tubes according to the principles of organic elemental analysis. The mass-spectrometric isotope ratio analysis is performed on the products CO_2, N_2 and H_2 (through reduction of H_2O from combustion) by means of high precision isotope ratio mass spectrometers. In general they have two or three fixed Faraday collectors for ions of adjacent masses and double inlet systems for the alternating measurement of samples and standards, which permits the determination of differences down to 0.1‰ (10^{-4} atom %).

A special form for the ^{15}N-analysis is the degradation of the organic material by a Kjeldahl-procedure and the oxidation of the resulting NH_3 by hypobromite [8]. Two main products of metabolism, urea and breath-CO_2, can be prepared for isotope analysis by special, simple techniques.

Urease can be used for the selective preparation of NH_3 and CO_2 from urea, and CO_2 from breath is isolated by condensation in liquid N_2. In very efficient mass spectrometers the direct isotope analysis on CO_2 in breath should be possible without isolation. Recent developments tend towards the automatization of the combustion and, in the case of breath-CO_2 measurement, microprocessor-controlled multisample analyzing [9]. A very promising supplementation of IRMS is the combination with gas chromatography [10, 11]: the fractions from the column pass a combustion unit, and the combustion products enter immediately the mass spectrometer. This technique eliminates the laborious purification of the substances and permits the diminution of the sample size to about 1/10 (0.1 mg).

SIM-GCMS implies per se the purification process, only nmol (μg) amounts of substances (in form of non-polar derivatives) are needed. However, the method is not suited to detect isotope enrichments below 0.1 atom-% excess, and hence it can only be used for the analysis of labeled molecules. On the other hand, the occurrence of defined fragments gives the opportunity to identify the site of a label (positional isotope analysis). Possibilities and application of the method have been presented in literature [12, 13] and are the subject of Dr. Matthew's contribution.

Let me, however, in this context point out a new, very powerful method suited for the in vivo investigation of the dynamics of metabolism by means of ^{13}C-labeled compounds: ^{13}C-NMR was used by N. Matwiyoff's group to control the gluconeogenesis in perfused liver from ^{13}C-alanine. The decrease of the ^{13}C-NMR-signals of the amino acid carbon atoms and the simultaneous increase of signals of glucose carbon atoms were registered as a function of time [14].

Influence of Diet and Exogenous Energy Sources on the $\delta^{13}C$-Value of Breath-CO_2

Most of the natural isotope variations mentioned before have a practical value only for food assignments and adulteration control [15, 16]; carbon isotope abundance variations are, in addition, of importance in context with investigations in the nutrition sciences. As shown in table II the $\delta^{13}C$-values of common foodstuffs cover a large area. Especially products originating directly or indirectly from corn or seafood differ from the

Table II. $\delta^{13}C$-values of some foodstuffs (‰$_{PDB}$) [16–18] (values in parentheses from US-originating products)

Vegetables, Fruits, and Cereals			Fats and Oils		Meat, Fish, and Dairy		
Potato	– 26.7	(– 25.8)	Sunflower oil	– 29.0	Beef*	– 23.2	(– 13.9)
Cabbage	– 27.4	(– 24.8)	Coconut oil	– 27.5	Pork*	– 24.8	(– 13.6)
Bean	– 24.0	(– 22.9)	Corn germ oil	– 14.3	Chicken*	– 19.6	(– 15.9)
Apple, Orange	– 25.3	(– 25.4)	Cod-liver oil	– 26.5	Fish	– 23.1	(– 16.8)
Corn flour	– 12.3	(– 10.7)	Peanut butter	– 24.9	Milk	– 25.3	(– 17.5)
Wheat flour	– 25.2	(– 22.7)	Butter	– 28.6	Cheese	– 26.2	(– 20.0)
Rice	–26.0	(– 24.2)	Pork lard	– 27.9	Eggs	– 18.1	(– 16.2)

* protein carbon only

others, and lipids are more depleted in ^{13}C than proteins and carbohydrates from the same origin [16–18].

Diet is the source of breath-CO_2. Due to an isotope discrimination of the metabolism, the $\delta^{13}C$-value of breath-CO_2 is slightly (~ 2‰) more negative than the average $\delta^{13}C$-value of the actual diet. The mean value for Europeans is near −26‰. However, even with normal nutrition, individual and long-term variations between −28 and −22‰ are observed. The effect of orally applied, naturally ^{13}C-enriched products depends on the kind and amount of the components, on the nutrition state, and the activity of the person under investigation. The examples in figure 1/table III have been obtained with healthy persons after overnight fast and during performance of light work.

Exogenous carbohydrates are rapidly absorbed and can be immediately metabolized up to 50% [19], thus being responsible for up to 65% of the actual breath-CO_2 produced. Therefore corn and cane carbohydrates have a dramatic effect on the basic $\delta^{13}C$-value of the breath-CO_2 and can seriously interfere with breath tests. Proteins do not have much influence, and probably the raise of the curve in figure 1 observed after the egg meal is mainly due to the digestion of the egg yolk.

The absorption of fats proceeds more slowly and over a longer period. Therefore there is no danger of a large and serious general interference of fats with breath tests. However, in the case of investigations with ^{13}C-labeled fats, one has to take into consideration the natural isotope content of the fat used as a carrier. In the examples given in table III 70 g of corn germ oil had a rise of breath-CO_2 δ-value equivalent to that after the application of 200 mg of ^{13}C-labeled trilinoleate (96 atom-% ^{13}C in the

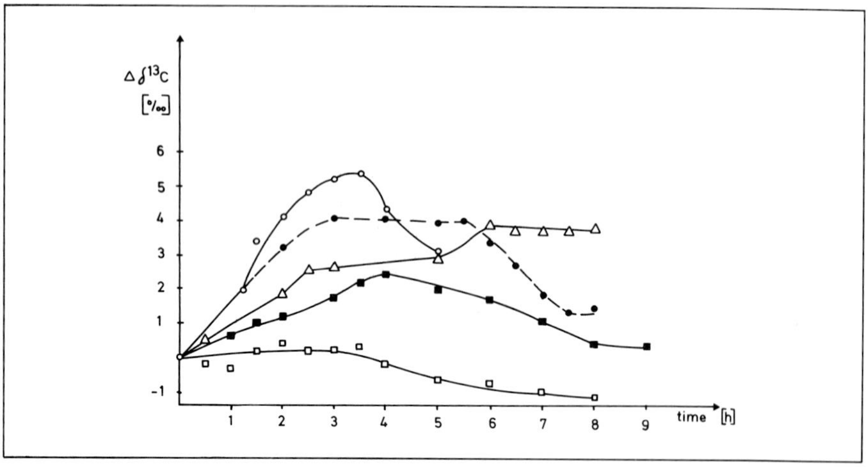

Fig. 1. $\delta^{13}C$ in breath CO_2 after oral administration per person of ○—○ corn glucose + flour, △—△ corn germ oil, ●---● labeled fat emulsion, ■—■ whole eggs (40% fat in dry matter), □—□ egg white.

carboxyl groups) in an emulsion of 5 g soja lipids ($\delta^{13}C = -29‰$). If the same amount of tracer had been applied in corn germ oil, the total turnover of the tracer calculated by integration of the breath curve would have been different.

Many preparations used for formula diets or for parenteral nutrition are based on corn [18–20]. When corresponding carbohydrates are used as main energy supply, they could provoke a shift of the base line of the breath-CO_2 δ-value from −26‰ to −18‰ within a few hours. While the average $\delta^{13}C$-value of amino acid solutions is not very far from that of a

Table III. Effect of orally applied, naturally ${}^{1}{}_{3}C$-enriched poroducts obtained with healthy persons after overnight fast and during performance of light work

	$\delta^{13}C$ (‰)	amount (g)	energy (kJ)
Corn glucose + flour	− 14.0	100	1700
Corn germ oil	− 14.3	70	2660
Labeled fat emulsion	+ 46.9	50 (6)*	274
Whole eggs (40% fat in dry matter)	− 15.7	220 (50)*	2390
Egg white	− 18.5	287 (37.3)*	650

* values in parentheses: dry matter (g)

Table IV. Mean $\delta^{13}C$-value ($‰_{PDB}$) of substances used in formula diets and in infusions for parenteral nutrition [18, 20]

Dextropur® (corn glucose)	– 10.2	Mazola (corn oil)	– 14.8
Maltodextrin® (corn based)	– 10.0	Lipomul® (corn based)	– 14.4
Mondamin® (corn flour)	– 10.4	Lipofundin® (soja based)	– 29.3
Sucrose (cane)	– 12.9	Intralipid® (soja based)	– 29.0
Sucrose (beet)	– 25.5	Casein (C_3-fed cows)	– 26.0
Nutricomp F® (tube feeding)	– 16.6	Soja protein	– 23.5
Sterofundin® (mixed carbohydrate)	– 18.9	Aminoplasmal® (amino acid mixture)	– 22.4

normal C_3-diet, individual amino acids may diverge by large values; according to our experience between −12.5 and −35.5‰. As most lipid emulsions for parenteral nutrition are based on soja lipids, they would not interfere with breath tests except in cases where the δ-base line of the subject is more positive than −24‰ (table IV).

After a longer fast, a shift of the ^{13}C-base value of the breath-CO_2 up to 3.5‰ can be observed, caused by the enhanced oxidation of endogenous lipids [21], and exercise or any other change of the physiological state can have similar changes [22].

Breath Tests with Naturally Labeled Carbohydrates

As a deduction of the results mentioned before, 'naturally labeled' carbohydrates should be suitable for the performance of certain breath tests. 100 g C_4-glucose contains the same amount of ^{13}C as 100 g C_3-glucose mixed with 25 mg uniformly labeled or 150 mg C-1-labeled glucose (90 atom-% ^{13}C). If 65% of the actual breath-CO_2 can originate from the oxidation of exogenous glucose, a maximum rise of about 10‰ in the $\delta^{13}C$ value of breath-CO_2 should be expected from a load of 100 g corn glucose. 6–7‰ is actually observed. This is sufficient for the investigation of many questions of carbohydrate metabolism. Examples for corresponding applications of naturally labeled carbohydrates are shown in table V.

Ravussin et al. [23], in studying the carbohydrate metabolism in obese subjects, found that they show an impairment of glucose utilization probably caused by an increased availability of free fatty acids, which favors lipid oxidation. The group of Lefebvre [24–27] found a diminution

Table V. Problems investigated and results obtained with the use of naturally labeled carbohydrates (C_4-products) in ^{13}C-breath tests

Problems	Results	Reference
Oral glucose tolerance tests in healthy subjects, diabetics, and obese subjects	correlations between dose, blood concentration, and oxidation rate of glucose	[23–25]
Blood glucose oxidation under the influence of antidiabetic drugs	no significant difference in comparison to reference	[26]
Exogenous and endogenous glucose, contribution to energy turnover under various physical exercises	total and exogenous consumption depend on exercise intensity, no influence of training on oxidation rate	[27–30]
Total starch ingestion in infants	development of digestion enzymes	[31]

of the $\delta^{13}C$-values in the expired air of diabetics, compared to healthy persons, and a small increase of the oxidation of exogenous glucose by obese subjects and diabetics after the application of an antidiabetic drug. An extensive field for the use of naturally labeled glucose is the determination of the contribution of exogenous glucose to energy production under various conditions of physical exercise. Pirnay et al. [28–30] found a 55% contribution of exogenous glucose to the overall carbohydrate utilization during a prolonged exercise. The $\delta^{13}C$-value showed a maximum

Table VI. Influence of diet composition on $\delta^{13}C$-values (‰$_{PDB}$) of body proteins

Subjects	Diet	$\delta^{13}C$ [‰]	Material analyzed	$\delta^{13}C$ [‰]	Reference
US-Americans	preferably C_4-based (corn, cane sugar)	– 18.8	hair	– 16.4	[17]
Japanese	C_3/C_4-mixed + seafood	– 21.2	hair	– 18.0	[17]
Europeans	preferably C_3-based (potatoes, cereals)	– 23.6	hair	– 20.4	[17]
Eskimos (present and prehistoric)	seafood	– 17.5	bone collagen	– 20.4	[37, 38]
North American Indians (< 500 AD)	preferably C_3 (gatherers)	– 25.0	bone collagen	– 21.0	[34]
North American Indians (> 1000 AD)	C_3/C_4-mixed (farmers)		bone collagen	– 10.0	[34]
Gerbils	change from C_4 to C_3		different tissues	– 12 to – 18	[39]
Europeans	change from C_3 to C_4		serum proteins	– 22 to – 18	this paper
Cows	change from C_3 to C_4		milk	– 22 to – 14	this paper

90 min after a load of 100 g C_4-glucose. Measuring the influence of 6 weeks' physical training on metabolic and hormonal response to a load of 100 g naturally labeled glucose, Krzentowski and coworkers [27] could not find a significant improvement of glucose oxidation. While the insulin response was decreased, the glucose tolerance showed no change. With the use of naturally labeled carbohydrates Shulman et al. [31] investigated the development of pancreatic amylase activity and cereal utilization by 1-month-old infants.

Natural Isotope Abundance in Food Chain Detection

You are what you eat (plus 3‰) [32]. While carbohydrates serve as main energy source, diet proteins are preferably used for the biosynthesis of body mass. This is connected to different isotope fractionation patterns and generally results in an enrichment of heavy isotopes in the body protein (collagen is 5‰ 'heavier' than diet) [33]. Correspondingly Nakamura et al. [17] found a shift of 3‰ between diet protein and that of human hair. A change in diet had as an immediate consequence a change in the δ-value of beard hair. The moving of Europeans to the United States (higher part of corn products in diet) could be recognized in a change of the $\delta^{13}C$-values of their serum proteins (table VI).

The shift of the $\delta^{13}C$-value of bone collagen was used as an indicator for the change of prehistoric diet, especially for the beginning of corn cultivation in America [34]. Correspondingly a shift of the $\delta^{15}N$-value of bone collagen could be used for the dating of the cultivation of beans by the Indians in the Tehuacan valley [35]. In similar studies nitrogen [36] and carbon isotope abundances [37, 38] were used to identify seafood as prehistoric diet. Investigations of Tieszen et al. [39] with animals showed that a change from C_3- to C_4-products as diet caused different shifts in individual organs, which indicates different half-lives for the proteins of these organs. On the other hand, an immediate maximum shift of the δ-value of milk was observed after changing the cows' feed from C_3- to C_4-diet. At present it is being investigated if these shifts can be used for the determination of protein half-lives.

An even more promising field is the investigation of the isotope distribution within organic substances. Any organism is in a dynamic equilibrium with mass fluxes in many directions, metabolic cycles with many turns and scrambling effects, to which isotope effects are connected. This has consequently a nonstatistical isotope distribution [2, 40]. The elucidation of some of the intercorrelations will help us to understand more about the dynamic state of the metabolism.

References

1 Hoefs, J.: Stable isotope geochemistry (Springer, Berlin, Heidelberg, New York 1980).

2 Galimov, E. M.: The biological fractionation of isotopes (Academic Press, Orlando 1985).

3 Schmidt, H.-L.; Winkler, F. J.: Einige Ursachen der Variationsbreite von $\delta^{13}C$-Werten bei C_3- und C_4-Pflanzen. Ber. dt. Bot. Ges. *92:* 185–191 (1979).

4 Monson, K. D.; Hayes, J. M.: Biosynthetic control of the natural abundance of carbon-13 at specific positions within fatty acids in saccharomyces cerevisiae. J. biol. Chem. *257:* 5568 (1982).

5 Melzer, E.: Kinetische Isotopeneffekte enzymatischer Pyruvat- und Lactat-Spaltungen: Ein Beitrag zur Untersuchung der Reaktionsmechanismen; diss. München-Weihenstephan (1985).

6 Schmidt, H.-L.: Analyse von stabil-isotop markierten Verbindungen; in Simon, Messung von radioaktiven und stabilen Isotopen, vol. II, pp. 291–400 (Springer, Berlin 1974).

7 Wolfe, R. R.: Tracers in metabolic research radioisotope and stable isotope/mass spectrometry methods; in Laboratory and research methods in biology and medicine, vol. 9, p. 190 (Alan R. Liss, New York 1984).

8 Medina, R.; Hoppe, W.; Schmidt, H.-L.: Memory-freie Routine-Aufbereitung biologischer Proben für die ^{15}N-Analyse. Z. analyt. Chem. *292:* 403–407 (1978).

9 Schoeller, D. A.; Klein, P. D.: Microprocessor controlled mass spectrometer for the fully automated purification and isotopic analysis of breath carbon dioxide. Biomed. Mass Spectrom. *6:* 350–355 (1979).

10 Matthews, D. E.; Hayes, J. M.: Isotope-ratio-monitoring gas chromatography-mass spectrometry. Analyt. Chem. *50:* 1465–1473 (1978).

11 Barrie, A.; Bricout, J.; Koziet, J.: Gas chromatography – stable isotope ratio analysis at natural abundance levels. Biomed. Mass Spectrom. *11:* 583–588 (1984).

12 Caprioli, R. M.; Bier, D. M.: Use of stable isotopes; in Waller, Dermer, Biochemical application of mass spectrometry; 1st supplement, pp. 895–925 (J. Wiley and Sons, New York 1980).

13 Matthews, D. E.; Bier, D. M.: Stable isotope method for nutritional investigations. Ann. Rev. Nutr. *3:* 309–339 (1983).

14 Brainard, J. R.; Hutson, J. J.; London, R. E.; Matwiyoff, N. A.: ^{13}C-enriched substrates for in situ and in vivo metabolic profiling studies by ^{13}C NMR; in Turnlund, Johnson, Stable isotopes in nutrition, ACS Symposium Series No. 258, pp. 157–174 (Am. Chem. Soc., Washington 1984).

15 Winkler, F. J.: Application of natural abundance stable isotope mass spectrometry in food control; in Frigerio, Milon, Chromatography and mass spectrometry in nutrition science and food control, p. 173 (Elsevier, Amsterdam 1984).

16 Winkler, F. J.; Schmidt, H.-L.: Einsatzmöglichkeiten der ^{13}C-Isotopen-Massenspek-

trometrie in der Lebensmitteluntersuchung. Z. Lebensm. Unters. Forsch. *171:* 85–94 (1980).
17 Nakamura, K.; Schoeller, D. A.; Winkler, F. J.; Schmidt, H.-L.: Geographical variations in the carbon isotope compositions of the diet and hair in contemporary man. Biomed. Mass Spectrom. *9:* 390–394 (1982).
18 Schoeller, D. A.; Klein, P. D.; Watkins, J. B.; Heim, T.; MacLean Jr., W. C.: ^{13}C-abundance of nutrients and the effect of variations in ^{13}C isotopic abundance of test meals formulated for $^{13}CO_2$ breath tests. Am. J. clin. Nutr. *33:* 2375–2385 (1980).
19 Wolfe, R. R.; Wolfe, M. H.; Shulman, G.: Glucose metabolism in humans, studied with stable isotopes and mass spectrometric analysis; in Turnlund, Johnson, Stable isotopes in nutrition, ACS Symposium Series No. 258, pp. 175–187 (Am. Chem. Soc., Washington 1984).
20 Metzler, S.; Stobbe, E.; Kranz, Ch.; Schmidt, H.-L.; Winkler, F. J.; Wolfram, G.: Einfluß des natürlichen Isotopengehaltes von Nährstoffen auf den Untergrund bei ^{13}C-Atemtests. Z. ErnährWiss. *22:* 107–115 (1983).
21 Schoeller, D. A.; Brown, C.; Nakamura, K.; Nakagawa, A.; Mazzeo, R. S.; Brooks, G. A.; Budinger, T. F.: Influence of metabolic fuel on the $^{13}C/^{12}C$ ratio of breath O_2. Biomed. Mass Spectrom. *11:* 557–561 (1984).
22 Wolfe, R. R.; Shaw, J. M. F.; Nadel, E. R.; Wolfe, M. H.: Effect of substrate intake and physiological state on background $^{13}CO_2$ enrichment. J. appl. Physiol. *56:* 230–234 (1984).
23 Ravussin, E.; Doerner, A.; Acheson, K. J.; Pahud, P.; Arnaud, M. J.; Jéquier, E.: Carbohydrate utilization in obese subjects after an oral load of 100 g naturally-labelled ^{13}C-Glucose. Br. J. Nutr. *43:* 281 (1980).
24 Lacroix, M.; Mosora, F.; Pontus, M.; Lefebvre, P.; Luyckx, A.; Lopez-Habib, G.: Glucose naturally labelled with carbon-13: Use for metabolic studies in man. Science *181:* 445 (1973).
25 Lefebvre, P. J.; Lacroix, M.; Luyckx, A.; Lopez-Habib, G.; Pontus, M.: Naturally labelled ^{13}C-glucose: Metabolic studies in normal and diabetic subjects. Diabetes *22:* 291 (1973).
26 Lefebvre, P.; Luyckx, A.; Mosora, F.; Lacroix, M.; Pirnay, F.: Oxidation of an exogenous glucose load using naturally labelled ^{13}C-glucose. Diabetologia *14:* 39–45 (1978).
27 Krzentowski, G.; Pirnay, F.; Luyckx, A.; Lacroix, M.; Mosora, F.; Lefebvre, P. J.: Effect of physical training on the oxidation of an oral glucose load at rest: A naturally labeled ^{13} C-glucose study. Diabetes & Metabolism *9:* 112–115 (1983).
28 Pirnay, F.; Crielaard, J. M.; Pallikarakis, N.; Lacroix, M.; Mosora, F.; Krzentowski, G.; Luyckx, A.; Lefebvre, P. J.: Fate of exogenous glucose during exercise of different intensities in humans. J. appl. Physiol. *53:* 1620–1624 (1982).
29 Pirnay, F.; Lacroix, M.; Mosora, F.; Lefebvre, P. J.: Effect of glucose ingestion on energy substrate utilization during prolonged muscular exercise. Eur. J. appl. Physiol. *36:* 247–254 (1977).
30 Pirnay, F.; Lacroix, M.; Mosora, F.; Luyckx, A.; Lefebvre, P.: Glucose oxidation during prolonged exercise evaluated with naturally labeled ^{13}C-glucose. J. appl. Physiol. *43* (2): 258–261 (1977).
31 Shulman, R. J.; Wong, W. W.; Irving, C. S.; Nicols, W. L.; Klein, P. D.: Dietary cereal utilization in young infants. J. pediat. Res. *103* (1): 23 (1983).

32 DeNiro, M. J.; Epstein, S.: You are what you eat (plus a few ‰): The carbon isotope cycle in food chains. Geol. Soc. Am. Abs. Prog. *8:* 834–835 (1976).

33 Krueger, H. W.; Sullivan, C. H.: Models for carbon isotope fractionation between diet and bone; in Turnlund, Johnson, Stable isotopes in nutrition, ACS Symposium Series No. 258, p. 205 (Am. Chem. Soc., Washington D.C. 1984).

34 Boutton, T. W.; Klein, P. D.; Lynott, M. J.; Price, J. E.; Tieszen, L. L.: Stable carbon isotope ratios as indicators of prehistoric human diet; in Turnlund, Johnson, Stable isotopes in nutrition, ACS Symposium Series No. 258, p. 191–204 (Am. Chem. Soc., Washington, D.C. 1984).

35 DeNiro, M.; Epstein, S.: Influence of diet on the distribution of nitrogen isotopes in animals. Geochim. Cosmochim. Acta *45:* 341–351 (1981).

36 Schoeninger, M. J.; DeNiro, M. J.: Stable nitrogen isotope ratios of bone collagen reflect marine and terrestrial components of prehistoric human diet. Science *220:* 1381–1383 (1983).

37 Tauber, H.: ^{13}C-evidence for dietary habits of prehistoric man in Denmark. Nature *292:* 332–333 (1981).

38 Crisholm, B. S.; Nelson, D. E.; Schwarcz, H. P.: Stable carbon isotope ratios as a measure of marine versus terrestrial protein in ancient diets. Science *216:* 1131–1132 (1982).

39 Tieszen, L. L.; Boutton, T. W.; Tesdahl, K. G.; Slade, N. A.: Fractionation and turnover of stable carbon isotopes in animal tissues. Implications for δ^{13}C analysis of diet. Oecologia *57:* 32–37 (1983).

40 Macko, S. A.; Estep, M. L. F.; Hare, P. E.; Hoering, T. C.: Stable nitrogen and carbon isotopic composition of individual amino acids isolated from cultured microorganisms; in Annual Report of the Director, Geophysical Laboratory 1982–1983, p. 404 (Carnegie Institution of Washington Year Book 1982).

Prof. Dr. H.-L. Schmidt, Lehrstuhl für Allgemeine Chemie und Biochemie der TU München, D-8050 Freising-Weihenstephan (FRG)

Dietze, Grünert, Kleinberger, Wolfram (eds.), Clinical Nutrition and Metabolic Research. Proc. 7th Congr. ESPEN, Munich 1985, pp. 169–177 (Karger, Basel 1986)

The $^2H_2{}^{18}O$ Method for Energy Expenditure Measurements – Clinical Possibilities, Necessary Assumptions and Limitations

W. A. Coward, S. B. Roberts, A. M. Prentice, A. Lucas

Medical Research Council, Dunn Nutrition Laboratory and Dunn Clinical Nutrition Centre, Cambridge, UK

Introduction

Quite rightly, the prospect of being able to make non-invasive measurements of energy expenditure by using the stable isotopes ^2H and ^{18}O has excited both clinicians and nutritionists. Much of this interest is, of course, justified but I want to use this opportunity of describing the method, and its potential, to also explain its limitations.

The Model

When water labelled with ^2H is given to a subject, it is observed that isotope disappearance to base-line values is exponential. If water labelled with ^{18}O is used, disappearance is again exponential but the biological half-life of the isotope is shorter than for ^2H. Single exponential disappearance curves do not prove a model (the model has to make physiological sense by itself) but Lifson and McClintock [5] explained that these observations are compatible with a situation in which:

(1) body-water is the single compartment which the isotopes label and from which the isotopes are lost;

(2) ^2H is lost, only as water,

(3) ^{18}O is lost, both as water and carbon dioxide, transference of oxygen between water and carbon dioxide being the consequence of a rapid exchange promoted by carbonic anhydrase;

(4) fractional output rates of water and carbon dioxide output are constant;

(5) water and carbon dioxide loss occurs at the same enrichment as that coexisting in body-water;

(6) background isotope intake rates are constant.

With these assumptions, the isotope procedure has, as its basis, the measurements of the rate constants kd and ko for ^2H and ^{18}O disappearance, and isotope distribution volumes, Vd and Vo.

Precision: Theoretical Considerations

Rate Constants and Isotope Distribution Spaces

It will become evident later that estimates of rate constants and volumes have to be made with a precision of about 1% to ensure reasonable degrees of precision on the final calculation of carbon dioxide production rate. The question is, how can this be achieved? Schoeller [7, 10] has tackled this problem theoretically and practically. Taking into account mass-spectrometric precision within individual background variation, and the costs involved in dosing human subjects with ^{18}O-labelled water, it was shown that for initial enrichments of about 500–900‰ for ^{2}H and 90–170‰ for ^{18}O acceptable degrees of precision would be observed on rate constants if measurements were made during 2 biological half-lives for the isotopes. This is a useful general rule and in ideal circumstances (outflow rates for water and carbon dioxide constant), estimates of rate constants could be made by the interpolation of single exponentials between two points this length of time apart without reference to the influence of variations of outflow rates on the precision of estimates of the rate constants. However, an inevitable limitation of the model is that outflow rates are not constant in nature and it would seem sensible, particularly at this stage in the method's development, to obtain estimates of precision on the slopes of disappearance curves by making several measurements in the investigation period [2, 3]. The same sort of arguments apply with respect to the measurement of distribution volumes. These could be obtained by single point determinations, perhaps with some allowance for isotope disappearance prior to sampling [8–10] or better, by extrapolating isotope disappearance curves to zero time [2, 3]. This is a useful approach because the errors on exponential slopes and intercepts are correlated so that errors on slopes and zero-time distribution volumes are inversely correlated. These correlations improve the precision on estimates of the products kdVd and koVo.

Fractionation

If the assumption that all sources of isotope egress from the body occurs at the same level of isotopic enrichment as in body-water, the equations:

$$kdVd = F_{H_2O}$$
$$koVo = F_{H_2O+CO_2}$$
$$0.5\ (koVo–Vd) = F_{CO_2} \qquad F = \text{outflow rate}$$

could be written immediately. It is, however, known that some water losses and CO_2 losses are fractionated. This leads to an alternative series of equations:

$$kdVd = x \times f_1 \times F_{H_2O} + (1–x)F_{H_2O}$$
x = proportion of water loss fractionated
f_1 = fractionation factor for fractionated ^2H_2O loss
$$koVo = 2f_3F_{H_2O} + f_2 \times x \times F_{H_2O} + (1–x)F_{H_2O}$$
f_2 = fractionation factor for $H_2{}^{18}O$ loss
f_3 = fractionation factor for $C^{18}O_2$ loss

In order to apply the equations, we need to know the appropriate values of the fractionation factors and the proportion of the losses to which they need to be applied.

In practice, likely physiological variations from the values (f_1 = 0.93, f_2 = 0.99, f_3 = 1.04) generally used will make very little difference to values for calculated carbon dioxide production rates. It is, however, important to consider the effects of an inadequate knowledge of the proportion of total water losses that are fractionated. The general points are illustrated in figure 1. If the increment that is carbon dioxide production

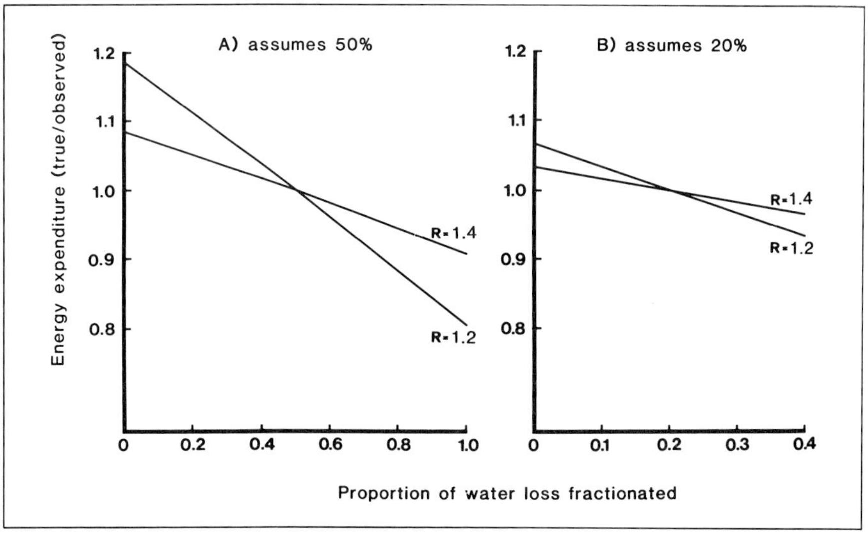

Fig. 1. Effect on energy expenditure measurements of variations in the proportion of water output fractionated (R = koVo/kdVd).

on water production is small (koVo/kdVd = R; R → 1), errors can be large. However, from our studies with premature babies and Gambian women, we have observed that reductions in values for R are the consequence of substantial increments in unfractionated water losses, i.e. high rates of urine output in premature babies and high rates of sweating in Gambian subjects (sweat is not fractionated). In these circumstances, a reasonable assumption to make about the proportion of water loss fractionated becomes smaller and the consequences of inadequate assumptions become less important.

Respiratory Quotient

Conversion of data for carbon dioxide production rate to energy expenditure measurements requires a knowledge of the metabolic mixture burnt. If respiratory quotient (RQ) was assumed to be 0.85 when in fact it was 0.8, an error of 5% would be generated (fig. 2).

RQ can vary substantially in the short-term but averaged over long periods for individuals in balance will resemble the RQ of the diet. The important point to consider is the amount of dietary observation required to predict dietary RQ. In fact, within individuals there appears to be little daily variation in dietary RQ (CV = 0.7% for Cambridge women) and even between individuals the variation is small (CV = 1.5%). Figure 2 indicates the effect of this level of error.

A further consideration with respect to RQ is the consequence of fat gains or losses in the experimental period. Again, predictions are possible (fig. 3) but only in exceptional circumstances will total ignorance of these changes contribute substantially to error.

Fig. 2. Effect of RQ assumptions on energy expenditure measurements. RQ assumed equal to 0.85. The brackets indicate ± 2 SD for Cambridge women.

Fig. 3. Effect of fat gain or loss on energy expenditure measurements in relation to dietary RQ.

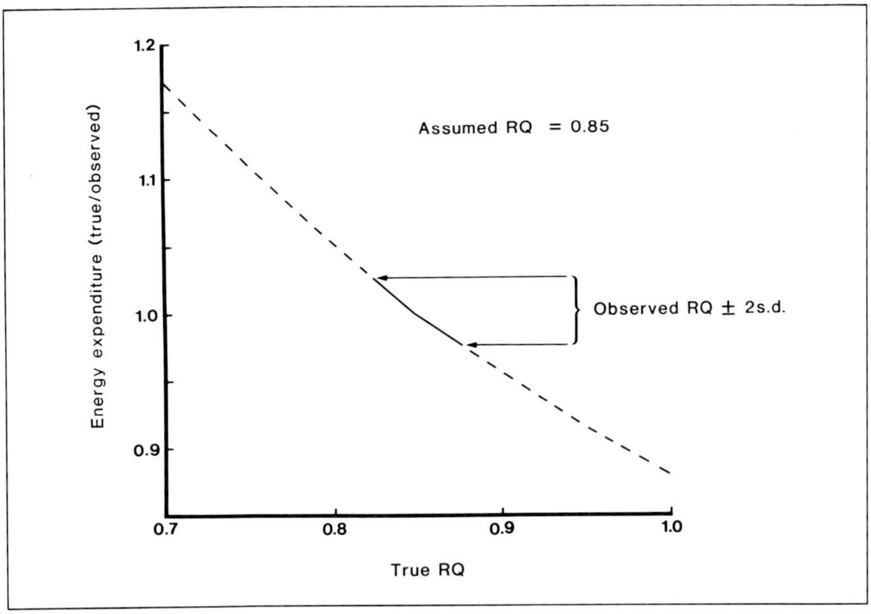
Energy expenditure (true/observed)
1.2
1.1
1.0
0.9
Assumed RQ = 0.85
Observed RQ ± 2s.d.
0.7
0.8
0.9
1.0
True RQ

2

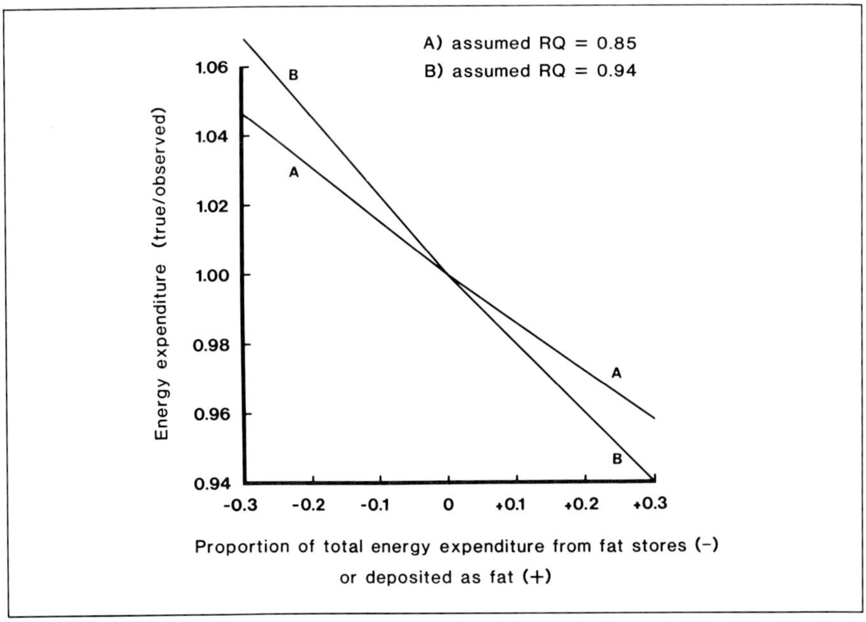
A) assumed RQ = 0.85
B) assumed RQ = 0.94
Energy expenditure (true/observed)
1.06
1.04
1.02
1.00
0.98
0.96
0.94
A
B
-0.3
-0.2
-0.1
0
+0.1
+0.2
+0.3
Proportion of total energy expenditure from fat stores (–)
or deposited as fat (+)

3

Changes in Isotope Distribution Volumes

For subjects not in balance, pool sizes will change during a measurement period, and isotope disappearance curves will reflect both turnover and volume change. Appropriate corrections are available [1].

Precision: Practical Considerations

It is instructive to examine the practical cumulative effect of the aforementioned errors and this can be done by examining a recent validation study in premature babies. Table I shows data taken from one of four infants studied. Despite the fact that precision on the estimates of slopes and intercepts was better than 1%, propagation of these values through the calculations produces an apparent precision of 6.3%. This is merely the consequence of the need to determine a small difference (F_{CO_2}) between two relatively large values ($F_{H_2O+CO_2}$ and F_{H_2O}). In practice, however, these values are highly correlated since one forms a large part of the other and this correlation will at least halve the error or F_{CO_2} to give acceptable precision on carbon dioxide production measurements. Table II shows the practical consequences of using assumptions about the proportion of water vapour fractionated and RQ. Use of group means (17% fractionated water loss) rather than values observed (range

Table I. Precision of estimates of carbon dioxide production rate in a single individual (subject 4, table II)

	Observed precision of estimate (CV %)
kd	0.92
Vd	0.67
ko	0.80
Vo	0.66
F_{H_2O}	0.50*
$F_{H_2O+CO_2}$	0.42*
F_{CO_2}	6.3$^+$

* k and V correlation improves precision on F estimates
$^+$ no allowance made for correlation between F_{H_2O} and $F_{H_2O+CO_2}$

Table II. Accuracy (% error) of estimates of carbon dioxide production rate and energy expenditure in a study with four preterm infants

Subject	1	2	3	4
(1) CO_2 production	+ 5.7	+ 6.6	− 10.4	− 10.0
(2) CO_2 production	− 2.9	+ 5.8	− 4.8	− 3.5
(3) Energy expenditure	+ 4.5	+ 10.9	+ 6.0	+ 6.5
(4) Energy expenditure	− 2.1	+ 4.0	− 0.6	− 0.1

(1) Group means for fractionation assumptions
(2) Observed values for fractionation assumptions
(3) Dietary RQ = 0.84 applied to CO_2 data from [2]
(4) RQ = 0.91 – literature figure for preterm infants

6–33%) is not entirely satisfactory and in these subjects dietary RQ (0.84) is an inappropriate approximation.

Applications and Limitations

Despite the success of most validation studies [3, 4, 8, 9, 11, 12], I have sometimes noticed that at workshops where this methodology has been discussed, that potential users are alarmed by the hostages to precision and accuracy I have described, but as far as studies of the type done in our laboratories are concerned, that is to say observations on free-living, normal populations [6], we must ask, what are the alternatives? Alternatives do exist in the form of activity diaries and the integration of the energy costs of recorded activities, or intake-balance methods but precision and accuracy is very difficult to define for these procedures. Precision will improve if many observations are made but increasing the number of observations is likely to interfere grossly with the subject's life-style. Observations may therefore be precise but are unlikely to represent the free-living situation. Potential for error undoubtedly exists in the double-labelled water method but these errors are all capable of objective definition and resolution provided that it is understood that a reasonable familiarity with the physiology of the subjects should be acquired. The method is not for indiscriminate application and indeed, it is probably fortunate that cost prevents its indiscriminate application.

In nutritional work I would anticipate that the method's main application would be at least to reinforce data available from dietary data and at best to provide information in circumstances where it is impossible to obtain information in any other ways (e.g. expenditure-balance studies in breast-fed babies).

As yet, little use of the method has been made in a clinical setting and it would be nonsense to apply it in circumstances in which short-term changes as a consequence of acute illness, or treatment, were of interest; calorimetry is a simpler and cheaper option. On the other hand, the method is suitable for long-term measurements in the chronically sick. There is no need for me to be specific; any disorder in which the clinical problem is failure to maintain energy balance should be amenable to investigation.

References

1 Coward, W. A.; Cole, T. J.; Gerber, H.; Roberts, S. B.; Fleet, I.: Water turnover and the measurement of milk intake. Pflügers Arch. *393:* 344–347 (1982).

2 Coward, W. A.; Prentice, A. M.: Isotope method for the measurement of carbon dioxide production rate in man. Am. J. clin. Nutr. *41:* 659–661 (1985).

3 Coward, W. A.; Prentice, A. M.; Murgatroyd, P. R.; Davies, H. L.; Cole, T. J.; Sawyer, M.; Goldberg, G. R.; Halliday, D.; Macnamara, J. P.: Measurement of CO_2 and water production rates in man using ^{2}H, ^{18}O-labelled H_2O. Comparisons between calorimeter and isotope values; in van Es, Euro. Nut. report 5. Human energy metabolism: Physical activity and energy expenditure measurements in epidemiological research based upon direct and indirect calorimetry, pp. 126–128 (CIP-gegevens Koninklijke Bibliotheek, Den Haag 1985).

4 Klien, P. D.; James, W. P. T.; Wong, W. W.; Irving, C. S.; Murgatroyd, P. R.; Cabrera, M.; Delosso, H. M.; Klien, E. R.; Nichols, B. L.: Calorimetric validation of the doubly labelled water method for determination of energy expenditure in man. Hum. Nutr. Clin. Nutr. *38C:* 95–106 (1984).

5 Lifson, N.; McClintock, R.: Theory of use of the turnover rates of body water for measuring energy and maternal balance. J. theor. Biol. *12:* 46–74 (1966).

6 Prentice, A. M.; Coward, W. A.; Davies, H. L.; Murgatroyd, P. R.; Black, A. E.; Goldberg, G. R.; Ashford, J.; Sawyer, M.; Whitehead, R. G.: Unexpectedly low levels of energy expenditure in healthy women. Lancet *i:* 1419–1422 (1985).

7 Schoeller, D. A.: Energy expenditure from doubly labelled water: Some fundamental considerations in humans. Am. J. clin. Nutr. *38:* 999–1005 (1983).

8 Schoeller, D. A.; Kushner, R.: Comparison of $^{2}H_2{}^{18}O$ with intake/balance in patients receiving parenteral nutrition; in van Es, Euro. Nut. report 5. Human energy metabolism: Physical activity and energy expenditure measurements in epidemiological research based upon direct and indirect calorimetry, pp. 132–135 (CIP-gegevens Koninklijke Bibliotheek, Den Haag 1985).

9 Schoeller, D. A.; van Santen, E.: Measurement of energy expenditure in humans by doubly labelled water method. J. appl. Physiol. *53:* 955–959 (1982).
10 Schoeller, D. A.; Slater, R.; Taylor, P.: Reproducibility of the $^2H_2{}^{18}O$ method in free-living subjects; in van Es, Euro. Nut. report 5. Human energy metabolism: Physical activity and energy expenditure measurements in epidemiological research based upon direct and indirect calorimetry, pp. 121–125 (CIP-gegevens Koninklijke Bibliotheek, Den Haag 1985).
11 Schoeller, D. A.; Webb, P.: Five-day comparison of the doubly labelled water method with respiratory gas exchange. Am. J. clin. Nutr. *40:* 153–158 (1984).
12 Westerterp, K. R.; Schoffelen, P. F. M.; Saris, W. H. M.; ten Hoor, F.: Measurement of energy expenditure using doubly labelled water, a validation study; in van Es, Euro. Nut. report 5. Human energy metabolism: Physical activity and energy expenditure measurements in epidemiological research based upon direct and indirect calorimetry, pp. 129–131 (CIP-gegevens Koninklijke Bibliotheek, Den Haag 1985).

W. A. Coward, Dunn Nutrition Laboratory and Dunn Clinical Nutrition Centre, Milton Road, GB-Cambridge CB4 1XJ (UK)

Dietze, Grünert, Kleinberger, Wolfram (eds.), Clinical Nutrition and Metabolic Research. Proc. 7th Congr. ESPEN, Munich 1985, pp. 178–191 (Karger, Basel 1986)

The Use of Stable Isotopes in the Measurement of Whole-Body Protein Turnover in the Human Neonate

D. J. Millward[a], *B. De Benoist*[a], *D. Halliday*[b]

[a] Nutrition Research Unit, Dept. of Human Nutrition, London School of Hygiene and Tropical Medicine, St. Pancras Hospital, London, UK
[b] Clinical Research Centre, Northwick Park Hospital, Harrow, UK

Introduction

The measurement of the dynamic aspects of protein metabolism is an essential step in the understanding of the regulation of growth and protein balance in the body. The recognition of this has resulted in the development of a number of methods involving stable isotopes which are more or less universally applicable [1], and several of these methods have been applied to the study of protein turnover in the neonate [2]. The results obtained to date are summarised in table I. The purpose of this paper is to highlight some of the particular problems associated with the study of protein turnover in the neonate and to present and discuss the limitations of one particularly noninvasive approach which we have used.

[^{15}N] Methods: General Principles

The most widely used methods have been based on the use of [^{15}N] usually in the form of [^{15}N]glycine, but [^{15}N]lysine [3] and yeast protein [4] have also been used (see table I). The methods generally involve study of the transfer of the isotope from the administered amino acid to an end product (urea and/or ammonia) in the urine. As extensively discussed

Table I. Estimated rates of whole-body protein synthesis in human infants

Reference	Population	Tracer	Sampling pool	Protein synthesis
[3]	4 term	[^{13}C]Leu	plasma leucine	5 ± 1
	4 term	[^{15}N]Lys	plasma lysine	6 ± 1
[17]	24 premies	[^{15}N]Gly	urinary urea	8 ± 1
[4]	3 infants	[^{15}N]Gly	urinary nitrogen	7 ± 1
	3 infants	[^{15}N]Yeast	urinary nitrogen	7 ± 1
[10]	5 premies	[^{15}N]Gly	urinary nitrogen	
[11]			38 weeks (age)	8 ± 1
			34 weeks	12 ± 3
			32 weeks	14 ± 4
[13]	3 premies	[^{15}N]Gly	urinary ammonia	11 ± 3
[20]	7 premies	[^{13}C]Leu	urinary leucine	11 ± 1
[12]	3 premies	[^{15}N]Gly	urinary urea	13 ± 2
	3 premies	[^{15}N]Gly	urinary ammonia	15 ± 2
[16]	4 premies	[^{15}N]Gly	urinary urea	14
[18]	20 premies	[^{15}N]Gly	urinary urea	14 ± 4
	20 premies	[^{15}N]Gly	urinary ammonia	18 ± 5
[14]	5 premies	[^{15}N]Gly	urinary urea	26 ± 7

elsewhere [1], the measurements can involve constant infusion of the isotope with measurement of the plateau enrichment of the end product or a single dose with measurement of the amount of the dose which is excreted in the end product [5]. Thus the flux (Q) is either calculated from the dilution of the tracer measured at plateau during the constant infusion or from the proportion of tracer excreted over the experimental period (i.e., $Q = E_a \cdot d/e_a$, where E_a is the rate of total N excretion, d is the dose of isotope, and e_a is the amount of ^{15}N excreted in the end product).

In this stochastic approach, it was originally assumed that there was a single metabolic pool exchanging with the body protein pool into which the isotope enters and from which it is excreted. In this case, the proportion of the administered tracer, which is excreted in the end product, is the same as the proportion of the amino acid nitrogen flux excreted as the end product.

However, the main problems arise with this assumption of a single metabolic pool throughout which there is complete equilibration of the administered isotope. It is obvious that the free amino acid pool in the body is not a single pool since there is compartmentation both within and between individual cells and tissues [1]. In practice, compartmentation with respect to the source of the end products is indicated by the fact that the transfer of isotope to the end products varies considerably according to the choice of administered amino acid and this involves not only variation in the proportion of total isotope excreted but also in the relative distribution between the end products; i.e., the enrichment of urinary ammonia is usually different from that of urea [5, 6]. Furthermore these differences are more marked in the fed state and when isotope is given via an intravenous rather than intragastric route. Thus intravenous infusion of glycine resulted in a 15% lower flux (calculated on urinary urea labelling) than oral administration [7, 8]. A single dose of glycine given intravenously in the fed state results in flux values which are 25% lower based on ammonia and 20% higher based on urea than values indicated by intragastric administration [5]. Furthermore, when glycine and [^{15}N] labelled wheat were compared, ammonia was more highly labelled than urea when glycine was given and less highly labelled by the wheat [9]. Because of these factors, the range of calculated flux values is large, ranging in a single adult from 20 g/12 h with glutamine to 1300 g/12 h with lysine [6].

Although the metabolic basis of these differences is not fully understood, it would appear that amino acids like glutamine and alanine, which are metabolically close to the end products, transfer more isotope to urea and ammonia than those such as lysine which are metabolically remote. Glycine, which has been used in most studies, appears to be, more by accident than design, a fortunate choice since it not only gives values in the middle of the range compared with other amino acids, but gives values comparable to those obtained with [^{13}C]leucine [6]. However, this is only the case when account is taken of excretion of isotope in both end products. Fern et al. [5] noted that there often appears to be a reciprocal relationship between the partition of the isotope between the two routes and argue that it would be better if average values are calculated from the ammonia and urea labelling. This does remove the effect of the route of administration on the calculated value. Their arguments are based on a two pool model for the amino acid pool which takes into account the fact that urea precursors are generally within the splanchnic bed whilst ammonia precursors arise from the muscle pool via glutamine. This has been incorporated into the metabolic model shown in figure 1. There is no doubt that this end-product averaging does reduce variability and, although it is strictly empirical, it is probably the best method for dealing with the results.

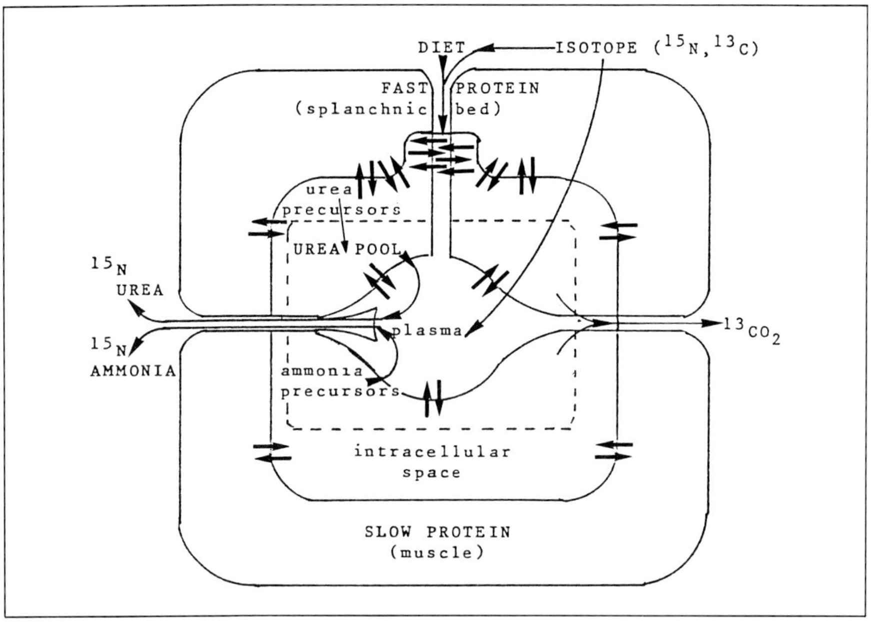

Fig. 1. General model of whole-body protein metabolism as applied to isotopic studies of protein turnover.

Measurements on Neonates – Special Problems

End-product averaging has not been done in neonate studies, except where cumulative total isotope excretion has been measured [4, 10, 11]. As shown in table I, with the exception of the study of Nicolson [12] who reported both values and Jackson [13] who argued for the ammonia value, other authors have generally ignored the ammonia labelling and calculated flux values from the urea enrichment [14–18]. It seems to us that whatever objections might be levelled at this end-product averaging, it is essential that some effort must be made to recognise and deal with the two possible end-product values.

In the present context, however, measurements of protein turnover in the neonate with [^{15}N]glycine appears to be associated with additional problems to those encountered in other studies. As indicated in table I, initial values reported for protein turnover in the preterm infant were very much higher than subsequent values [14]. Whilst the explanation for this may simply indicate termination of the infusion before the plateau was reached, another problem was raised by Jackson et al. [13] who showed in studies on premature infants that in some cases there was very little transfer of [^{15}N] from glycine to urea which markedly elevated the apparent flux (although the values based on ammonia were not especially high, table I). They suggested that glycine requirements may be so high in the neonate that transfer of [^{15}N] to the metabolic pool was limited. Clearly, the low glycine content of milk-based formulas does mean that [^{15}N]glycine might not be the appropriate tracer. This particular aspect is discussed in detail elsewhere [19].

Another special problem arises in those important studies which attempt to evaluate the nutritional merits of various formulas in comparison to human milk. Pencharz et al. [15] investigated the effects of human milk and 2 similar low protein formulas, based on either whey or casein, on growth and protein turnover in neonates. Whilst they reported identical growth rates and nitrogen retention, protein turnover was quite suprisingly 50% higher in the infants fed human milk (table II), implying either that human milk has special properties which influence protein metabolism, or that there are specific methodological errors associated with the feeding of human milk when end-product analysis is used. According to Pencharz et al. [15], the explanation offered by Jackson et al. [13] that dietary glycine was limiting was unlikely to account for the results since glycine intakes were the same in their children fed on the human milk and the two formulae.

However, as shown in table II, other studies have not found this apparent property of human milk. A second problem not generally appreciated is that in infants fed on human breast milk there will be a

Table II. Rates of whole-body protein synthesis (g/kg/d) in preterm infants fed on human milk or a formula

Reference	Method	Formula	Human milk
[15]	[^{15}N]Gly infusion	(A) 13.1 ± 3.1	
	Urea labelling	(B) 12.4 ± 3.2	18.4 ± 4.8
[10]	[^{15}N]Gly single dose	8.0 ± 2.1	7.9 ± 2.7
	Cumulative excretion in urinary nitrogen		
[20]	[^{13}C]Leu infusion	(A) 11.2 ± 0.6	
		(B) 13.0 ± 1.1	10.6 ± 2.2

Table III. Problem of dietary urea in ^{15}N methods based on analysis in urea

(1)	Human milk: 12% nitrogen intake (approximately) is urea
(2)	Net nitrogen utilisation = 75% (approximately) so that 25% dietary N excreted as (mainly) urea
(3)	Thus of the excreted urea: 50% diet, 50% endogenous (i.e. dilution of tracer $\times 2$, flux (increased) $\times 2$)

substantial dietary intake of urea [21]. Since the protein utilisation will generally be high, the dietary urea could constitute a substantial proportion of the excreted urea, and since it is unlabelled, it would lower the enrichment of the urea and elevate the apparent flux. The magnitude of the error (see table III) is such that the flux can be overestimated by a factor of 2, according to the extent of the intestinal hydrolysis and utilisation of dietary urea as ammonia. The extent of this is probably low since although there is an intestinal metabolism of endogenous urea [22], and although protein isolated from the intestinal flora of infants given [^{15}N] urea was enriched with the isotope, the enrichment was low [23]. Furthermore, recent experiments with dilabelled urea given to neonates show that it is absorbed and excreted largely unchanged (Foman, Matthews and Bier, personal communication). Thus, there can be no doubt that the flux calculated from urea enrichment will be overestimated and calculation of some average value (by including the ammonia value), invalid. All that can be done is to calculate the values based on the ammonia, even though they will indicate lower values (as in [16]). In other studies, a similar comparison of human milk and a formula in preterm infants has been made with [^{15}N]glycine and the flux calculated from the cumulative total excretion of isotope [10]. In this case, the effect of dietary urea is probably much less. It would not influence the cumulative excretion of isotope, but it would increase nitrogen excretion and increase the calculated flux because of this. However, any effect must have been small since no differences in rates of protein turnover were observed in the 2 groups (see table II). These authors have most recently used this approach to examine protein turnover in very small premature infants fed breast milk and report values for protein synthesis of 14.3 g/kg/d falling to 7.75 g/kg/d at term [16].

Without more information of the actual amount of dietary urea and the extent of its metabolism and excretion in comparison with endogenous production, it is difficult to determine the extent of this particular problem in these latter studies. However, it does seem to me that, in addition to the general problems associated with use of [^{15}N], the problem of dietary urea in human milk does mean that methods based on [^{15}N] are particularly problematical in studies which involve such feeds.

[^{13}C] Studies: General Considerations

Clearly the use of carbon-labelled tracers excludes end-product analysis since there is no carbon end product which derives exclusively from protein. Thus studies involving CO_2 are limited to measurements of amino acid oxidation rates. However, [^{13}C] studies lend themselves very well to the measurement of the turnover of individual amino acids such as leucine. The approach, developed by Waterlow (see [1]), involves the constant infusion of the labelled amino acid, (at a rate = i), so that a plateau enrichment of the free amino acid is achieved (A_{max}) when the incorporation into protein equals the infusion rate. Protein turnover is calculated from the amino acid flux (Q) and this is usually calculated (as $Q = i/A_{max}$) on the basis of a two pool model comprising a single homogeneous pool of amino acids and body protein. The components of the flux, dietary input (D), protein degradation (B), amino acid oxidation (O), and protein synthesis (S) are related according to the equation

$$Q = D + B = O + S$$

Of course the parameters calculated in this way will be in amounts (μmols) of amino acid and this means that some factor must be used to convert this to protein (in theory, the average amino acid content of the protein actually turning over weighted according to its turnover rate), and this poses problems which are often not appreciated [24].

The primary problem with this method also derives from compartmentation of body protein and amino acids, and the inadequacy of a two pool model. In theory, the true flux is that calculated from the weighted average value of the labelling of the actual amino acid precursors for protein synthesis (the amino-acyl tRNA), which will probably in most tissues be closer to the intracellular pool shown in figure 1. Since proteolysis occurs predominantly in the intracellular compartment and amino-acid transport into cells takes a finite time, there will be dilution of label intracellularly which will vary between cells and tissues according to the relative rates of proteolysis and transport. In practice, the appropriate values cannot be determined for the whole body in human studies and usually no attempt is made to correct plasma values so that flux will be underestimated. In the case of leucine, one partial solution is to sample its transamination product in the plasma, ketoisocaproate (KIC), which can be measured by mass spectrometry without particular difficulties [25, 26]. This is formed intracellularly and therefore has an enrichment similar to intracellular leucine in those tissues where leucine is transaminated. Such measurements generally indicate that plasma leucine flux is some 80% of 'true' flux.

This problem of the actual precursor enrichment is also important in the calculation of the oxidation rate, but since KIC is the precursor for CO_2 production from leucine, there should be much less uncertainly in this case. However, as discussed below, the oxidation rate must also take into account the extent of CO_2 retention in the body.

The extent to which the route of administration influences the results has also been investigated with this approach. Hoerr et al. [28] have simultaneously infused [^{3}H]leucine intravenously and [^{13}C]leucine intragastrically in the fed and fasted state and have shown that the route results in a 20% lower flux in the fasted state rising to a 30% underestimation in the fed state. As indicated in the model (fig. 1), it must be assumed that with an oral infusion the initial entry of the isotope into the compartments of the system, which contain the most rapidly turning over proteins (i.e., the splanchnic bed), results in a more rapid loss of isotope, (a better mixing?), and consequently higher flux than when entry is intravenous. Indeed, Bier and Young [2] report convincing data showing the need to consider splanchnic metabolism since the leucine flux in young adults based on intravenous administration was not only too low but was actually less than the leucine intake in subjects on a high protein diet. Thus protein degradation (flux-intake) was negative, an impossible result.

Measurements on the Neonate with [^{13}C]Leucine

Clearly all of the general problems mentioned above which derive from studies on adults apply to the neonate but there is the obvious additional problem posed by the clinical management and handling of the babies. Thus the intravenous catheterization and blood sampling, which is part of the method as applied to adults [29], is much more difficult in the neonate or preterm infant. Since feeding is often by continuous intragastric infusion, administration of isotope by this route is obviously much more convenient. For this reason, we investigated whether measurements of whole body protein turnover could be made in preterm infants with a minimum of invasive procedures by measuring the enrichment of urinary leucine during an intragastric infusion of [^{13}C]leucine [20].

The measurement of the enrichment of urinary amino acids can be made without difficulty on the GC-MS although no previous measurements had been reported. Amino acids in the urine are most likely to arise from the plasma ultrafiltrate. The only other possible source would be the degradation of proteins in the kidney liberating amino acids into the lumen of the tubule against the normal flow. If this unlikely event occurred, it would result in a markedly lower labelling of leucine.

In fact, our experiments showed that enrichments of urinary and plasma leucine were generally the same (see fig. 2). The fact that they were not always identical is not unexpected. The leucine in the kidney ultrafiltrate is arterial leucine and this may have a slightly different enrichment from that in venous blood. However, if the main source of variability in enrichment of plasma leucine is variability in the infusion rate or intestinal absorption rate, then the urinary leucine enrichment (the average

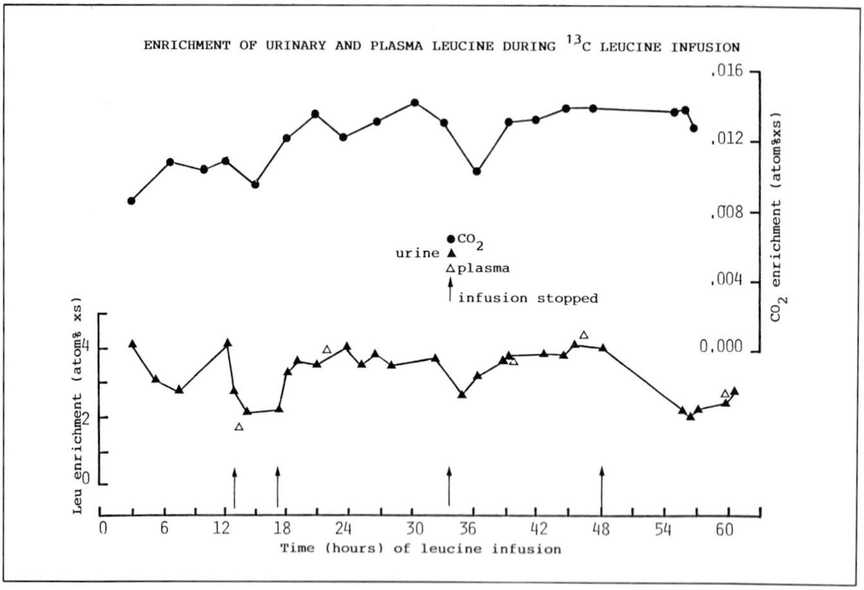

Fig. 2. Time course of changes in plasma and urinary leucine and CO_2 enrichment during an intragastric infusion of a preterm neonate [20].

value of that excreted over periods lasting up to 120 min) should be the preferred value.

The variability of the plateau labelling of leucine as illustrated by the results in figure 2 means that it is preferable to prolong the infusion longer than the few hours necessary for a primed-dose intravenous infusion of labelled amino acids [29], and one approach which we have examined is administration of isotope with the feed throughout the night with collection of urine and expired CO_2 during the following day time. The length of the infusion in figure 2 was specifically longer than we consider necessary to enable the stability of the plateau to be examined. It is shown that when the infusion was stopped to allow patient manipulation although there was a prompt fall in the labelling, the plateau was quickly resumed.

As discussed above, the true flux is likely to be higher than that calculated on the plasma enrichment. Since the enrichment of KIC was 78% of the leucine, the true flux would be 28% higher. This is similar to the values found for KIC enrichment in other studies [25–26].

Leucine Oxidation and Protein Synthesis

A second problem inherent in calculating protein turnover from the leucine flux is that the rate of protein synthesis is dependent on the measurement of the leucine oxidation rate from the rate of [$^{13}CO_2$] excretion. This latter value not only is subject to similar problems relating to the determination of the true value of the enrichment of the precursor for oxidation but, in addition, is also subject to errors associated with the assumed value for the extent of retention of enriched CO_2. In most studies a single value is assumed. It has been shown that the recovery of labelled CO_2 in obese adults did not vary with feeding or fasting, or with alterations of the dietary composition, but the point was made there that recovery rates ought to be measured rather than assumed [27]. Indeed, in the preterm infant, disturbances of acid-base status are likely and this could alter the extent of CO_2 retention. Recent studies on the kinetics of the HCO_3^-/CO_2 in the infant have indicated not only greater retention than in adults (57% [30]), but also have shown that the retention is variable according to the food intake [31]. For these reasons, the leucine oxidation rate is subject to two sources of error which could seriously influence the final value.

The extent of the errors in practice can be determined since the leucine oxidation rate (converted to nitrogen excretion) can be compared with the rate of nitrogen excretion. This comparison is best done indirectly since the amount of leucine oxidized will only bear a constant relationship to the amount of nitrogen excreted if the leucine content of the deposited tissue and dietary protein is the same. The high leucine content of the dietary protein in milk protein (about 10% compared with the 8% assumed for tissue protein) will increase the ratio of leucine oxidation to N excretion.

We attempted to minimize this particular difficulty by comparing leucine retention converted to nitrogen retention, with the measured nitrogen retention from the nitrogen balance study, and we showed that, when the leucine content of tissue protein was assumed to be 8%, the nitrogen retention calculated from leucine retention was remarkably similar to the measured nitrogen balance.

Rates of whole-body protein synthesis and degradation and retention calculated from the leucine flux are shown in table IV. A single value for protein degradation is shown calculated as leucine flux-intake, converted into protein assuming that body protein which is participating in protein turnover contains 8% leucine. However, two values are shown for protein synthesis. These values are calculated either as flux-leucine oxidation, or degradation + nitrogen retention, (which is normally numerically equal to flux-nitrogen excretion, but is theoretically more acurate if there is dietary nitrogen such as urea which is not metabolised).

As already shown in table II, there was no suggestion that the infants fed on breast milk had higher turnover rates and the average values for all the children is shown. Because of the similarity of the values for nitrogen retention calculated from leucine oxidation and directly from nitrogen balance, the two values for protein synthesis shown in table IV are very

Table IV. Rates of whole-body protein synthesis, degradation, and retention in 7 preterm infants (g/d/kg) [20]

Degradation	9.54 ± 0.55
Retention	
leucine oxidation	1.87 ± 0.24
N balance	1.94 ± 0.28
Synthesis	
leucine oxidation	11.48 ± 0.67
N balance	11.32 ± 0.78

similar. In fact, since the only problems associated with the measurement of nitrogen balance are technical rather than theoretical, it seemed to us that the measurement of leucine oxidation could be dispensed with in the present clinical context where a nitrogen balance is likely to be part of the study. Thus protein synthesis would be calculated from the leucine flux and nitrogen retention. This would simplify the procedure considerably, dispensing with not only the need to measure and collect CO_2 but also with the isotope-ratio mass-spectrometer. A suggested protocol could be the infusion of the leucine during the second day of a 3-day balance period so that the frequent sampling of the urine during the infusion would not interfere with the nitrogen balance, which would be measured on the first and third days of the study.

Conclusions

The measurement of whole-body protein turnover involves several assumptions which vary according to the method used, and as recently concluded [2], none of the simplified models designed to understand metabolic events can account entirely for the observed data which all must be analysed with caution. In the very particular case of the human infant, in addition to the usual problems, studies involving human milk can pose particular problems when measurements are made with [^{15}N]glycine, not only because the low dietary levels of glycine relation to needs could reduce metabolic mixing of the nitrogen pool, but also because of the presence of dietary urea. In contrast, measurements with [^{13}C]leucine seem to result in no particular additional problems and, in our opinion, have the advantage that the analytical model, whilst a gross simplification, is nevertheless less empirical and more open to investigation and verification. Clearly only with the increased availability and application of stable isotope facilities will completely satisfactory methods be designed.

References

1 Waterlow, J. C.; Garlick, P. J.; Millward, D. J.: Protein turnover in mammalian tissues and in the whole body; chapter 8 (Elsevier/North Holland, Amsterdam 1978).

2 Bier, D. M.; Young, V. R.: Assessment of whole body protein-nitrogen kinetics in the human infant; in Foman, Heird, Protein and energy needs of the infant (Academic Press, New York, in press).

3 Frazer, T. E.; Bier, D. M.: Essential amino acid turnover in the human newborn. Pediat. Res. *14:* 571 (1980).

4 Wutzke, K.; Heine, W.; Drescher, U.; Richter, I.; Plath, C.: ^{15}N-labelled yeast protein – A valid tracer for calculating whole body protein parameters in infants: A Comparison between [^{15}N]-yeast protein and [^{15}N]-glycine. Hum. Nutr. Clin. Nutr. *37C:* 317–327 (1983).

5 Fern, E. B.; Garlick, P. J.; McNurlan, M. A.; Waterlow, J. C.: The excretion of isotope in urea and ammonia for estimating protein turnover in man with [^{15}N]glycine. Clin. Sci. mol. Med. *61:* 217–228 (1981).

6 Fern, E. B.; Garlick, P. J.; Waterlow, J. C.: Apparent compartmentation of body nitrogen in one human subject: Its consequences in measuring the rate of whole-body protein synthesis with [^{15}N]. Clin. Sci. mol. Med. *68:* 271–282 (1985).

7 Picou, D.; Taylor-Roberts, T.: The measurement of total protein synthesis and catabolism and nitrogen turnover in infants in different nutritional states and receiving different amounts of dietary protein. Clin. Sci. *36:* 283–289 (1969).

8 Steffe, W. P.; Goldsmith, R. S.; Pencharz, P. B.; Scrimshaw, N. S.; Young, V. R.: Dietary protein intake and dynamic aspects of whole body nitrogen metabolism in adult humans. Metabolism *25:* 281–289 (1976).

9 Fern, E. B.; Garlick, P. J.: The rate of nitrogen metabolism in man measured with [^{15}N]glycine and uniformly labelled [^{15}N]-wheat. Hum. Nutr. Clin. Nutr. *37C:* 91–107 (1983).

10 Heine, W.; Plath, C.; Richter, I.; Wutzke, K.; Towe, J.: ^{15}N-tracer investigations into the nitrogen metabolism of preterm infants fed mothers' milk and a formula diet. J. pediat. Gast. Nutr. *2:* 606–612 (1983).

11 Plath, C.; Heine, W.; Krienke, L.; Richter, I.; Wutzke, K.; Towe, J.; Krawielitski, K.: ^{15}N-tracer kinetic studies on the nitrogen metabolism of very small preterm infants on a mothers' milk diet. Hum. Nutr. Clin. Nutr. (in press 1985).

12 Nicholson, J. F.: Rate of protein synthesis in premature infants. Pediat. Res. *4:* 389–396 (1970).

13 Jackson, A. A.; Shaw, J. C. L.; Barber, A.; Golden, M. H. N.: Nitrogen metabolism in preterm infants fed human donor breast milk: The possible essentiality of glycine. Pediat. Res. *15:* 1454–1461 (1981).

14 Pencharz, P. B.; Steffee, W. P.; Cochran, W.; Scrimshaw, N. S.; Rand, W. M.; Young, V. R.: Protein metabolism in human neonates: Nitrogen-balance studies, estimated obligatory losses of nitrogen and whole-body turnover of nitrogen. Clin. Sci. mol. Med. *52:* 485–498 (1977).

15 Pencharz, P. B.; Farri, L.; Papageorgiou, A.: The effects of human milk and low protein formulae on the rates of total body protein turnover and urinary 3-methylhistidine excretion of preterm infants. Clin. Sci. mol. Med. *64:* 611–616 (1983).

16 Schutz, Y.; Catzeflis, C.; Gudinchet, F.; Micheli, J.; Welsch, C.; Arnaud, M. J.; Jequier, E.: Energy expenditure and whole body protein synthesis in very low birth weight infants. Experientia (suppl.) *44:* 45–56 (1983).

17 Duffy, B.; Gunn, T.; Collinge, J.; Pencharz, P.. The effect of varying protein quality and energy intake on the nitrogen metabolism of parenterally fed very low birth weight infants. Pediat. Res. *15:* 1040–1045 (1981).

18 Pencharz, P.; Masson, M.; Desgranges, F.; Papageorgiou, A.: Total body protein turn-

over in human premature neonates: Effects of birth weight, intra-uterine nutritional status and diet. Clin. Sci. mol. Med. *61:* 207–212 (1981).

19 Golden, M. H. N.; Jackson, A. A.: Assumptions and errors in the use of [^{15}N]-excretion data to estimate whole body protein turnover; in Waterlow, Stephen, Nitrogen metabolism in man; chapter 27 (Applied Science Publishers, London 1981).

20 De Benoist, B.; Abdulrazzak, Y.; Brooke, O. G.; Halliday, D.; Millward, D. J.: Measurement of whole body protein turnover in the preterm infant with intragastric infusion of [1-^{13}C]leucine and sampling of the urinary leucine pool. Clin. Sci. mol. Med. *66:* 155–164 (1984).

21 Hambraeus, L.: Proprietary milk versus human breast milk in infant feeding. Pediat. Clins N. Am. *24,* 1: 17–36 (1977).

22 Walser, M.: Urea metabolism; in Waterlow, Stephen, Nitrogen metabolism in man, pp. 229–246 (Applied Science Publishers, London 1981).

23 Heine, W.; Tiess, M.; Stolpe, H. J.; Wutzke, K.: Urea utilisation by the intestinal flora of infants fed mothers' milk and a formula diet as measured with the ^{15}N-tracer technique. J. Pediat. Gast. Nutr. *3:* 709–712 (1983).

24 Reeds, P. J.; Harris, C. I.: Protein turnover in animals: Man in his context; in Waterlow, Stephen, Nitrogen metabolism in man, pp. 391–408 (Applied Science Publishers, London 1981).

25 Rennie, M. J.; Edwards, R. H. T.; Halliday, D.; Matthews, D. E.; Wolman, S. L.; Millward, D. J.: Muscle protein synthesis measured by stable isotope techniques in man: The effects of feeding and fasting. Clin. Sci. mol. Med. *63:* 519–523 (1982).

26 Matthews, D. E.; Schwarz, H. P.; Yang, R. D.; Motil, K. J.; Young, V. R.; Bier, D. M.: Relationship of plasma leucine and alpha-ketoisocaproate during a L-(1-^{13}C)leucine infusion in man: A method for measuring the intracellular leucine tracer enrichment. Metabolism *31:* 1105–1112 (1982).

27 Clugston, A. G.; Garlick, P. J.: Recovery of infused [^{14}C] bicarbonate as respiratory $^{14}CO_2$ in man. Clin. Sci. mol. Med. *64:* 231–233 (1983).

28 Hoerr, R. A.; Mattews, D. E.; Bier, D. E.; Blackburn, G. L.; Young, V. R.: Splanchnic bed metabolism of leucine in man measured by simultaneous intravenous and intragastric infusion of stable isotope tracers of leucine. Am. J. clin. Nutr. *36:* 687–693 (1984).

29 Matthews, D. E.; Motil, K. J.; Rohrbaugh, D. K.; Burke, J. F.; Young, V. R.; Bier, D. M.: Measurement of leucine metabolism in man from a primed continuous infusion of L-[1-^{13}C]leucine. Am. J. Physiol. *238:* E473–E479 (1980).

30 Van Aerde, J. E. E.; Sauer, P. J. J.; Pencharz, P. B.; Canagaraya, U.; Beesley, J.; Smith, J. M.; Swyer, P. R.: Effect of energy intake and expenditure on the recovery of the parenterally fed neonate during a primed constant infusion of $NaH^{13}CO_3$. Pediat. Res. *19:* 806–810 (1985).

31 Irving, C. S.; Lifschitz, C. H.; Wong, W. W.; Bouton, T. W.; Nichols, B. L.; Klein, P. D.: Characterisation of HCO_3^-/CO_2 pool sizes and kinetics in infants. Pediat. Res. *19:* 358–363 (1985).

D. J. Millward, Dept. of Human Nutrition, London School of Hygiene and Tropical Medicine, St. Pancras Hospital, 4, St. Pancras Way, GB-London NW1 2PE (UK)

Dietze, Grünert, Kleinberger, Wolfram (eds.), Clinical Nutrition and Metabolic Research. Proc. 7th Congr. ESPEN, Munich 1985, pp. 192–207 (Karger, Basel 1986)

$^{13}CO_2$-Breath Tests in Nutritional Diagnosis: Present Applications and Future Possibilities

Y. Ghoos, P. Rutgeerts, G. Vantrappen

Dept. of Medicine and Medical Research, Gastrointestinal Research Center, University Hospital St. Rafaël-Gasthuisberg, Leuven, Belgium

Since their introduction more than 40 years ago by Schoenheimer [1], stable isotopes are finding more and more application in nutritional and gastroenterological research. This is due not only to the absence of radiation risks, but to the potentials offered by newly developed stable isotope technology [2–7].

Breath tests measuring the respiratory excretion of $^{14}CO_2$ following the administration of ^{14}C-labelled substrates have been used since the early 1960s for the study of gastroenterological and hepatic functions [8]. The radiation hazard restricts the application of these tests in infants, children, and women of child-bearing age. During the seventies, the basic methodology was developed to perform CO_2-breath tests by means of isotope ratio mass spectrometry of the nonradioactive isotope ^{13}C [9–11].

Both ^{14}C- and ^{13}C-breath tests are carried out using interval breath sampling. To calculate the dilution of the tracer in the total amount of CO_2, it is assumed that the CO_2 production in resting subjects is constant and equals of 9 mmol/kg/h or 300 mmol/BSA/h. This assumption may not always be valid.

The aims of our studies were (1) to render the $^{13}CO_2$-breath tests more quantitative; this was achieved by measuring the CO_2 output by the Ar/CO_2 method and spirometry [12], and (2) to make these tests suitable for routine clinical diagnosis. During the past few years new pancreatic function breath test, i.e. the ^{13}C-mixed triglyceride breath test was developed in our laboratory [13]. For the diagnosis of disaccharidase deficiency we have combined the ^{13}C-lactose breath test with measurement of H_2-excretion in breath [14].

Principles of the Test

All $^{13}CO_2$-breath tests share the common characteristic of requiring a substrate whose structure contains a ^{13}C-labelled functional group that may be enzymatically cleaved under specific conditions. Cleavage may occur during the passage of the substrate down the gastrointestinal tract, during its absorption, or in later metabolic processes. After enzymatic cleavage of the target bond linking the labelled group to the remainder of the substrate, the cleaved portion undergoes metabolic processes that ultimately result in the release of ^{13}C-labelled carbon dioxide in the expired air [5]. Schematically, this principle can be summarized as follows:

$$^{13}\text{C-substrate} \xrightarrow[\text{enzyme studied}]{} {}^{13}\text{C-portion} \longrightarrow {}^{13}\text{CO}_2$$

In table I, the ^{13}C-breath tests, used on a routine basis in our laboratory for the diagnosis of various gastrointestinal, hepatic, and metabolic functions are summarized.

Methods

Test Procedure, Sample Collection, and Handling

All ^{13}C-breath tests are carried out in the same manner. After an overnight fast breath samples are obtained from patients in basal conditions 15 and 5 min before the test meal. Expired air is collected by blowing in a 3 l-balloon. After ingestion of the labelled substrate,

Table I. ^{13}C-breath tests

^{13}C-substrate	Function tested	Disease	References
Mixed triglyceride	luminal lipase activity	pancreatic insufficiency	[13, 15, 16]
Glycocholic acid	enterohepatic circulation of conjugated bile acids	ileal dysfunction bacterial overgrowth of jejunum	[10, 17, 18]
Lactose-sucrose	disaccharidase activity of brush border	lactose or sucrose malabsorption	[19–21]
Glucose-fructose	hexose absorption and oxidation	diabetes mellitus	[22–27]
Aminopyrine	microsomal demethylation and oxidation in the liver cell	liver cell injury	[28–33]

breath samples are obtained with 30 min intervals for 4 to 6 h. Pure CO_2 samples are obtained by passage of the air from the balloon through a −196 °C liquid nitrogen trap (cryogenic CO_2).

Measurement of ^{13}C-Enrichment

Small excesses of $^{13}CO_2$ arising from oxidation of the labelled substrate are calculated from the increase in the ratio of $^{13}CO_2$ (mass 45) to $^{12}CO_2$ (mass 44). However, since mass 45 not only comprises $^{13}C^{16}O_2$ but also $^{12}C^{17}O^{16}O$, the contribution of the oxygen-17 isotope must be substracted from the measured $^{13}C/^{12}C$ ratio in the standard and in the sample. In practice, this correction is achieved by also taking into account the amount of oxygen-18 present as $^{12}C^{18}O^{16}O$, mass 46 [34]. The results of this differential measurement are expressed as delta pro mille (δ‰) difference between the $\frac{^{13}CO_2}{^{12}CO_2}$ ratio of the sample (R_{sa}) and the standard (R_s).

$$\delta\ ^{13}C = \left(\frac{R_{sa}}{R_s} - 1\right) \times 1000$$

In $^{13}CO_2$-breath tests, the delta value is analogous to a molar specific activity.

The results are expressed as percentage ^{13}C-recovery per hour, following the formula of D. Schoeller et al. [17], and the cumulative excretion of $^{13}CO_2$ over the test period is calculated by addition of the values obtained at each sampling period.

Before $^{13}CO_2$-breath tests could be used for clinical diagnosis, the limitations and possible sources of error of these tests required investigation. A major problem with $^{13}CO_2$-breath tests arises from the large natural abundance of ^{13}C (1.1%).

The concentration of natural ^{13}C-abundance represents a relatively high background that will affect the accuracy of the $^{13}CO_2$-breath test. Moreover, the natural ^{13}C-background in breath is not constant. The ^{13}C-enrichment in the expired CO_2 depends on the diet, because the $^{13}C/^{12}C$ ratio depends on the ingredients of the plants taken with the meal [35–37]. In plants, fractionation of carbon is brought about primarily by carbon dioxide assimilation in photosynthesis and is due to preferential utilization of ^{12}C and exclusion of ^{13}C. Higher plants which fix carbon dioxide by way of the Calvin-Benson C_3-cycle pathway differ in $^{13}C/^{12}C$ ratios from plants which fix carbon dioxide through the C_4-dicarboxylic acid Hatch-Slack pathway [38]. As the C_4-plants show a natural enrichment in ^{13}C [39], the consumption of the ingredients of these plants will enhance the test signal after administration of the ^{13}C-labelled substrate in $^{13}CO_2$-breath tests.

Each laboratory has to study the food-related natural variations in the isotope ratios of breath CO_2 in the population they serve. We have extensively studied the natural variations on fasting and with normal eating patterns in the Belgian population.

The mean δ-value after an overnight fast amounted to −25.829 ± 0.519 (SD) and the mean variation between fasting values averaged 0.212 δ.

In figure 1 the changes of δ-values of 9 normal subjects are summarized throughout a 6-h study period, including fasting and postprandial periods (breakfast and lunch).

The δ-value decreased below the fasting level in all subjects with a maximal decrease of 0.929 at 6 h.

When foods containing naturally enriched carbons are ingested during the study period the δ-value increases. This is not always an unwanted interference. Lacroix and coworkers [9] used naturally enriched glucose derived from corn starch to study glucose oxidation in

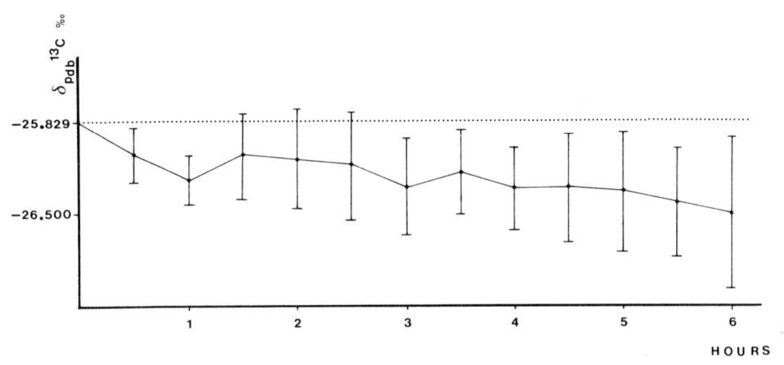

Fig. 1. Mean δ-value of the $^{13}CO_2$ in breath after an overnight fast for 9 normal volunteers, and time course of δ-variation during 6-h period, including postprandial period after non-^{13}C-enriched food intake.

diabetics by a $^{13}CO_2$-breath test. We used the same method to study glucose oxidation in patients after partial gastrectomy [26]. These observations clearly indicate that clinical tests have to be carried out after an overnight fast and that multiple breath samples have to be obtained before the test meal, in order to obtain a mean basal value with high confidence. Moreover, food must be withheld from the patients throughout the test period and the standard meal used should not include naturally enriched carbons.

Calculation of % Dose Recovery

In $^{13}CO_2$-breath tests, the endogenous production of CO_2 should be kept constant as the isotope dilution, and consequently the measured δ-value depends on the mixing of $^{13}CO_2$, resulting from oxidation of the labelled substrate, with the (background-labelled) CO_2-pool in the body. To assure constant CO_2-production, the metabolic activity of the organism should be maintained at a constant oxidation rate by keeping the patients in complete rest during the test. In this condition, a constant CO_2-production of 9 mmol CO_2/kg/h [40] or 300 mmol CO_2/BSA/h [17] is accepted for the computation of $^{13}CO_2$-dilution.

We have developed and validated a new method for measuring the CO_2 concentration and total CO_2 output in mass spectrometric analyses [41]. Argon, an inert gas, that is present in air in a constant concentration of 0.923%, was used as an internal standard. By determining the ratio of CO_2 (mass 44) to Ar (mass 40) in the breath samples, the CO_2 concentration can be read from a standard curve relating CO_2 concentration to CO_2/Ar ratio. By combining mass spectrometric determination of CO_2 concentration in breath with spirometric measurement of expired volumes, the CO_2 production is determined. Application of this method in 67 normal subjects at rest showed that although the mean CO_2 production rate (8.86 mmol/kg/h) is close to the assumed 9 mmol/kg/h, there are marked interindividual variations in the actually measured rates, ranging from 5.31 to 13.46 mmol/kg/h. As differences in CO_2 production may be so important it is clear that calculation of label recovery after ingestion of a labelled test meal is only semi-quantitative [42].

Mixed Triglyceride Breath Test

The ^{13}C-mixed triglyceride breath test was developed in our laboratory to study intraluminal lipase activity, the main parameter in fat digestion. The test molecule 1,3-distearyl-2-(carboxyl-^{13}C)-octanoyl glycerol (= S*OS) consists of a medium chain fatty acid in the 2-position and long chain fatty acids in the 1- and 3-positions. The rationale of the test is that the two stearyl groups have to be split off the glycerol by lipase before ^{13}C-octanoyl monoglyceride or ^{13}C-octanoate, a medium chain fatty acid, is absorbed, transported via the portal vein to the liver where it is rapidly metabolized to $^{13}CO_2$ (fig. 2).

The ^{13}C-mixed triglyceride we use (IRE, Fleurus, Belgium) is 91% ^{13}C-enriched, and the chemical purity exceeds 98%. The test meal consists of 100 g of toast with 0.25 g of butter per kg of body weight, to which 16 mg of S*OS per gram of butter is added.

The cumulative $^{13}CO_2$ excretion during a 6-h period reflects intraluminal lipase activity. In figure 3, a typical $^{13}CO_2$ excretion curve (in % dose/h) is given for a normal individual. In figure 4, the cumulative $^{13}CO_2$-excretion over 6 h is shown for normal subjects and for a patient with chronic pancreatitis. The 6-h cumulative $^{13}CO_2$ excretion correlates closely with duodenal outputs of lipase in normal subjects and in patients with pancreatic disease.

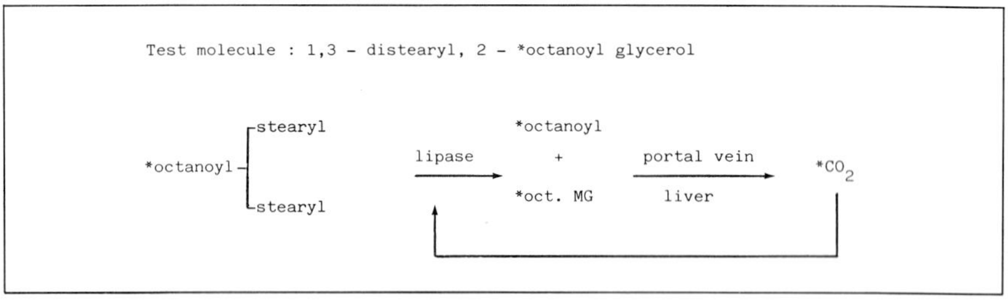

Fig. 2. Principle of the mixed triglyceride breath test. The glycerol moiety of the triglyceride is esterified with stearic acid in the 1- and the 3-positions. ^{13}C-labelled octanoic acid is esterified in the 2-position of glycerol. Upon hydrolysis of the triglyceride by luminal lipase, the octanoic acid portion of the triglyceride is absorbed and rapidly converted to $^{13}CO_2$ by the liver.

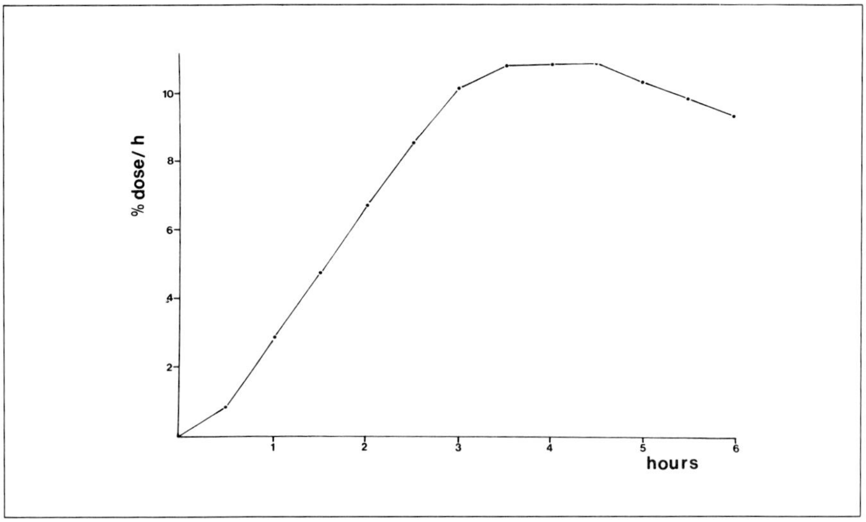

Fig. 3. Time course of $^{13}CO_2$-excretion (in % of dose/h) in normal men upon administration of the ^{13}C-mixed triglyceride.

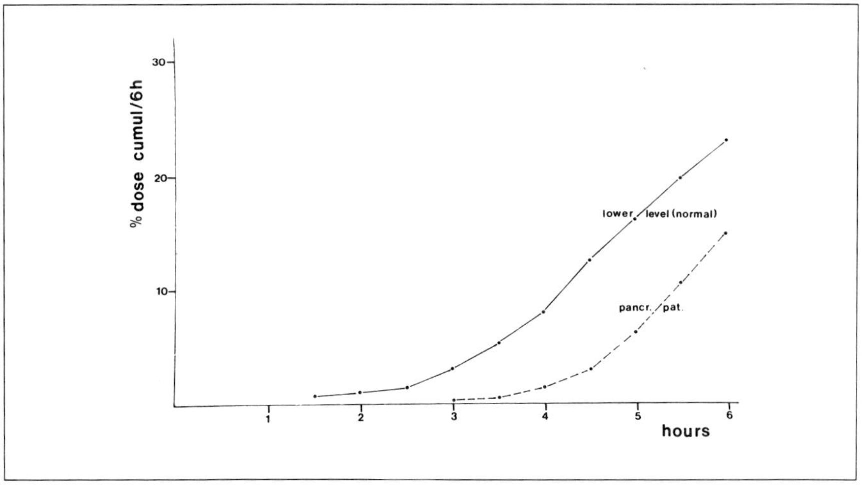

Fig. 4. Cumulative $^{13}CO_2$-excretion over a 6-h period after the intake of the ^{13}C-mixed triglyceride is shown for normal men and for pancreatic patients.

This mixed triglyceride breath test is a sensitive pancreatic function test that is particularly suitable for the follow-up of pancreatic function in patients with pancreatic disease.

^{13}C-Aminopyrine Breath Test

An important function of the liver is to metabolize endogenous and exogenous lipophylic compounds to more hydrophylic substances. The cytochrome P-450 dependent monooxygenases (localized in hepatic microsomes) catalyze the metabolism of many such compounds by reactions that usually involve oxidation or reduction. ^{13}C-aminopyrine is demethylated and the methyl group is subsequently oxidized to $^{13}CO_2$ by this system. The principle of the ^{13}C-aminopyrine breath test is shown in figure 5.

The test molecule, 60% ^{13}C-enriched aminopyrine (IRE, Fleurus, Belgium), is administered to the patient (after an overnight fast) in a dose of 2 mg/kg. Dissolved in water, the molecule is rapidly absorbed and metabolized. Breath sampling for 2 h allows to differentiate between normal individuals and patients with impaired liver cell function. In figure 6, the excretion pattern of $^{13}CO_2$ (in % dose, cumulative) is given for normal individuals and cirrhotic patients.

The ^{13}C-aminopyrine breath test has a good prognostic value in the follow-up of liver cell function. It can show restitution of liver cell function in alcoholic liver disease after abstinence. Further impairment of micro-

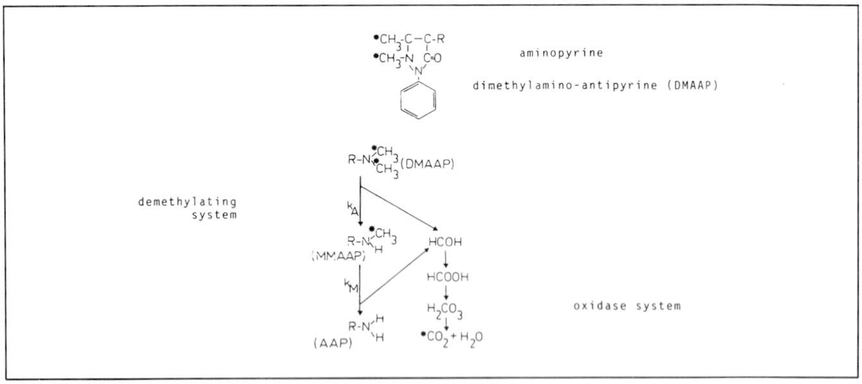

Fig. 5. Principle of the ^{13}C-aminopyrine breath test. By intact microsomes of the liver cell the CH_3-group of aminopyrine are demethylated and oxidized to $^{13}CO_2$.

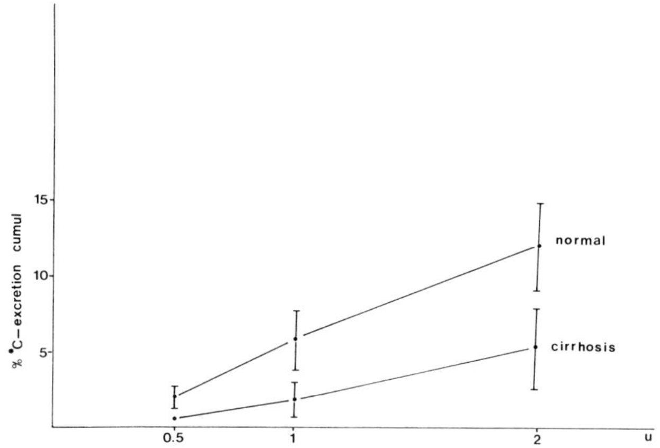

Fig. 6. The cumulative $^{13}CO_2$-excretion is shown over a 2-h period after the intake of ^{13}C-aminopyrine in normal subjects and in patients with liver cirrhosis.

somal liver cell function, as demonstrated by decreasing ^{13}C-aminopyrine demethylation and oxidation, predicts evolution to coma and death in chronic hepatitis and cirrhosis.

^{13}C-Glycocholate Breath Test

^{13}C-glycocholic acid, labelled on the carboxyl carbon atom of the glycine moiety, mixes with the bile acid pool after oral intake. The glycine moiety is liberated only when the amine bond, linking the glycine to the bile acid, is hydrolized by intestinal bacteria, either in the presence of small intestinal bacterial overgrowth or when the nonabsorbed conjugated bile acid is exposed to the colonic flora because of bile acid malabsorption. The ^{13}C-glycine, liberated by bacterial deconjugation, is readily metabolized by bacteria or in the body to $^{13}CO_2$, which is excreted in expired air (fig. 7).

The test molecule, ^{13}C-glycocholic acid (99% ^{13}C-enriched, chemical purity $> 98\%$; IRE, Fleurus, Belgium), is administered to the patient in a dose of 6 mg ^{13}C-glycocholic acid/kg wt.

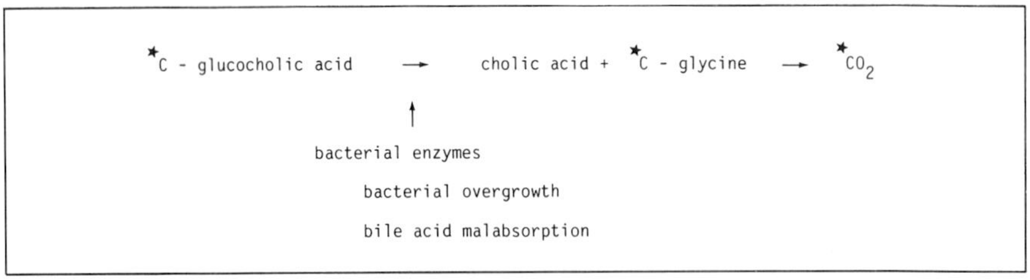

Fig. 7. Principle of the ^{13}C-glycocholate breath test. The ^{13}C-labelled glycine moiety of the molecule is split off only by bacterial enzymes. This can either be due to small intestinal bacterial overgrowth or to bile acid malabsorption by the ileum.

Figures 8 and 9 show the $^{13}CO_2$ excretion pattern in % dose/h of a normal individual, a patient with bacterial overgrowth, and a patient with bile acid malabsorption, respectively.

The ^{13}C-glycocholic acid breath test is very useful for the diagnosis of ileal dysfunction due to ileal disease or resection, and for the diagnosis of jejunal bacterial overgrowth, due to various intestinal diseases, e.g. diverticulosis of the small bowel, achlorhydria, blind loop syndrome. Elderly subjects, aged 70 or more, frequently have abnormal bile acid breath tests, due to bacterial overgrowth that may remain without symptoms, but occasionally may lead to malabsorption and weight loss [43].

^{13}C-Lactose Breath Test

Lactose, the main carbohydrate of milk, is a disaccharide in which galactose is bound with a β,1 → 4 link to glucose. Lactose is hydrolized by lactase before absorption and metabolization occur. Lactase is a brush border enzyme and is present mainly in the proximal small intestine.

When ^{13}C-lactose is administered with a load of unlabelled lactose, the excretion of $^{13}CO_2$ in the breath reflects the hydrolysis, absorption, and oxidation of ^{13}C-lactose. Decreased $^{13}CO_2$ excretion reflects malabsorption of the labelled lactose.

The test molecule, β-D-galactosyl-(1-4)-α-D-^{13}C-glucose (90% ^{13}C-enriched; MSD-Isotopes, Montreal, Canada), is administered to patients in a dose of 4 mg/kg wt, after mixing with lactose to a maximal dose of 50 g (for children 2 g/kg wt).

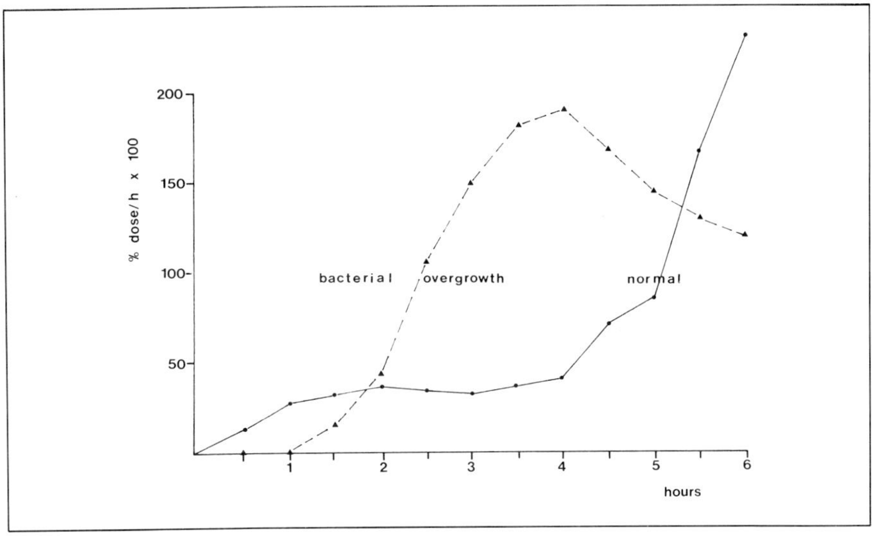

Fig. 8. In case of bacterial overgrowth there is an increase of $^{13}CO_2$-excretion (in % dose/h) around 3 h after the intake of ^{13}C-glycocholic acid.

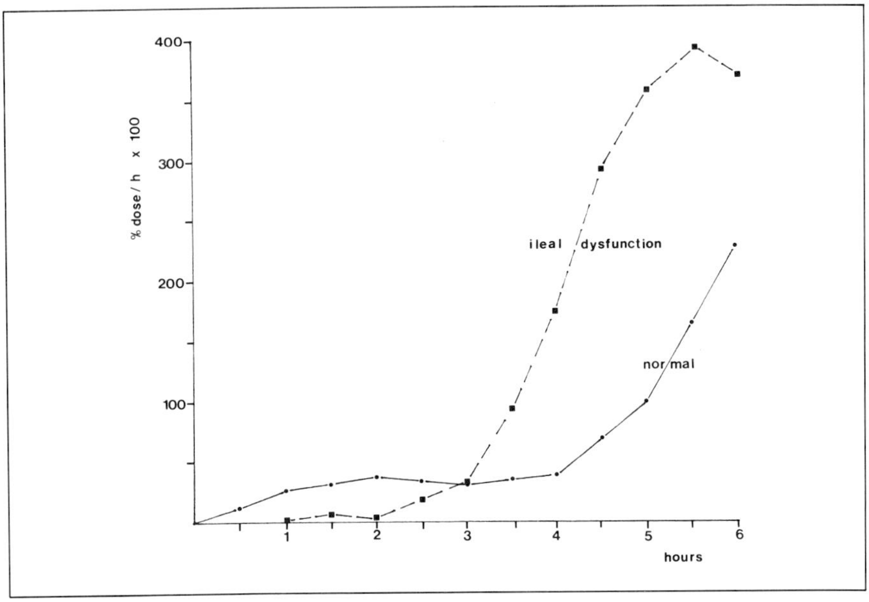

Fig. 9. In case of ileal bile acid malabsorption, the typical excretion pattern of $^{13}CO_2$-excretion (in % dose/h) shows an increase 4 h after the administration of ^{13}C-glycocholic acid.

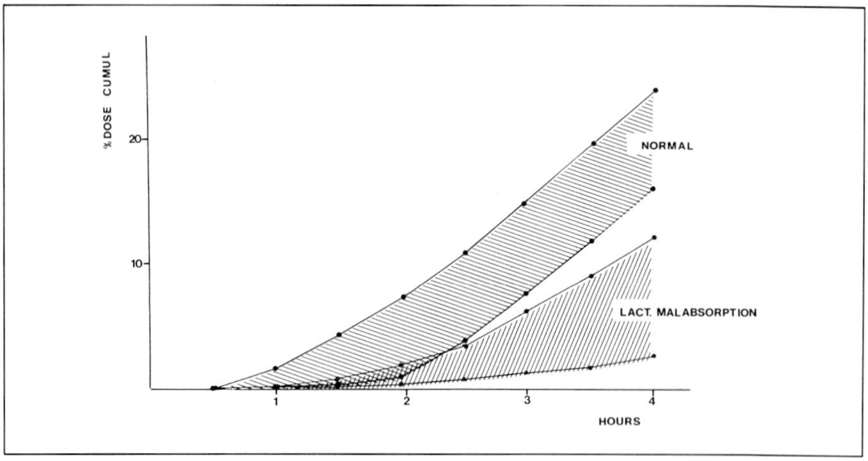

Fig. 10. $^{13}CO_2$-excretion pattern is given in cumulative values for normal men and for lactose intolerant patients.

In figure 10 the cumulative % $^{13}CO_2$ is given for normal subjects and for patients with lactose intolerance.

Lactose malabsorption can also be detected by breath hydrogen measurement after administration of a load of lactose. The lactose that enters the colon is fermented by bacterial enzymes to short chain fatty acids and H_2 (fig. 11). 2 to 17% of patients, however, do not produce hydrogen. In children hydrogen production is absent when the colonic pH decreases due to the presence of fatty acids. Moreover, breath hydrogen excretion can be falsely elevated in patients having bacterial overgrowth of the small bowel.

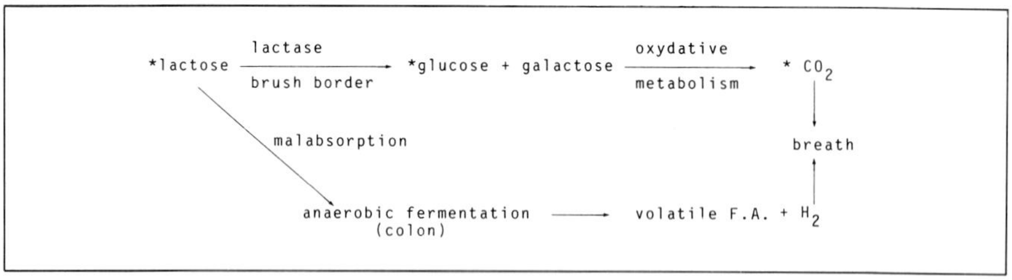

Fig. 11. Principle of $^{13}CO_2$-lactose and H_2-lactose breath test. ^{13}C-lactose, a galactose-glucose dissaccharide, is split by brush border lactase. The hexoses are absorbed and metabolized to $^{13}CO_2$. Lactose, which is not absorbed, enters the colon and is anaerobically metabolized to H_2, which is partly expired in the breath.

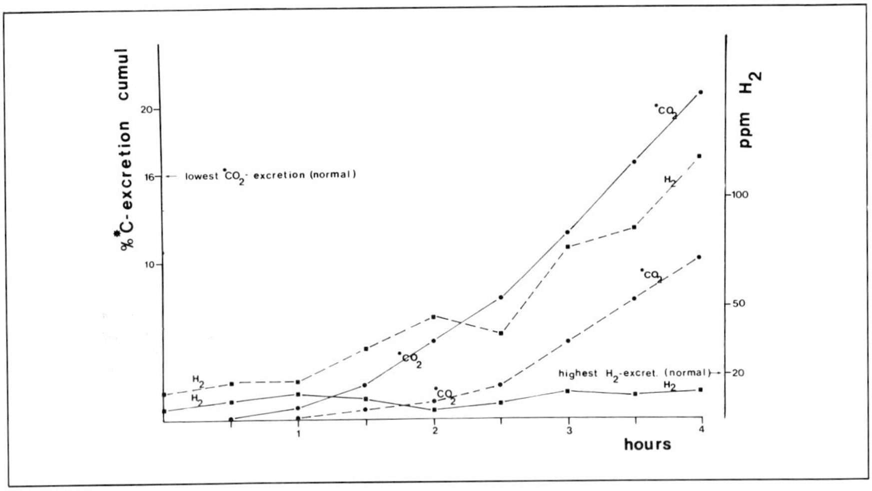

Fig. 12. The combined $^{13}CO_2$- and H_2-excretion after the intake of ^{13}C-lactose. Normals (full line) excrete high $^{13}CO_2$- and low H_2-levels, whereas lactose intolerant patient (dotted line) excrete low $^{13}CO_2$- and high H_2-levels (more than 20 ppm H_2 above background level).

We therefore combined the ^{13}C-lactose breath test with the H_2-breath test (fig. 12). The combination of these two breath tests allows us to make a diagnosis of lactose malabsorption as well as to identify conditions interfering with the normal metabolism of lactose, including bacterial overgrowth and diabetes.

Conclusions

$^{13}CO_2$-breath tests have emerged as an exciting new tool in the diagnosis of various gastrointestinal and liver diseases. Metabolic processes such as bacterial overgrowth, ileal malabsorption, lactose intolerance are more easily quantitated by $^{13}CO_2$-tests than by any other means.

Although we already disposed of $^{13}CO_2$-breath tests for the study of fat digestion, bile acid metabolism, carbohydrate digestion, and absorption and hepatic microsomal function, the search for other useful breath tests needs to be continued.

There is still a wide field open for breath test investigation. A protein breath test has been reported [35]. Labelled amino acids may be used for $^{13}CO_2$ breath test to explore their metabolism in different diseases [44, 45]. Biochemical reactions, in which a vitamin is the rate-limiting determinant, should be explored to be useful as CO_2-breath tests in the study of vitamin bioavailability.

More research is also needed when different ^{13}C-substrates already exist for the same function, as is the case for liver function [33, 46].

The development of $^{13}CO_2$-breath test can also be hampered by the fact that no ^{13}C-analog is available for the ^{14}C-substrate as shown by ^{14}C-xylose [47], which is considered as a good substrate for demonstrating small intestine epithelium integrity and for bacterial overgrowth.

Is there a future for ^{13}C-breath tests? The answer appears to be a guarded yes, as the above described tests have already proved to be very useful in the clinical diagnosis of gastrointestinal functions and diseases. The tests are simple, non-invasive, and easy to perform. The patients do not need to be hospitalized; the tests can be done in an ambulatory way. This is important because it lowers the cost of the tests. If more diagnostic centers for $^{13}CO_2$-breath tests become available, the search for naturally ^{13}C-labelled substrates is stimulated [48]. ^{13}C-substrates prices will also decrease, and central laboratory facilities circumvent the costs of isotope measurements. The use of $^{13}CO_2$-breath tests offers a unique technique for in vivo determination of kinetics of important metabolic functions, especially in infants, children, and pregnant women.

References

1 Schoenheimer, R.: The dynamic state of body constituents, pp. 13–78 (Harvard University Press, Cambridge 1942).

2 Halliday, D.; Lockhart, I.: The use of stable isotopes in medicinal chemistry; in Ellis, West, Progress in medicinal chemistry, pp. 2–86 (Elsevier Biomedical Press, Amsterdam 1978).

3 Barr, R.; Perman, J.; Schoeller, D.; Watkins, J.: Breath tests in pediatric gastrointestinal disorders: New diagnostic opportunities. Pediatrics *62:* 393–401 (1978).

4 Halliday, D.; Rennie, M.: The use of stable isotopes for diagnosis and clinical research. Clin. Sci. mol. Med. *63:* 485–496 (1982).

5 Klein, P.: Clinical applications of $^{13}CO_2$ measurements. Fed. Proc. *41:* 2698–2701 (1982).

6 Ghoos, Y.; Rutgeerts, P.; Vantrappen, G.; Habfast, K.: Atemgas-Analysen mit Stabilisotopen in der Diagnostik des Magen-Darm-Traktes. Labor Praxis *1:* 20–24 (1983).

7 Wolfe, R.: Tracers in metabolic research – Radioisotope and stable isotope/mass spectrometry methods; in Laboratory and research methods in biology and medicine, vol. 9, pp. 179–187 (Alan R. Liss, New York 1984).
8 Caspary, W.: Breath tests. Clin. Gastroenterol.: 351–374 (1978).
9 Lacroix, M.; Mosora, F.; Pontus, M.; Lefebvre, P.; Luyckx, A.; Lopez-Habib, G.: Glucose naturally labelled with carbon-13; Use for metabolic studies in man. Science *181:* 445–446 (1973).
10 Solomons, N.; Schoeller, D.; Wagonfeld, J.; Ott, D.; Rosenberg, I.; Klein, P.: Application of a stable isotope (^{13}C)-labelled glycocholate breath test to diagnosis of bacterial overgrowth and ileal dysfunction. J. Lab. clin. Med. *90:* 431–439 (1977).
11 Watkins, J.; Schoeller, D.; Klein, P.; Ott, D.; Newcomer, A.; Hofmann, A.: ^{13}C-trioctanoin: A nonradioactive breath test to detect fat malabsorption. J. Lab. clin. Med. *90:* 422–430 (1977).
12 Ghoos, Y.; Rutgeerts, P.; Vantrappen, G.: Measurement of ^{13}C-glucose oxidation rate using mass spectrometric determination of the CO_2/Ar ratio and spirometry. Biomed. Mass Spectr. (in press).
13 Rutgeerts, P.; Vantrappen, G.; Ghoos, Y.: The quantitative ^{13}C mixed triglyceride breath test is a good pancreatic function test. Gastroenterology *86:* 1227 (1984).
14 Rutgeerts, P.; Ghoos, Y.; Vantrappen, G.: Combined ^{14}C-lactose and H_2-breath test for the diagnosis of lactose malabsorption. Gastroenterology *84:* 1291 (1983).
15 Ghoos, Y.; Vantrappen, G.; Rutgeerts, P.; Schurmans, P.: A mixed-triglyceride breath test for intraluminal fat digestive activity. Digestion *22:* 239–247 (1981).
16 Watkins, J.; Klein, P.; Schoeller, D.; Kirschner, B.; Park, R.; Perman, J.: Diagnosis and differentiation of fat malabsorption in children using ^{13}C-labelled lipids: Trioctanoin, triolein and palmitic acid breath test. Gastroenterology *82:* 911–917 (1982).
17 Schoeller, D.; Klein, P.; MacLean, W.; Watkins, J.; Van Santen, E.: Fecal ^{13}C analysis for the detection and quantitation of intestinal malabsorption. J. Lab. clin. Med. *97:* 439–448 (1981).
18 Sasaki, Y.; Oh-hara, H.; Takahashi, S.; Someya, K.: ^{13}C-breath test for detection of bacterial deconjugation of bile salts: Studies using an animal model; in Klein, Klein, Stable isotopes. Proceedings of the Third International Conference, pp. 527–532 (Academic Press, New York 1979).
19 MacLean, W.; Fink, B.; Schoeller, D.; Wong, W.; Klein, P.: Lactose assimilation by full-term infants: Relation of [^{13}C] and H_2-breath tests with fecal [^{13}C] excretion. Pediatr. Res. *17:* 629–633 (1983).
20 McGill, D.: Diagnostic tests for lactase deficiency; in Delmont, Milk intolerance and rejection, pp. 35–41 (Karger, Basel 1983).
21 Rating, D.; Gryzewski, N.; Burger, W.; Jacobs, C.; Weber, B.; Helge, H.: The effect of acarbose on sucrose absorption measured by the ^{13}C-sucrose breath test; in Schmidt, Förstel, Heinzinger, Stable isotopes, pp. 359–366 (Elsevier Scientific Publ., Amsterdam 1982).
22 Pirnay, F.; Lacroix, M.; Mosora, F.; Luyckx, A.; Lefebvre, P.: Glucose oxidation during prolonged exercise evaluated with naturally labelled ^{13}C-glucose. J. appl. Physiol. *43:* 258–261 (1977).
23 Helge, H.; Gress, B.; Gregg, C.; Knies, S.; Nötges-Borgwardt, I.; Weber, B.; Neubert, D.: $^{13}CO_2$-breath test in normal and diabetic children following ingestion of ^{13}C-

glucose; in Baillie, Stable isotopes. Applications in pharmacology, toxicology and clinical research, pp. 227–239 (MacMillan Press, London 1978).

24 Ravussin, E.; Dörner, A.; Acheson, K.; Pahud, P.; Arnaud, M.; Jéquier, E.: Carbohydrate utilization in obese subjects after an oral load of 100 g naturally labelled ^{13}C-glucose. Br. J. Nutr. *43:* 281–288 (1980).

25 Wolfe, R.: Tracers in metabolic research – Radioisotope and stable isotope/mass spectrometry methods; in Laboratory and research methods in biology and medicine, vol. 9, pp. 113–130 (Alan R. Liss, New York 1984).

26 Vantrappen, G.; Rutgeerts, P.; Ghoos, Y.: Quantitative measurements of ^{13}C-glucose oxidation in patients following gastric surgery. Gastroenterology *84:* 1341 (1983).

27 Ravich, W.; Bayliss, T.; Thomas, M.: Fructose: Incomplete intestinal absorption in humans. Gastroenterology *84:* 26–29 (1983).

28 Wildgrube, H.; Stang, H.: Zur diagnostischen Relevanz des Aminopyrin-Atemtests bei Lebererkrankungen. Z. Gastroenterologie *20:* 667–672 (1982).

29 Jäger-Roman, E.; Rating, D.; Platzek, T.; Helge, H.: Development of N-demethylase activity measured with the ^{13}C-aminopyrine breath test. Pediatrics *139:* 129–134 (1982).

30 Breyer-Pfaff, U.; Harder, M.; Egberts, E.: Plasma levels of parent drug and metabolites in the intravenous aminopyrine breath test. Eur. J. clin. Pharmacol. *21:* 521–528 (1982).

31 Haustein, K.; Hüller, G.; Sensing, H.: The determination of aminopyrine elimination for control of the metabolic capacity of the liver in man. Eur. J. clin. Invest. *12:* 157–164 (1982).

32 Zahlten, R.: Letter to the Editor. Hofmann, A.: Reply. Hepatology *3:* 463–464 (1983).

33 Baker, A.; Kotake, A.; Schoeller, D.: Clinical utility of breath tests for the assessment of hepatic function. Sem. Liver Dis. *3:* 318–329 (1983).

34 Mook, W.; Grootes, P.: The measuring procedure and corrections for the high-precision mass spectrometric analysis of isotopic abundance ratios, especially referring to carbon, oxygen and nitrogen. Int. J. Mass Spectr. Ion Phys. *12:* 273–298 (1973).

35 Schoeller, D.; Klein, P.; Watkins, J.; Heim, T.; MacLean, W.: ^{13}C-abundances of nutrients and the effect of variations in ^{13}C-isotopic abundances of test meals formulated for $^{13}CO_2$-breath tests. Am. J. clin. Nutr. *33:* 2375–2385 (1980).

36 Metzler, S.; Stobbe, E.; Kranz, C.; Schmidt, H.; Winkler, F.; Wolfram, G.: Einfluß des natürlichen Isotopengehaltes von Nährstoffen auf den Untergrund bei ^{13}C-Atemtests. Z. ErnährWiss. *22:* 107–115 (1983).

37 Schoeller, D.; Brown, C.; Nakamura, K.; Kakagawa, A.; Mazzeo, R.; Brooks, G.; Budinger, T.: Influence of metabolic fuel on the $^{13}C/^{12}C$ ratio of breath CO_2. Biomed. Mass Spectr. *11:* 557–561 (1984).

38 Hatch, M.; Slack, C.: Photosynthetic CO_2-fixation pathways. Annu. Rev. Plant Physiol. *21:* 141–162 (1970).

39 Smith, B.; Epstein, S.: Two categories of $^{13}C/^{12}C$ ratios for higher plants. Plant Physiol. *47:* 380–384 (1971).

40 Fromm, H.; Hofmann, A.: Breath test for altered bile acid metabolism. Lancet *ii:* 621–625 (1971).

41 Ghoos, Y.; Rutgeerts, P.; Vantrappen, G.: A new method for quantitative CO_2 measurement in $^{13}CO_2$ breath tests. Gastroenterology *82:* 1062 (1982).
42 King, C.; Toskes, P.: Alterations of CO_2-production during nonfasting isotopic CO_2 breath tests: Concise communications. J. nucl. Med. *22:* 955–963 (1981).
43 Hellemans, J.; Joosten, E.; Ghoos, Y.; Carchon, H.; Vantrappen, G.; Pelemans, W.; Rutgeerts, P.: Positive $^{14}CO_2$ bile acid breath test in elderly people. Age Ageing *13:* 138–143 (1984).
44 Read, W.; Read, M.; Rennie, M.; Griggs, R.; Halliday, D.: Preparation of CO_2 from blood and protein-bound amino acid carboxyl groups for quantification and ^{13}C-isotope measurements. Biomed. Mass Spectr. *11:* 348–352 (1984).
45 Wolfe, R.: Tracers in metabolic research – Radioisotope and stable isotope mass spectrometry methods; in Laboratory and Research Methods in Biology and Medicine, vol. 9, pp. 151–173 (Alan R. Liss, New York 1984).
46 Schneider, J.; Schoeller, D.; Schreider, B.; Kotake, A.; Hachey, D.; Klein, P.: Use of ^{13}C-phenacetin and ^{13}C-methacetin for the detection of alterations in hepatic drug metabolism; in Klein, Klein, Stable isotopes. Proceedings of the Third International Conference, pp. 507–516 (Academic Press, New York 1979).
47 King, E.; Toskes, P.; Guilarte, T.; Lorentz, E.; Welkos, S.: Comparison of the one-gram d (^{14}C) xylose breath test to the (^{14}C) bile acid breath test in patients with small-intestine bacterial overgrowth. Dig. Dis. *25:* 53–58 (1980).
48 Jung, G.; Jüttner, F.: Herstellung stabil markierter (^{15}N, ^{13}C, ^{2}H) Naturstoffe mit Hilfe autotropher Algenkulturen und neue Anwendungen stabiler Isotope in den Biowissenschaften. Chem. Zeit. *96:* 603–611 (1972).

Dr. Y. Ghoos, Labo Gastrointestinale Fysiopathologie, U. Z. St. Rafaël-Gasthuisberg, Herestraat, 49, B-3000 Leuven (Belgium)

Dietze, Grünert, Kleinberger, Wolfram (eds.), Clinical Nutrition and Metabolic Research. Proc. 7th Congr. ESPEN, Munich 1985, pp. 208–222 (Karger, Basel 1986)

Amino Acid and Substrate Turnover in Man Using GCMS

D. E. Matthews

Dept. of Medicine, Washington University School of Medicine, St. Louis, Mo., USA

Introduction

Although both radioactive and stable isotopes have been used since the 1930s to study in vivo metabolism, the advent of gas chromatography-mass spectrometry (GCMS) as a biomedical tool introduced many new applications in the 1970s for stable isotopes as metabolic tracers. During the past decade, research dealing with GCMS and stable isotopes has greatly expanded beyond a few centers to the point where GCMS facilities are available at almost every major university. In this paper I would like to discuss first the strengths and weaknesses of GCMS before discussing its applications. Too many important metabolic studies using stable isotopes and GCMS have been reported by too many laboratories to mention more than a few here, and the interested reader is referred to other reviews of the stable isotope tracer field which discuss in more detail the full range of applications and research [1, 2, 13, 22].

Why Use GCMS?

GCMS measures isotopic enrichment in a complementary fashion to conventional isotope ratio mass spectrometry (IRMS) [1, 22]. The primary strengths of GCMS are sensitivity and selectivity. Typically if a nmole to a few pmoles of a metabolite are available, an isotopic enrichment can be determined by GCMS; in contrast, IRMS requires μmol amounts of compound which can be readily isolated and converted to CO_2

or N_2. GCMS provides selectivity both from the temporal, chromatographic resolution of components by the gas chromatograph and from the generation of ions in the mass spectrometer, uniquely relating each compound to its molecular weight and fragmentation pattern. Furthermore, several different ionization modes (electron impact ionization, chemical ionization, and both positive and negative ion generation) have been developed for the mass spectrometer which can often be used to provide information specific to a given atom in a molecule. For example, different ionization modes have been used to distinguish [^{15}N]leucine from [1-^{13}C]leucine (two tracers with identical mass), and thereby simultaneously determine leucine transamination rates (via the ^{15}N tracer) and α-ketoisocaproate (KIC) decarboxylation rates (via the ^{13}C tracer) in man [17, 19, 26].

Because most biological molecules are too polar to pass through the gas chromatograph directly, they must be first chemically modified ('derivatized') to block the polar groups. Fortunately, most of the chemical reactions have been worked out for rapid micro-scale derivatization of entire lots of samples using prepackaged commercial reagents and micro-sample vials [16]. What would appear to be a nuisance – the derivative preparation step – can often be an additional step for adding selectivity to the GCMS assay. For many different classes of compounds, derivatives specific to them are available [16]. Thus, other interfering compounds can often be removed by judicious choice of derivative type.

Although GCMS is far more selective and sensitive to the compound being measured when compared to IRMS, GCMS is much less sensitive to measuring the tracer. GCMS can typically measure one labeled molecule in the presence of 1000 unlabeled molecules, whereas IRMS, designed for isotope sensitivity, can distinguish one labeled atom in 10^6. Note that GCMS measures molecules or large fragments thereof, but IRMS measures essentially atoms. Stable isotopes by their very nature are naturally occurring, so that when a stable isotope tracer is added to a biological system, we are measuring the tracer 'in excess' of the natural abundance 'background' stable isotopes [2, 22]. This measured enrichment is usually expressed in percent enrichment above natural abundance as 'atom % excess' or 'mole % excess' (the latter term evolves from GCMS applications). Thus, GCMS sensitivity for tracer enrichment is about 0.1 mole % excess, while IRMS can measure ca. 0.0001 atom % excess tracer.

Which technique, GCMS or IRMS, is most appropriate in stable isotope tracer studies of human metabolism? Both are necessary [2, 18].

Figure 1 illustrates the situation for administration of a labeled amino acid. When a ^{15}N or ^{13}C labeled amino acid is infused intravenously, the labeled amino acid is diluted in the blood with the unlabeled amino acids entering the free amino acid pool from protein breakdown and dietary intake. Conversely, amino acids are removed from the pool for protein synthesis and oxidation to the end products, CO_2 and urea. With infusion of tracer, the enrichment of the infused amino acid rises to plateau (isotopic steady state) in blood. The flux (or 'turnover') of the amino acid being studied is simply calculated from the tracer infusion rate divided by the amino acid tracer enrichment in blood. To keep the labeled amino acid a 'tracer' it must be infused slowly compared to amino acid turnover. Although there are no hard definitions, a tracer dose is generally considered an infusion rate less than 10% of the flux. Because GCMS will optimally measure a 2–5 mole % excess enrichment, the infusion rate is usually set to produce this level of enrichment.

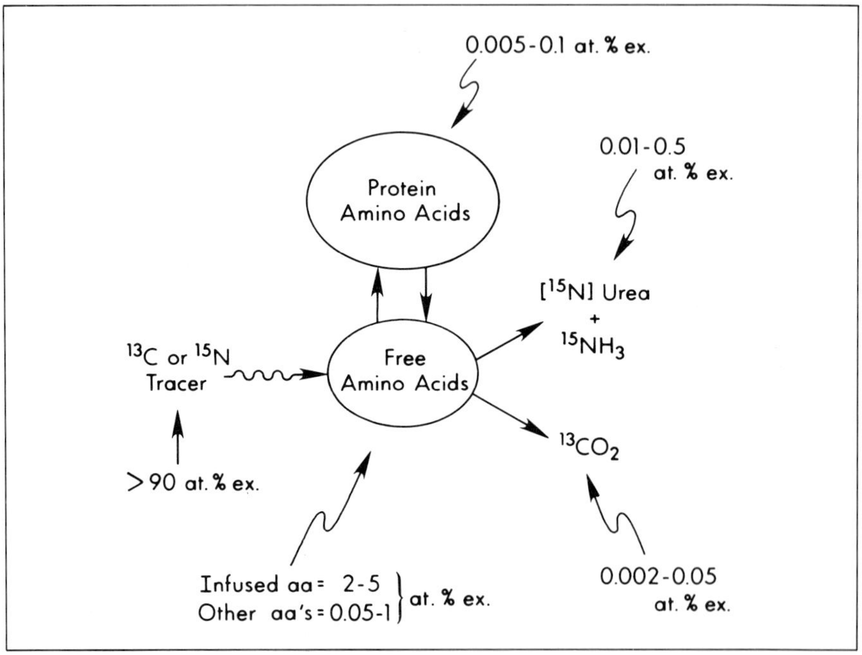

Fig. 1. Typical dilutions of an amino acid stable isotope tracer infused intravenously. The labeled amino acid is infused into the blood at a slow rate to produce only 'tracer' level of enrichment. From here the tracer undergoes several of further levels of dilution.

If label is transferred to other compounds (e.g., amino acid transamination), the label will be diluted, but usually at an enrichment level which can still be measured by GCMS. Important kinetic information about precursor-product relationships, e.g., what fraction of glucose production comes from alanine [10], can be obtained from measuring the transfer of label to other compounds.

Amino acid oxidization sends the label into a pathway of high throughput: urea production for a ^{15}N label and CO_2 production for a ^{13}C label resulting in 100–1000 fold dilutions (fig. 1). Incorporation of labeled amino acid into most proteins is slow compared to the duration of the tracer infusion, resulting in a very low enrichment in most protein amino acids. Both of these pathways result in tracer dilutions far too severe for measurement by GCMS. Thus, IRMS is generally required for measurement of tracer in either metabolic end products or in proteins [24].

Why Choose a Stable Isotope Tracer instead of a Radiotracer?

The development of the modern scintillation counter made the radioactive isotopes very easy to use, but ethical considerations greatly limit radiotracer use with human subjects. The importance of stable isotopes to study children and infants [8, 10, 22] is obvious. However, table I presents, comparing ^{13}C and ^{14}C leucine tracers, more subtle differences that are not usually considered. For example, stereoisomer impurities, which are often overlooked or are difficult to work around with radioisotopes, are easily determined for stable isotopes using chiral gas chromatographic columns. With the present availability of stable isotopes, 'grams' of stable isotopically labeled compounds rarely cost more than the comparable amount of radioisotope by the μCurie. By adding deuterated internal standards to blood samples at collection, GCMS can be used to quantitate substrate levels simultaneously with determination of isotopic enrichment [6, 20, 22], and the GCMS quantitation is often more precise and interference free than can be obtained with conventional methods [4, 20]. Finally, without a dose limit for stable isotopes, the same subjects can be studied serially on separate days with multiple tracer infusions per study.

Not mentioned in table I is a major drawback for GCMS: its limited ability to measure isotopic dilution. The bounds of GCMS measurement

Table I. ^{13}C vs. ^{14}C: Comparison of whole body leucine kinetics in man

	Tracer	
	L-[1-^{13}C]leucine	L-[1-^{14}C]leucine
Detect D-isomer contamination?	yes	difficult
Subject population that can be studied:		
> 40 years old	yes	yes
20–40 years old	yes	sometimes
Children	yes	no
Infants	yes	no
Isotope dose for 70 kg adult:	200 mg	50 μCi
Cost of isotope for a single infusion:	$50	$100
Number of infusions per subject:	numerous	1–2 limit
Number of tracers per infusion:	numerous	1–2 limit
Blood sample size:	0.2	> 2.0
Sample analysis time (min):		
^{13}C or ^{14}C	10	30
Leucine concentration	0	30
N kinetics?	yes, with ^{15}N	no

are the GCMS detection limit (ca. 0.1 mole % excess) at the low end and the maximum enrichment allowed that would be considered a tracer dose (ca. 10 mole % excess) at the high end. Thus, the dynamic range for GCMS measurement of stable isotopes as tracers is 100-fold or less. Figure 2 illustrates this situation both for a primed, infusion study and for a pulse-dose study. The infusion rate can be selected for optimal GCMS precision with the primed, infusion study, but with pulse-dose studies GCMS is extremely limited in following the tracer through more than one pool and one exponential disappearance parameter. For pulse-dose studies, ^{14}C is still superior to ^{13}C and GCMS.

GCMS to Measure Urea Production

Since the original study of human lysine turnover using a 30-h infusion of ^{14}C-lysine in 1967 [27], fluxes of individual amino acids have been determined primarily by the stochastic approach with the single amino acid pool model of Waterlow [28]. In contrast to radiotracer work, most of

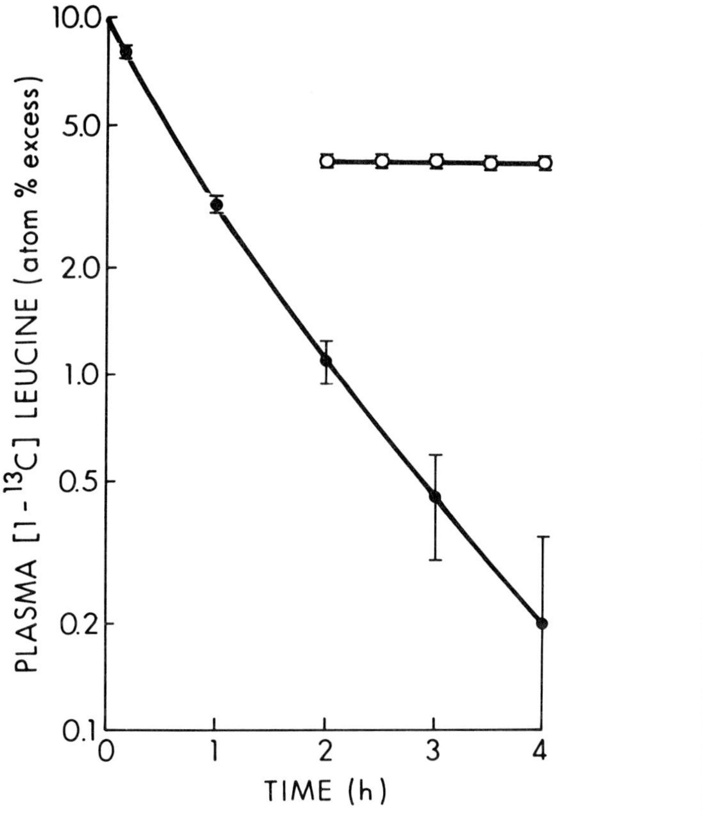

Fig. 2. GCMS measurement precision of a [1-^{13}C]leucine label in blood for a hypothetical single tracer dose (closed circles) or a primed infusion (open circles). Error bars represent typical standard error of measurement indicating the limited dynamic range of GCMS (Y-axis is logarithmic) in the 'tracer dose' range. With the primed infusion, the infusion rate can be set for optimal enrichment measurement, and the priming dose chosen to provide rapid attainment of isotopic steady state. See figure 3 for an exception to this rule.

the stable isotope tracer studies using GCMS have been infusion studies with priming doses. The priming dose can greatly shorten the time required to reach isotopic steady state ('plateau') in both the primary pool (the plasma amino acid) and secondary pools (e.g., breath CO_2) [22]. For example, we demonstrated that a primed infusion of [1-^{13}C]leucine can be completed in less than 4 h [18], and Wolfe and coworkers have reduced this infusion time to 2 h or less [9, 30].

There is a limit as to how short the infusion period can be, which is set by the kinetics of the system being studied, not by the GCMS measurement system. Surprisingly, this simple point can be overlooked. Measurement of urea production in man is a good example. The fractional turnover of urea in man is slow (ca. 8% d^{-1}), and without a priming dose almost 60 h of tracer infusion are required to reach an isotopic plateau in urea [23]. This infusion time frame presents no advantage over simple measurement of urinary urea excretion. However, a primed infusion approach using GCMS was reported measuring urea production in humans in less than 2 h [9, 30]. When we tried to duplicate this method, we noticed that the reported optimal priming dose of urea was about half of what we would have calculated based on the body urea pool size, and that different values for urea production rate could be obtained depending upon the priming dose chosen. Figure 3 illustrates the problem for two

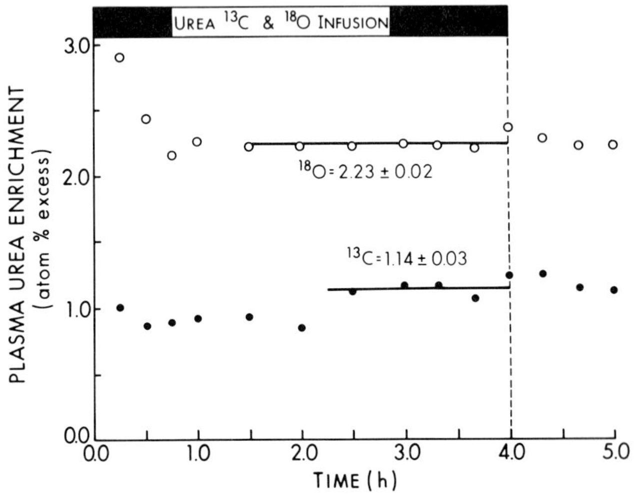

Fig. 3. Plasma urea enrichment during a primed 4-h infusion of [^{18}O]urea administered at a normal priming dose and [^{13}C]urea administered at a low priming dose. The infusion rates were identical for both tracers. The subject was an overnight-fasted healthy young man. Plasma [^{13}C]urea enrichments (closed circles) were almost half the [^{18}O]urea enrichments (open circles). This figure was reproduced from [23].

urea tracers which were infused at the same rate and should have given identical plasma enrichments. The only difference between the tracer infusions was the priming dose administered. The remarkable difference in the apparent enrichment plateaus (fig. 3) was, therefore, attributed to the two different priming dose sizes. Additional studies demonstrated that body urea is effectively divided between two nearly equal compartments, the second compartment probably being a slow mixing pool [23]. Administering a priming dose large enough for this entire system gives an initial appearance of overpriming (the open circles in figure 3) until the tracer distributes into both pools, whereas the lower priming dose initially appears appropriate because it just primes the sample compartment, but not the whole system (causing the falsely low plateau). The false plateau would have been recognized had the urea tracer infusion been continued. This problem demonstrates the failing of a primed infusion protocol performed more rapidly than the system being studied can respond. Urea metabolism can be determined by GCMS in a relatively short period, but using a single dose of labeled urea, rather than a primed infusion [23].

Measurement of urea production was presented as a 'worst case' examples for GCMS methodology to illustrate limitations that are often overlooked when expensive technology is applied. Most of the compounds important to energy and protein metabolism are readily studied with short duration infusion studies and GCMS. Three examples are glucose, palmitate, and leucine [11, 22, 29]. Since glucose exists as free glucose only in the extracellular space (intracellular glucose is phosphorylated or in glycogen), the infused glucose tracer mixes rapidly and completely with the unlabeled glucose tracee, such that minute by minute changes can be followed. Similarly rapid changes in fatty acid transport can be followed with a labeled palmitate infusion [11, 22, 29]. Leucine differs from the first two examples because it distributes throughout the intracellular pools as free leucine resulting in a variety of small intracellular/extracellular gradients. However, using a single leucine pool model, extensive leucine kinetics studies in man have been completed using leucine tracer infusions [1, 2, 8, 13, 14, 18, 19, 21, 22, 24–26, 28–31]. Intracellular-extracellular mixing of the leucine tracer has not been a significant problem since leucine is not concentrated within cells and mixes rapidly under most conditions [21]. In all three examples presented, both stable and radioisotopes have been used and the only reasons for choosing GCMS and stable isotopes are the points outlined in table I.

Glutamine and Glutamate Metabolism

Nonessential amino acids are not unimportant amino acids. Two excellent examples are glutamine and glutamate. Glutamate is the focal point amino acid for amino acid transamination in the body, and glutamine is the primary carrier of N from skeletal muscle. Both amino acids are highly concentrated within cells. Yet we know very little about the N kinetics of these amino acids in man. One study prior to 1984 has reported glutamine amide-N turnover in man [12]. The principal limitations to study of glutamine and glutamate kinetics has simply been methodological difficulties for both IRMS and GCMS. We recently devised and tested a scheme to permit isolation and measurement of glutamine separately from glutamate by GCMS [6]. This scheme includes the addition of deuterated glutamine and glutamate internal standards to the blood samples immediately upon collection. Because the deuterated glutamine and glutamate used have different masses from both the ^{15}N-labelled and unlabelled species, they can be measured simultaneously by GCMS when the glutamine or glutamate ^{15}N enrichments are determined. The deuterated internal standards also include correction for any glutamine degradation to glutamate during sample handling and storage [6].

Our first studies of glutamine and glutamate kinetics in man [7] used unprimed infusions of glutamine and glutamate ^{15}N tracers, because both amino acids have large intracellular pools and are likely to be compartmentalized within the body. The rate of rise to plateau in an unprimed infusion gives the same kinetic information that would be obtained from following tracer disappearance after administration of a single tracer dose. This point is often overlooked, but it is extremely useful with GCMS since it is difficult to follow tracer disappearance beyond a decade or two of dilution (fig. 2). With the unprimed infusion, the turnover is determined from the plateau, while rate constants and pool sizes are estimated from the rate of tracer enrichment rise to plateau.

The time courses of plasma glutamate ^{15}N and glutamine amino-^{15}N during separate infusions of the L-[^{15}N]glutamate and L-[2-^{15}N]glutamine tracers in young adult men are shown in figure 4. The ^{15}N enrichments rose rapidly to plateau in ca. 90 min for both amino acids. The fractional turnover rates of glutamine and glutamate were 170 and 480% h^{-1}, respectively. Considering the very large free glutamine and glutamate intracellular levels [3], these fractional turnover rates are remarkably fast: the tracer-miscible glutamate and glutamine pools were less 1 and 4%, respectively, the size of the estimated free pools. Thus, both amino acids are strongly compartmentalized between extracellular and intracellular matrices. Another demonstration that the [^{15}N]glutamate tracer mixes slowly with intracellular glutamate is the low level of ^{15}N enrichment appearing in plasma glutamine during the glutamate ^{15}N infusion (fig. 4). Because plasma glutamine is produced intracellularly from glutamate, its enrichment should reflect intracellular glutamate enrichment, and that enrichment was very low even after 4 h of glutamate ^{15}N infusion (ca. 5% that of the plasma glutamate enrichment).

The glutamate and glutamine amino-N fluxes measured from the respective ^{15}N plateau enrichments in figure 4 were 83 and 348 μmol $kg^{-1}h^{-1}$, respectively. These values are compared in table II with other amino acid fluxes measured under the similar conditions (healthy male subjects consuming a maintenance energy diet with > 0.8 g $kg^{-1}d^{-1}$ protein and infused in the postabsorptive state). The fluxes of the essential amino acids reflect a single inflow of amino acid from protein breakdown. Thus, it is not surprising that the different essential amino acid flux values are proportional to each amino acid's abundance in body protein, i.e.,

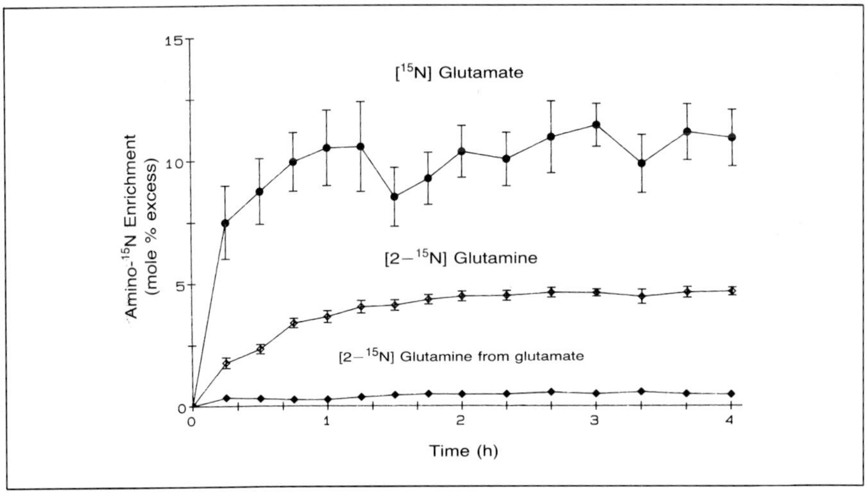

Fig. 4. Time course of plasma glutamate and glutamine amino-^{15}N enrichments during unprimed infusions of L-[^{15}N]glutamate or L-[2-^{15}N]glutamine. Five healthy young adult men were infused in the postabsorptive state. The closed circles are plasma glutamate ^{15}N, and the closed diamonds are plasma glutamine amino-^{15}N, both during infusion of [^{15}N]glutamate. The open diamonds are plasma glutamine amino-^{15}N during infusion of [2-^{15}N]glutamine. The error bars are ± 1 SE. The data are from [7].

Table II. Comparison of amino acid fluxes in healthy young adult men studied postabsorptively

Amino acid	Literature reference	Amino acid flux* (μmol $kg^{-1}h^{-1}$)
Glutamine amino-N	[7]	348
Glutamate N	[7]	83
Alanine N	[31]	256
Glycine N	[25]	240
Leucine	[24, 26, 31]	93
Valine	[26]	80
Lysine	[24]	78
Tyrosine	[5]	40
Phenylalanine	[5]	36

* Studies from the literature were chosen where subjects ate a standard weight-maintaining diet containing > 0.8 g $kg^{-1}d^{-1}$ of protein and were infused in the postabsorptive state. The four nonessential amino acid fluxes were determined for the amino-N; the five essential amino acid fluxes are for the carbon skeleton.

tyrosine and phenylalanine are half as abundant in protein as leucine or valine, and have flux rates which are also about half. The nonessential amino acid fluxes reflect a second inflow component: de novo synthesis, as shown by the higher glutamine, alanine, and glycine fluxes. For these amino acids, de novo synthesis is predominant. The obvious exception is the glutamate which appears to have very little de novo synthesis. Because glutamate is strongly compartmentalized between extracellular and intracellular spaces, the glutamate 'flux' reflects only glutamate appearance into plasma. Much of the glutamate metabolism in cells is missed when the glutamate tracer is infused into and sampled from the blood. Although the same is true of glutamine, glutamine's role in the body is largely interorgan transport, which the intravenously infused glutamine tracer will follow.

Study of Splanchnic Metabolism

The glutamine and glutamate tracer data emphasize the inherent limitations of both administering and sampling the tracer from the same compartment: blood. Some intracellular events are not observed. There are two schemes to address this problem. The first scheme follows intracellular events using an extracellular metabolite created in the cell from the infused tracer. Measurement of plasma glutamine ^{15}N during infusion of [^{15}N]glutamate is one example. Another example is assessment of intracellular leucine enrichment from the plasma KIC enrichment during infusion of labeled leucine [21].

The second scheme administers two tracers, one directly to the target organ and another to systemic circulation. This approach is ideal for studying splanchnic bed metabolism. One tracer is infused intravenously and the other is infused by an intragastric route. Any sequestration of intragastric tracer by the splanchnic bed will result in less tracer reaching the systemic circulation. For example, when subjects received L-[1-^{13}C]leucine intragastric and L-[5,5,5-$^{2}H_3$]leucine intravenous infusions in the postabsorptive state, a ca. 20% lower plasma enrichment was observed with the intragastric tracer versus the intravenous tracer [13]. This means that 20% of intragastric-administered leucine was sequestered (either oxidized or incorporated into protein) by the splanchnic bed before it could enter the systemic circulation. When subjects were also fed enterally, the portion of leucine sequestered by the splanchnic bed on the first pass rose to 30% [13]. These results demonstrate that leucine does not pass through the splanchnic bed untouched and that intragastric tracer administration is important in studying enterally fed subjects.

In feeding studies the labeled amino acid does not have to be administered as a 'tracer' dose. That is, the labeled amino acid or protein can be the 'meal'. This raises the upper limit of GCMS enrichment measurement, making single-dose studies practical. Because GCMS blood sample size requirements are very small, as many blood samples as are required to characterize the kinetics of the meal can be taken.

Digestion and absorption of nutrients using stable isotopically labeled compounds can be studied, either as individual components (e.g., free amino acids) or complex structures (e.g., entire labeled proteins). An example of this approach is presented in figure 5 from the Ph.D. thesis work of Robert Hoerr [15]. On one day a young healthy male adult was given an oral dose of L-[1-^{13}C]leucine in solution, and timed blood samples were collected for 3 h. On another day the subject was given an oral dose of uniformly labeled (> 90 atom % ^{15}N) protein harvested from yeast, and timed blood samples were obtained. Tracer enrichment was detectable in the blood within 5 min, the first sampling point, for both the free leucine and leucine from the yeast protein. The peak enrichment occurred by 30 min for both free leucine and leucine from yeast protein. The onset of protein hydrolysis occurred so rapidly that absorption was

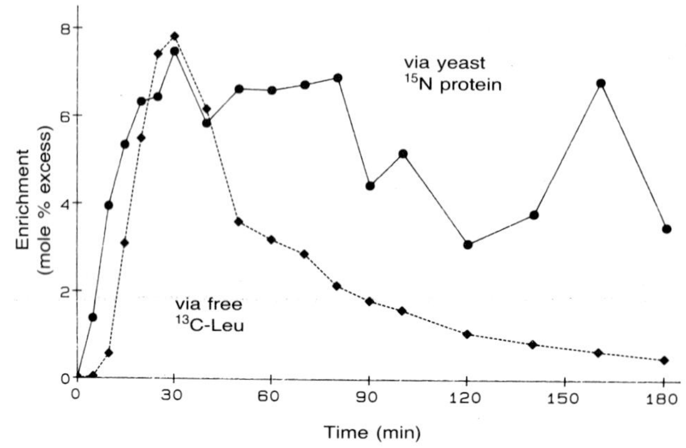

Fig. 5. Time course of plasma leucine enrichment following either an oral dose of L-[1-^{13}C]leucine or ^{15}N-labelled protein in a young male adult. The diamonds and dotted line are the plasma [1-^{13}]leucine enrichments following a single 0.4 g dose of [1-^{13}C]leucine. The circles and solid line are the mean ^{15}N branched-chain amino acid enrichments following a single 7 g dose of ^{15}N-labeled yeast protein. Data are from [15].

initially rate limiting, not digestion. The free leucine dose was almost completely absorbed by 30 min as noted by the exponentially declining disappearance curve after 30 min while the branched-chain amino acid ^{15}N enrichment from the yeast protein remained elevated for ca. 90 min before a decline began. The peak in ^{15}N enrichment at 160 min appeared to be a second round of digestion. The time course for the ^{15}N enrichments of the other amino acids were also measured by GCMS [15]. Although the absolute enrichment levels varied, the enrichment pattern for the different amino acids, essential and nonessential, were nearly identical. This one simple experiment illustrates how a wealth of information concerning digestion and absorption of amino acids and protein can be obtained using GCMS and stable isotopes.

References

1 Bier, D. M.: Stable isotope methods for nutritional diagnosis and research. Nutr. Rev. *40:* 129–134 (1982).

2 Bier, D. M.; Matthews, D. E.: Stable isotope tracer methods for in vivo investigations. Fed. Proc. *41:* 2679–2685 (1982).

3 Bergstrom, J.; Furst, P.; Noree, L.-O.; Vinnars, E.: Intracellular free amino acid concentration in human muscle tissue. J. appl. Physiol. *36:* 693–697 (1974).

4 Bjorkhem, I.; Blomstrand, R.; Lantto, O.; Svensson, L.; Ohman, G.: Toward absolute methods in clinical chemistry: Application of mass fragmentography to high-accuracy analyses. Clin. Chem. *22:* 1789–1801 (1976).

5 Clarke, J. R. T.; Bier, D. M.: The conversion of phenylalanine to tyrosine in man. Direct measurement by continuous intravenous tracer infusions of L-[ring-$^{2}H_5$]phenylalanine and L-[1-^{13}C]tyrosine in the postabsorptive state. Metabolism *3:* 999–1005 (1982).

6 Darmaun, D.; Manary, M. J.; Matthews, D. E.: A method for measuring both glutamine and glutamate levels and stable isotopic enrichments. Analyt. Biochem. *147:* 92–102 (1985).

7 Darmaun, D.; Matthews, D. E.; Bier, D. M.: Glutamine and glutamate nitrogen metabolism in man. Am. J. clin. Nutr. *39:* 655 (1984).

8 De Benoist, B.; Abdulrazzak, Y.; Brooke, O. G.; Halliday, D.; Millward, D. J.: The measurement of whole body protein turnover in the preterm infant with intragastric infusion of L-[1-^{13}C]leucine and sampling of the urinary leucine pool. Clin. Sci. mol. Med. *66:* 155–164 (1984).

9 Dietz, W. H., Jr.; Wolfe, M. H.; Wolfe, R. R.: A method for the rapid determination of protein turnover. Metabolism *31:* 749–754 (1982).

10 Frazer, T. E.; Karl, I. E.; Hillman, L. S.; Bier, D. M.: Direct measurement of gluconeogenesis from [2,3-$^{13}C_2$]alanine in the human neonate. Am. J. Physiol. *240:* E615–E621 (1981).

11 Galster, A. D.; Clutter, W. E.; Cryer, P. E.; Collins, J. A.; Bier, D. M.: Epinephrine plasma thresholds for lipolytic effects in man: Measurements of fatty acid transport with [1-^{13}C]palmitic acid. J. clin. Invest. *67:* 1729–1738 (1981).

12 Golden, M. H. N.; Jahoor, P.; Jackson, A. A.: Glutamine production rate and its contribution to urinary ammonia in normal man. Clin. Sci. mol. Med. *62:* 299–305 (1982).

13 Halliday, D.; Rennie, M. J.: The use of stable isotopes for diagnosis and clinical research. Clin. Sci. mol. Med. *63:* 485–496 (1982).

14 Hoerr, R. A.; Matthews, D. E.; Bier, D. M.; Blackburn, G. L.; Young, V. R.: Splanchnic bed metabolism of leucine in man measured by simultaneous intravenous and intragastric infusion of stable isotope tracers of leucine. Am. J. clin. Nutr. *39:* 687 (1984).

15 Hoerr, R. A.: Gut and liver contributions to whole body leucine metabolism in man: A stable isotope tracer approach; PhD diss. Mass. Inst. Tech., Cambridge, Mass. (1986).

16 Knapp. D. R.: Handbook of analytical derivatization reactions (John Wiley, New York 1979).

17 Matthews, D. E.; Ben-Galim, E.; Bier, D. M.: Determination of stable isotopic enrichment in individual plasma amino acids by chemical ionization mass spectrometry. Analyt. Chem. *51:* 80–84 (1979).

18 Matthews, D. E.; Motil, K. J.; Rohrbaugh, D. K.; Burke, J. F.; Young, V. R.; Bier, D. M.: Measurement of leucine metabolism in man from a primed, continuous infusion of L-[1-^{13}C]leucine. Am. J. Physiol. *238:* E473–E479 (1980).

19 Matthews, D. E.; Bier, D. M.; Rennie, M. J.; Edwards, R. H. T.; Halliday, D.; Mill-

ward, D. J.; Clugston, G. A.: Regulation of leucine metabolism in man: A stable isotope study. Science *214:* 1129–1131 (1981).

20 Matthews, D. E.; Starren, J. B.; Drexler, A. J.; Kipnis, D. M.; Bier, D. M.: Picomole assay for N-methylhistidine by gas chromatography-mass spectrometry. Analyt. Biochem. *110:* 308–317 (1981).

21 Matthews, D. E.; Schwarz, H. P.; Yang, R. D.; Motil, K. J.; Young, V. R.; Bier, D. M.: Relationship of plasma leucine and α-ketoisocaproate during a L-[1-^{13}C]leucine infusion in man: A method for measuring human intracellular leucine tracer enrichment. Metabolism *31:* 1105–1112 (1982).

22 Matthews, D. E.; Bier, D. M.: Stable isotope methods for nutritional investigation. Annu. Rev. Nutr. *3:* 309–339 (1983).

23 Matthews, D. E.; Downey, R. S.: Measurement of urea kinetics in humans: A validation of stable isotope tracer methods. Am. J. Physiol. *246:* E519–E527 (1984).

24 Rennie, M. J.; Halliday, D.: The use of stable isotope tracers as metabolic probes of whole-body and limb metabolism. Proc. Nutr. Soc. *43:* 189–196 (1984).

25 Robert, J.-J.; Bier, D. M.; Zhao, X. H.; Matthews, D. E.; Young, V. E.: Glucose and insulin effects on de novo amino acid synthesis in young men: Studies with stable isotope labelled alanine, glycine, leucine, and lysine. Metabolism *31:* 1210–1218 (1982).

26 Staten, M. A.; Bier, D. M.; Matthews, D. E.: Regulation of valine metabolism in man: A stable isotope study. Am. J. clin. Nutr. *40:* 1224–1234 (1984).

27 Waterlow, J. C.: Lysine turnover in man measured by intravenous infusion of L-[U-^{14}C]lysine. Clin. Sci. *33:* 507-515 (1967).

28 Waterlow, J. C.; Garlick, P. J.; Millward, D. J.: Protein turnover in mammalian tissues and in the whole body (North-Holland, Amsterdam 1978).

29 Wolfe, R. R.: Stable isotope approaches for study of energy substrate metabolism. Fed. Proc. *41:* 2692–2697 (1982).

30 Wolfe, R. R.; Goodenough, R. D.; Wolfe, M. H.; Royle, G. T.; Nadel, E. R.: Isotopic analysis of leucine and urea metabolism in exercising humans. J. appl. Physiol. *52:* 458–466 (1982).

31 Yang, R. D.; Matthews, D. E.; Bier, D. M.; Wen, Z. M.; Young, V. R.: Response of alanine metabolism in humans to manipualtion of dietary protein and energy intakes. Am. J. Physiol. (in press).

D. E. Matthews, Ph.D., Metabolism Division, Washington University School of Medicine, 660 S. Euclid Avenue, St. Louis, MO 63110 (USA)

Dietze, Grünert, Kleinberger, Wolfram (eds.), Clinical Nutrition and Metabolic Research. Proc. 7th Congr. ESPEN, Munich 1985, pp. 223–235 (Karger, Basel 1986)

Protein Turnover after Operation

W. Hartig[a], *R. Matkowitz*[a], *H.-D. Czarnetzki*[b], *Ch. Metzner*[a], *R. Ritter*[a], *K. Jung*[c], *H. Faust*[c], *P. Junghans*[c]

[a] Surgical Clinic, Postgraduate Education Clinic, District Hospital St. Georg, Leipzig
[b] Surgical Clinic, District Hospital Rostock-Süd
[c] Central Institute of Isotope and Radiation Research, Academy of Sciences of GDR, Leipzig, GDR

Today we have effective and developed methods to take care of the postoperative or posttraumatic metabolism, based on a fairly good knowledge, for instance to prepare a patient for an extended operation and to support his postoperative course. On the basis of results obtained by our research in the last years we are now able to give a summary on postoperative protein metabolism.

1st Study

An elevated breakdown of body protein is a characteristic feature of postaggression metabolism. This could be demonstrated in rats, operated and nonoperated (fig. 1). These animals received twice a day for 5 days by tube an amino acid solution, labelled with ^{15}N-glycine as tracer. We measured excretion of total N and ^{15}N in urine. Using a mathematical model we could calculate breakdown of body protein of both groups of animals. Thereby we found a breakdown of 245 mg protein-N/day for operated rats and of 171 mg N/day for nonoperated animals.

It could be shown that skeletal muscle represents the main source for increased protein catabolism. Evidence for that is the 3-methyl-histidine elimination [2] though skeletal muscle is not the only source for 3-methylhistidine excretion.

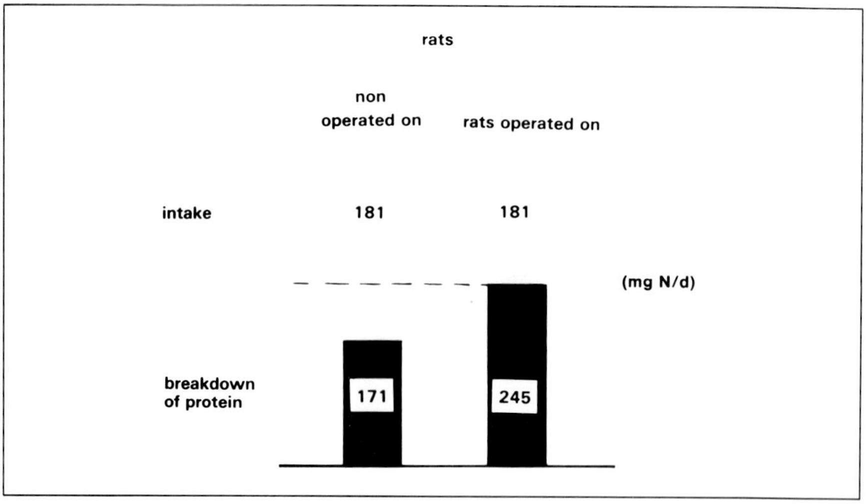

Fig. 1. Breakdown of protein (mg N/day) in nonoperated and operated rats fed with the same nutritional regimen [7, 8].

2nd Study

The more severe the trauma, the more pronounced is the loss of protein. This could be demonstrated in 3 groups of patients: patients without trauma, for instance patients before repair of an inguinal hernia; then patients after moderate, and patients after severe trauma. The differences are remarkable (fig. 2). Due to the fact that all patients were fasting, we can conclude: the higher the intensity of injury, the more intensive is the breakdown of body protein.

As we have seen, breakdown concerns preferably muscle protein. Amino acids arising from muscle enlarge the non-protein-nitrogen-pool (NPN-pool). It is the source for amino acids used for synthesis of protein in the viscera, especially in the liver. Due to this liver protein, synthesis is diminished only insignificantly or it is normal or even elevated.

So after trauma we can observe a new distribution of protein in the different pools of tissues and organs (fig. 3). This is an argument for the thesis that total body protein synthesis does not reveal alterations in all tissues, neither in quantity nor in direction. Estimation of total body protein gives only the sum of all processes in all tissues.

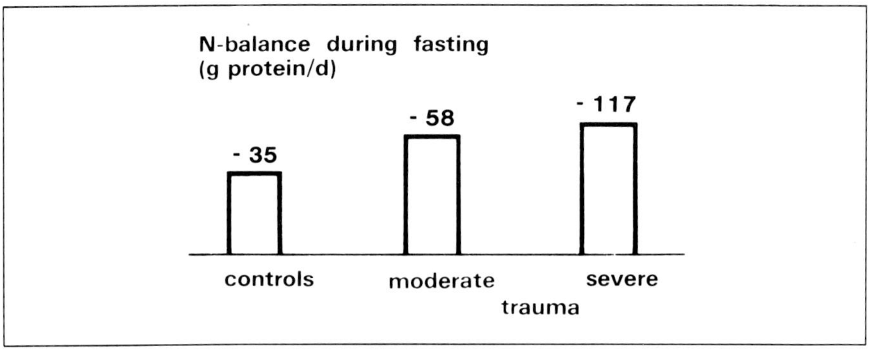

Fig. 2. N-balance during fasting in healthy persons and after moderate and severe trauma.

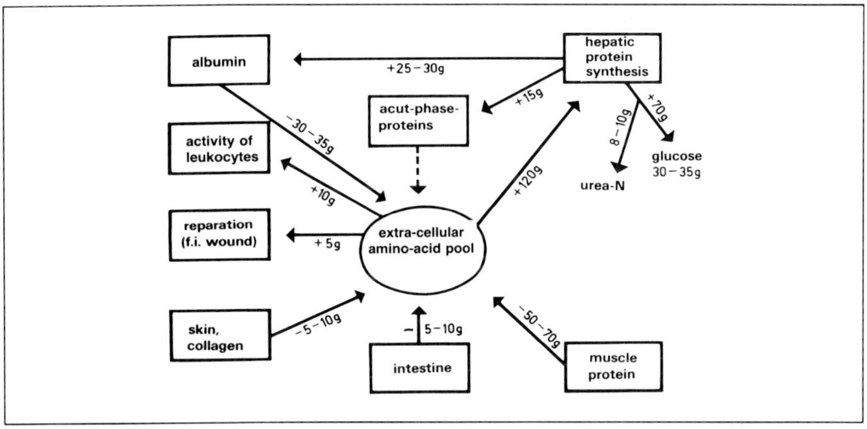

Fig. 3. Redistribution of body protein after injury [13, 14].

3rd Study

Application of amino acids or protein increases protein synthesis. Protein synthesis occurs in fasting patients too. The origin of amino acids available for protein synthesis in such patients is protein breakdown. But synthesis can be elevated by N-intake. Figure 4 demonstrates operated rats fed with 17 mg or with 181 mg amino-N/day. Rats on the small N-intake still synthesized 64 mg protein-N/day, but rats fed with the considerably higher amount synthesized 155 mg.

4th Study

It is interesting that a higher rate of nitrogen intake increases not only protein synthesis but also protein breakdown. Figure 5 shows operated rats on a small and operated rats on a higher amount of nutritional intake (17 mg/181 mg amino acid-N). The breakdown of protein increases in rats on a higher N-intake. But we have to consider the following: the stimulation of synthesis due to elevated food intake preponderates the breakdown (increase of synthesis: 91 mg protein-N; increase of breakdown: 27 mg protein-N). So N-balance improves due to a more pronounced increase of synthesis as opposed to breakdown. In this way a higher intake accelerates protein turnover (fig. 13).

5th Study

The same can be seen studying the protein pools in single organs. Though we are still in the beginning with these problems, we can show our first results. We studied in 13 pigs the influence of different L-amino-acid solutions after poisoning them with thioacetamide. Intermittent intraperitoneal application of thioacetamide provokes a reproducible liver damage. At the end of intoxication the animals were treated with infusion therapy: 4 animals received a balanced solution developed for healthy persons (Infesol); 5 animals a solution developed for liver insufficiency (Aminofusin hepar); 4 animals got oral food intake and as infusion only water and electrolytes. All solutions were labelled with ^{15}N-glycine. We estimated, besides other parameters, the incorporation of ^{15}N in liver proteins [15]. As result we found the lowest ^{15}N-enrichment in animals fed orally and infused only with water and electrolytes, and the highest rate in pigs which received the 'liver solution' (table II). A higher rate of ^{15}N-labelling of liver protein is an indicator for an elevated protein turnover and also for a better regeneration rate, which could be confirmed with other methods too (enzymes, histology, survival time).

6th Study

If we compare synthesis rates in operated and nonoperated individuals with the same intake of N and energy, then operated patients or

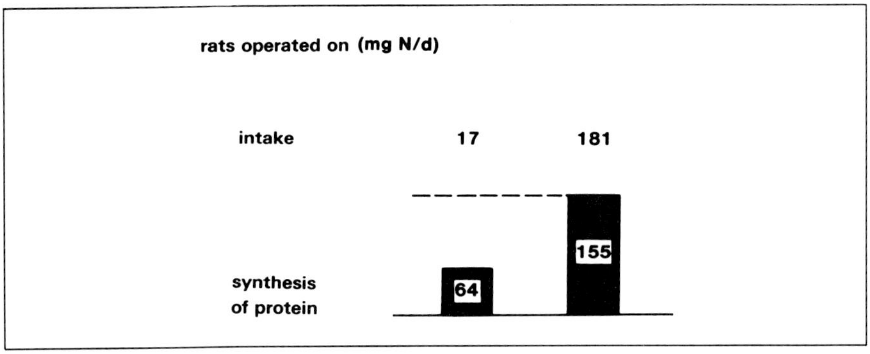

Fig. 4. Synthesis of body protein in rats on a minimal and on a high amino acid and energy intake [7, 8].

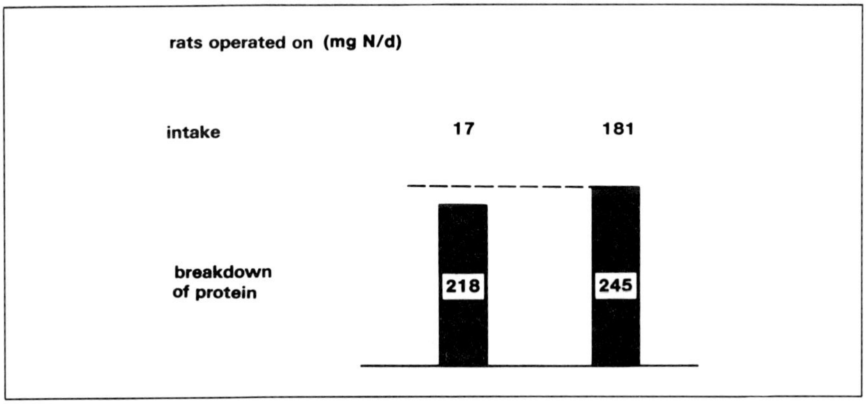

Fig. 5. Breakdown of body protein in rats on a minimal and on a high amino acid and energy intake [7, 8].

Table I. Protein synthesis in operated and nonoperated pigs on the same intake of amino acids and energy (plateau method B) (g protein/day/kg)

Control animals	Pigs operated on	Significance
8.2 ± 1.6	3.1 ± 1.3	< 0.1

Table II. ^{15}N-quantity in liver protein of pigs, poisoned by intermittent intraperitoneal application of thioacetamide and treated thereafter with 3 different infusion solutions labelled with ^{15}N-glycine

		mg protein-^{15}N/10 g tcaa-precipitated liver protein
'Normal' solution of amino acids	×	1.26
(Infesol)	r	1.10–1.60
	n	4
'Liver solution'	×	2.35
(Aminofusin hepar)	r	2.10–2.60
	n	4
Oral intake and infusion of	×	0.24
water and electrolytes	r	0.17–0.29
	n	3

animals show a smaller protein synthesis. We studied this in operated and nonoperated pigs (fig. 6). After a period of pre-balance, the animals were infused for 24 h with a labelled amino acid solution (Infesol 40). The elimination of N and ^{15}N in urine was measured. The results obtained were calculated using the 3-pool model (Sprinson and Rittenberg; fig. 7). Pool 1 includes the body protein, pool 2 all non-protein-N, and pool 3 nitrogen excreted in urine. With R we describe the N-streams: R_{10} = N-intake; R_{21} = protein-synthesis; R_{12} = protein breakdown, and R_{31} = N-excretion. The N-streams between the different pools can be described with mathematical equations. To simplify the evaluation we developed graphical methods which have been approved in the last time (fig. 8a–c).

We found a decreased protein synthesis in operated animals (amino acid and energy intake was the same in both animal groups; table I).

7th Study

The reason for the diminished efficiency of amino acids under stress condition is due to a higher rate of urea production, that means more amino acids are introduced into energy production. After operation the glucose output is elevated by 50 to 60%, the oxidation of glucose by 25% [4].

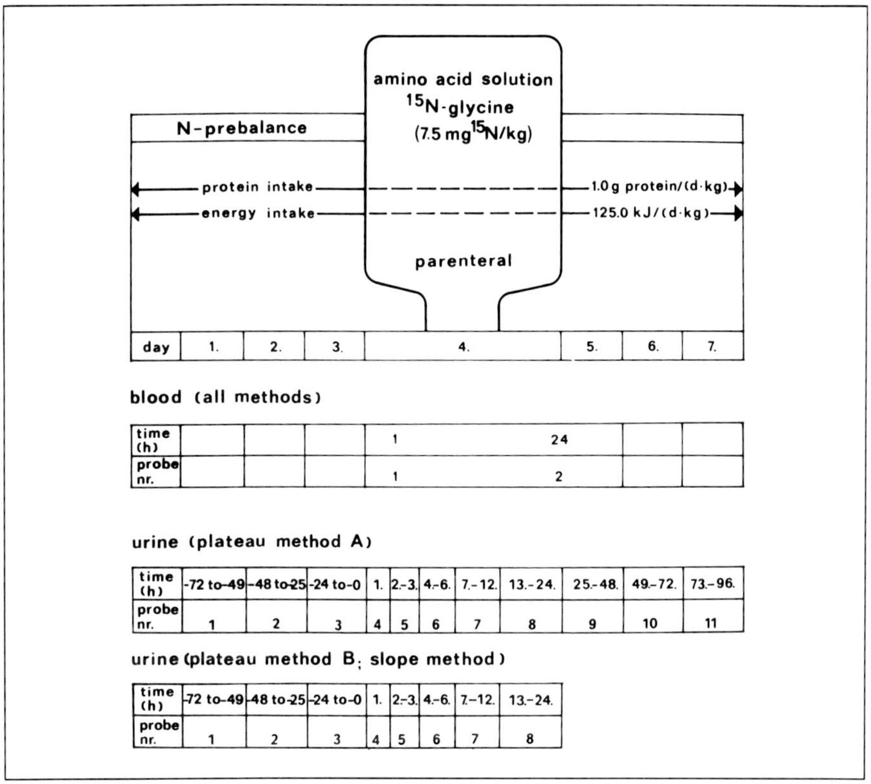

Fig. 6. Design of 'standardized infusion test' for calculation of total body protein synthesis.

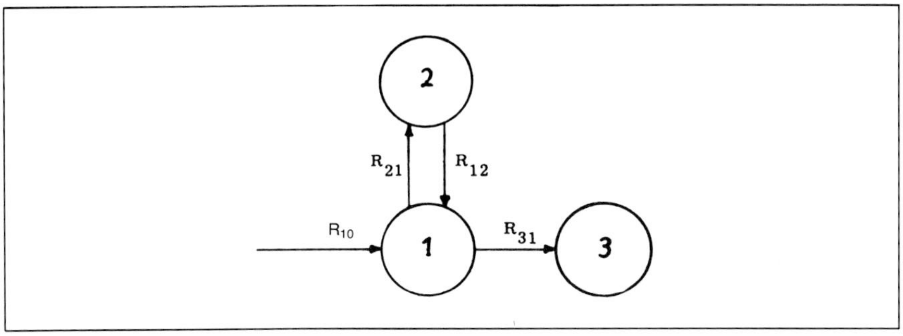

Fig. 7. 3-pool model of Sprinson and Rittenberg (explanation see text).

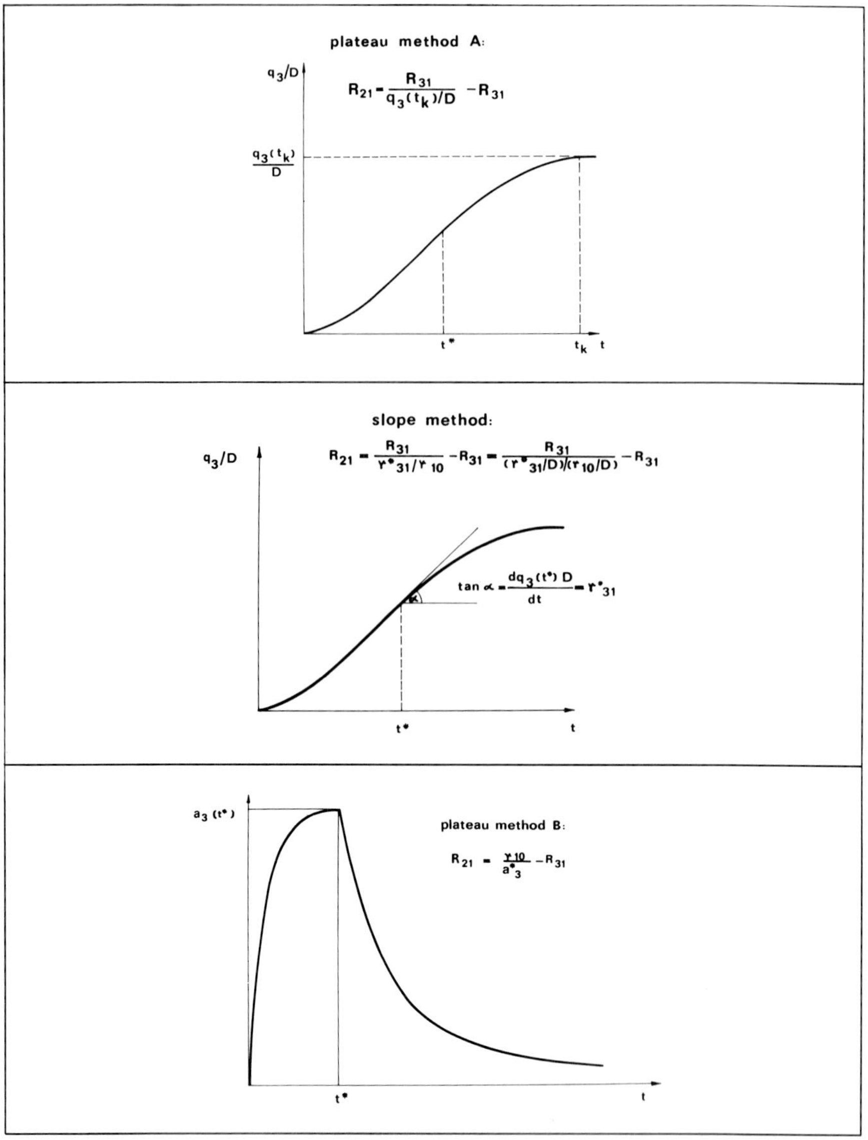

Fig. 8. Assessment of protein synthesis on the basis of graphical evaluation methods: *a* plateau method A (cumulative elimination of total ^{15}N in urine in % of uptake); *b* slope method (increase of ^{15}N-elimination in urine during infusion period); *c* plateau method B (abundance of ^{15}N in urine at the end of infusion period).

We have measured this in patients (fig. 9). We studied healthy persons and patients after cholecystectomy. For 48 h we infused an amino acid solution (labeled with ^{15}N-glycine) and carbohydrates. The relation of amino acids to energy was 1 g : 126 kJ. We estimated elimination of total-N, urea-N, and the ^{15}N-elimination with these N-fractions and calculated ^{15}N-excretion in percent of intake during steady state (36th–48th hour). What we found was the following (fig. 10): urea-production rate was 16% in healthy persons and 26% in operated patients. With other words, more amino acids were introduced into energy production in gluconeogenesis.

These values could be used for further calculations (fig. 11). In healthy persons, 72 to 77% of amino acids given are efficacious on N-balance. This corresponds to an angle of 37°. This angle describes the efficiency of an amino acid solution on N-balance. The angle is smaller in operated patients. In this way influence on N-balance is diminished in such patients. To achieve the same N-balance in operated patients as in healthy persons, more amino acids are necessary. Using this calculation we can conclude that patients after trauma need a higher amount of amino acids to achieve the same balance as healthy persons.

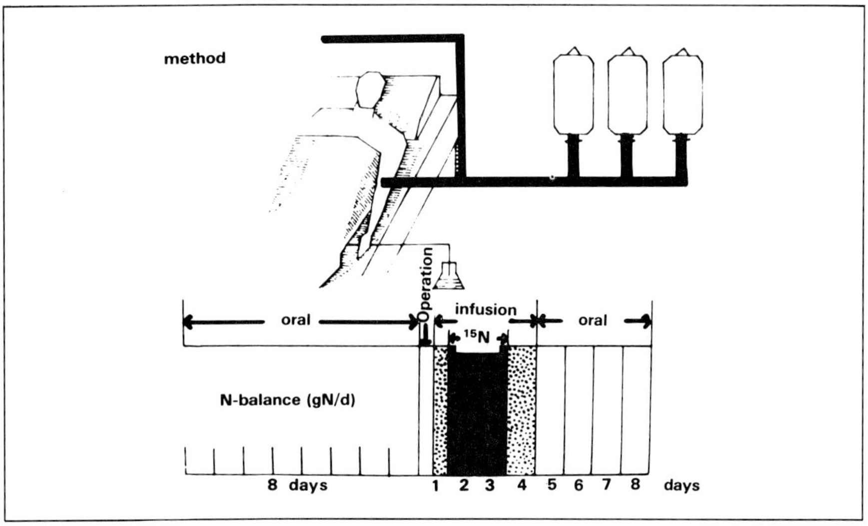

Fig. 9. Design of the study to estimate utilization of a ^{15}N-glycine labelled amino acid solution (infusion for 48 h) [10].

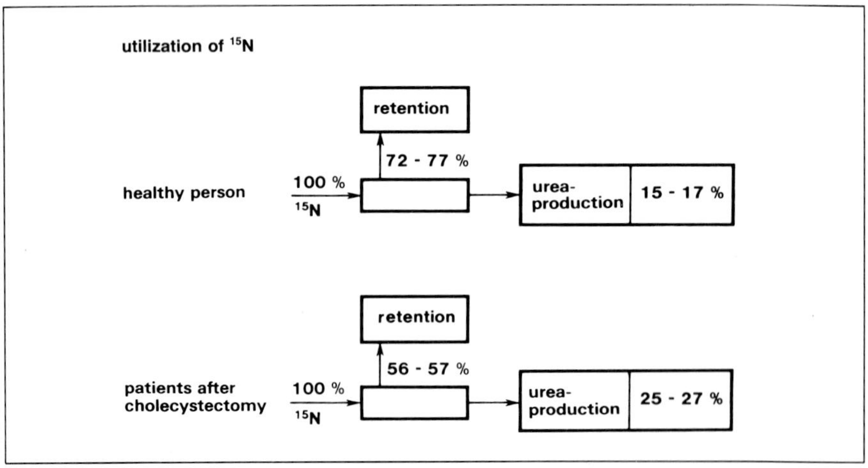

Fig. 10. Utilization of ^{15}N-glycine in healthy persons and patients after cholecystectomy in % of uptake (36th–48th hour of infusion period – quasi stationary condition) [10].

8th Study

With this series we studied another question: Should we add energy if we give amino acids to a patient? We examined two groups of rats fed parenterally over 5 days via a central venous catheter. One group received a solution containing only amino acids without energy, the second group amino acids and glucose (1 g amino acids to 126 kJ). The amino acids were labeled with ^{15}N-glycine. High loss of ^{15}N in rats only infused with amino acids could be shown (fig. 12). In this case amino acids were used to form glucose. The relation of protein synthesis to urea production has shifted to urea production.

Another important question concerns the composition of amino acid solutions. Many studies were done in the last years to get more information on this problem. Due to the time limit, these interesting questions cannot be answered in this paper.

Fig. 11. Mathematical derivations from results of the study: *a* 75 resp. 57% of ^{15}N infused is efficacious on N-balance. The balance-improving angle thereby is 37° resp. 30°; *b* to achieve the same N-balance more amino acids are to be given: 130%.

Fig. 12. Elimination of ^{15}N in % of uptake in rats during infusion of amino acids with and without energy [3].

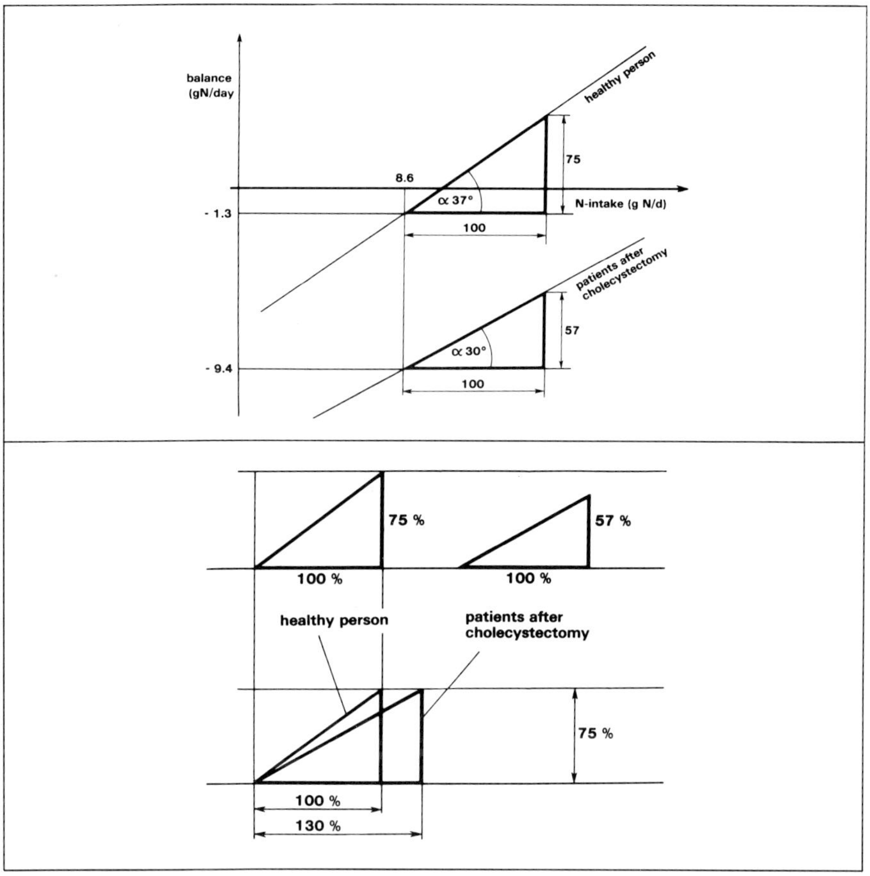
balance
(gN/day
healthy person
75
8.6
α 37°
N-intake (g N/d)
- 1.3
100
patients after
cholecystectomy
57
α 30°
- 9.4
100
75 %
57 %
100 %
100 %
healthy person
patients after
cholecystectomy
75 %
100 %
130 %

11

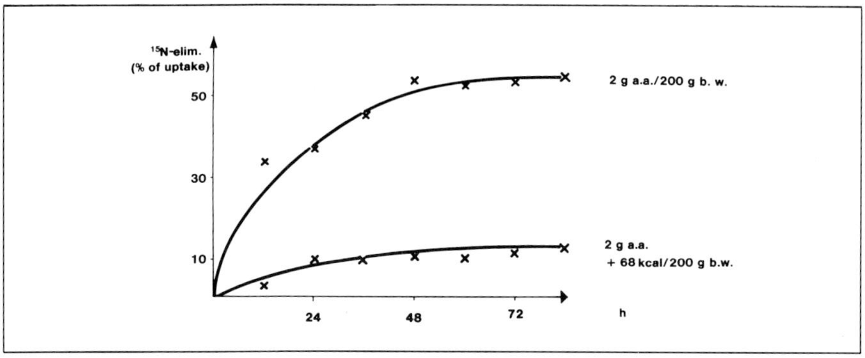
^{15}N-elim.
(% of uptake)
50
30
10
24
48
72
h
2 g a.a./200 g b. w.
2 g a.a.
+ 68 kcal/200 g b.w.

12

Conclusion (fig. 13)

Protein metabolism after injury is influenced by a lot of factors. Severity of injury is of special significance, since breakdown of muscle protein is especially stimulated. On the other hand, amino acid or protein intake, together with other sources of energy, are important for protein synthesis. Both N-streams determine N-balance. So giving nutrients is the most effective method to stimulate whole body protein synthesis. Protein breakdown is not lowered by giving nutrients, on the contrary, it is somewhat elevated. In this way protein turnover is accelerated, which seems useful as we could show in our experiments with liver diseases.

Breakdown of body protein for a longer time without giving nutrients lowers protein synthesis and also vital functions, for instance immunological defense mechanisms, wound-healing, respiration, etc. Optimal nutrition is, therefore, a useful tool to support the postoperative course of our patients.

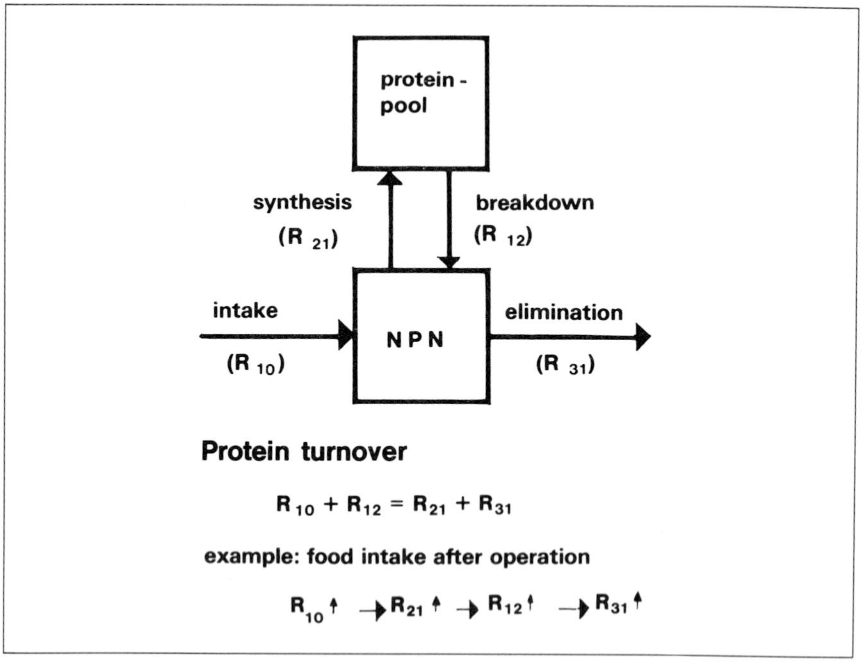

Fig. 13. Model of protein turnover.

References

1 Bürger, M.; Grauhan, M.: Über postoperativen Eiweißzerfall. Z. ges. exp. Med. *27:* 97–114 (1922).

2 Fürst, P.; Josephson, B.; Vinnars, E.: Die Aufnahme von ^{15}N im Muskeleiweiß von einem Patienten in katabolem Zustand. Anaesthesiologie und Wiederbelebung; in Stoffwechsel. Pathophysiologische Grundlagen der Intensivtherapie, vol. 58, pp. 115–124 (Springer, Berlin, Heidelberg, New York 1972).

3 Futtig, D.; Mory, M.: Tierexperimentelle Untersuchungen über Eiweißstoffwechselveränderungen im Streß unter Verwendung verschiedener Eiweiß-Kalorien-Relationen im Ernährungsplan; Diss. Leipzig (1981).

4 Gelfand, R. A.; de Fronzo, R. A.; Gusberg, R.: Metabolic alterations associated with major injury or infection; in Kleinberger, Deutsch, New aspects of clinical nutrition, pp. 211–239 (Karger, Basel 1983).

5 Hartig, W.: Untersuchungen über den Eiweißstoffwechsel in der frühen postoperativen Phase. Habschr. Leipzig (1966).

6 Hartig, W.: Der postoperative Eiweißstoffwechsel. Z. exp. Chir. u. chirurg. Forsch. *2:* 102–113 (1969).

7 Hartig, W.; Wetzel, K.; Gebhardt, G.; Czarnetzki, H.-D.; Hübner, G.: Der postoperative Eiweißstoffwechsel. Z. exp. Chir. u. chirurg. Forsch. *3:* 56–72 (1970).

8 Hartig, W.; Hübner, G.; Czarnetzki, H.-D.; Gebhardt, G.; Wetzel, K.: Der postoperative Eiweißstoffwechsel. Z. exp. Chir. u. chirurg. Forsch. *3:* 170–176 (1970).

9 Hartig, W.; Goyk, M.; Löbe, J.; Richter, D.: Der postoperative Eiweißstoffwechsel. Z. exp. Chir. u. chirurg. Forsch. *3:* 297–314 (1970).

10 Hartig, W.; Czarnetzki, H.-D.; Faust, H.; Fickweiler, E.: Zur Verwertung von Aminosäuren-Infusionslösungen beim Gesunden und bei Patienten im Streß, untersucht an ^{15}N-Glycin. Infusionstherapie *3:* 268–273 (1976).

11 Hartig, W.; Czarnetzki, H.-D.; Faust, H.; Martin, H.; Martin, R.; Wetzel, K.: Zur Utilisation von oral appliziertem ^{15}N-Glycin beim Menschen. Infusionstherapie *6:* 6–9 (1979).

12 Hartig, W.; Matkowitz, R.; Junghans, P.; Jung, K.; Faust, H.: Proteinsynthese nach experimentellem Trauma am Tiermodell Schwein. Ein Vergleich von Infusionslösungen mit unterschiedlichen Aminosäurenmustern. Infusionstherapie *10:* 276–279 (1983).

13 Löhlein, D.: Proteinsparende Mechanismen der parenteralen Ernährung. I. Grundlagen und Methodik. Infusionstherapie *11:* 90–99 (1984).

14 Löhlein, D.: Proteinsparende Mechanismen der parenteralen Ernährung. II. Klinische Aspekte. Infusionstherapie *11:* 114–128 (1984).

15 Metzner, Chr.; Hartig, W.; Graubaum, H.-J.; Matkowitz, R.; Jung, K.; Wagenknecht, C.; Ritter, R.: Wertigkeit verschiedener Aminosäurengemische für die Behandlung des chronischen Leberschadens (in press).

Prof. Dr. sc. med. W. Hartig, Chirurgische Klinik des Bezirkskrankenhauses St. Georg, Straße der DSF 141, DDR-7021 Leipzig (GDR)

Dietze, Grünert, Kleinberger, Wolfram (eds.), Clinical Nutrition and Metabolic Research. Proc. 7th Congr. ESPEN, Munich 1985, pp. 236–241 (Karger, Basel 1986)

Ketone Body Turnover Rates in the Human Neonate and Infant

P. F. Bougnères

National Institute of Health and Medical Research, Pediatric Endocrinology, Hospital Saint Vincent de Paul, Paris, France

Introduction

The human newborn develops accelerated lipid mobilization from its large fat stores in order to meet energy requirements. The release of fatty acids from adipose tissue occurs at a rate of ~ 4–5 g/kg/day during the first days of life, and serves a dual role in fuel homeostasis: it serves in substrate delivery both for direct energy supply and for ketogenesis. Because of the precarious balance between neonatal glucose production and the almost equal glucose utilization requirements of the 400-g newborn brain, there is an absolute need for alternative fuels capable of sparing (or replacing) glucose for cerebral nutrition. Free fatty acids, while providing several tissues with readily oxidizable substrates, cannot cross the blood-brain barrier to be utilized by the brain. However, their water-soluble derivatives, acetoacetate (AcAc) and 3-hydroxybutyrate (3-OHB), besides being used as fuel by tissues, have the unique capacity of replacing glucose for the energy needs of the central nervous system in humans. Since this capacity is already functional in the immature human brain, ketone bodies (KB) might play an important role in the caloric homeostasis of newly born infants. Whether fasted for the first 24 h of life or fed under current nursery practices, newborn infants have a degree of ketosis that is achieved by the adult only after 1–2 days of total starvation. We developed a gas chromatography-mass spectrometry (GCMS) approach using nonradioactive, deuterium-labeled 3-OHB tracer, which has allowed us to make measurements of KB transport in human neonates in an ethically acceptable fashion. In addition, ketone body turnover was also measured in older infants (1–6 months of age) to evaluate the quantitative importance of these substrates during short-term fasting.

Methods

Patients

Glucose and ketone body turnover rates were measured simultaneously in 6 newborns (group A) and 4 older infants (group B). Infants in group A were born at term and appropriate weight for gestational age. All infants were born after an uncomplicated pregnancy. 4 mothers had premature rupture of membranes and 1 mother had a temperature of 38.5 °C during labor. Thus, 5 of the newborns studied were receiving intravenous antibiotic therapy, but in none was infection confirmed by culture. At the time of the study, all infants were asymptomatic, resting comfortably in an isolette or a crib, and covered with a blanket to avoid hypothermia during the study. Medical care of each newborn was under control of the child's physician who designated the infant's feeding schedule according to his routine nursery practice, so that none of the infants was specifically fasted for the purpose of the tracer experiment. Subjects 1 and 2 had received no oral feedings before the study. These 2 infants, and the 4 others treated with intravenous antibiotics, received intravenous dextrose at a 'keep-open' rate of < 1 mg dextrose/kg/min. In each instance, the intravenous solution was switched to 0.45% saline a minimum of 3 h before starting the tracer experiment. Infants of group B were referred patients: 2 of them because of suspected but undocumented hypoglycemia (and later proved to be normal infants on a metabolic and endocrine basis), and the 2 others because of viral diarrhea with weight loss $< 10\%$ of body weight. Thus, subjects 7 and 8 were fasted as part of routine evaluation for hypoglycemia, while subjects 9 and 10 had resumed normal feeding for 2–3 days before the study.

Materials

D-(−)3-hydroxy(4,4,4-$^2H_3$)butyrate (92% atom % $^2H_3$), and D-(6,6-$^2H_2$) glucose (97 atom % $^2H_2$) were purchased from Merck, Sharp and Sohme Canada, Ltd., Montreal, Quebec, Canada, dissolved in 0.5 N saline and prepared from human use as described.

Procedural Methods

Infants were studied after obtaining parental consent according to protocols approved by the Saint-Vincent-de-Paul Hospital and Institut National de la Santé et de la Recherche Médicale (INSERM) Committees on Ethics in Human Experimentation. In all of the newborns, and in infants 9 and 10, the peripheral intravenous 'scalp vein' needle already in place for antibiotic or fluid administration was used for tracer infusion. In the remaining infants (numbers 7 and 8), a 25-gauge 'scalp vein' needle was inserted into a peripheral vein at least 2 h before the onset of the tracer infusion.

At time 0 of the study, we collected base-line samples (see below) and began continuous infusion of labeled tracers using a calibrated syringe pump at the rate of 0.266 ± 0.025

(SEM) μmol/kg/min D-(−)-3-hydroxy(4,4,4-$^2H_3$)butyrate ($^2H_3$)OHB and 0.446 ± 0.017 μmol/kg/min D-(6,6-$^2H_2$)glucose. These rates of infusion were maintained for 120 min in all studied infants. Before the start of the study, and every 10 min from 90 to 120 min, 500 μl 'heel stick' arterialized capillary blood samples were collected into iced heparinized tubes.

Analytical Methods

Blood glucose, acetoacetate, and D-(−)-3-hydroxybutyrate were measured spectrophotometrically by specific enzymatic micromethods within 12 h after collecting blood samples. Isotopic enrichments in circulating (6,6-$^2H_2$)glucose ($^2H_3$)OHB and in (4,4,4-$^2H_3$) acetoacetate (($^2H_3$)AcAc) were measured by selected ion monitoring GCMS as recently described. Plasma total free fatty acid (FFA) content was calculated from the summed individual fatty acid methyl ester gas chromatography peak areas referenced to heptadecanoic acid as internal standard.

Calculations

Blood total ketone body (AcAc + 3-OHB) inflow transport (or rate of appearance, Ra), rate of outflow (or disappearance, Rd), and clearance rate (Rc) were calculated from samples taken between 90 and 120 min of study. In all studied infants, both blood AcAc and 3-OHB content, and the ($^2H_3$) enrichment in each ketone remained reasonably constant (SD/mean < 0.15) and were considered at or near steady state. Treatment of kinetic data was carried out by the 'single pool' approach, with blood AcAc and 3-OHB pools being lumped as one.

There was rapid formation of ($^2H_3$) AcAc from ($^2H_3$)OHB, with both ketones retaining the deuterium atoms in position 4. Since, at steady state, ($^2H_3$) AcAc enrichment averaged 67.1 ± 3.5% (SE) that of the ($^2H_3$) OHB tracer, we considered that 3-OHB and AcAc were interconverted rapidly enough to minimize the error of considering them in the same pool.

Because each subject also achieved approximately constant values (SD/mean < 5%) for plasma glucose and (6,6-$^2H_2$)glucose enrichment, similar steady state equations were employed for the calculation of glucose turnover rate, as described. Total FFA inflow and outflow transport rates were estimated from plasma FFA concentrations and the established linear relationship between plasma FFA content and transport in newborn infants.

Results

Substrate Levels

In group A, none of the newborns was hypoglycemic, although number 5 had a plasma glucose level at the lower normal limit at the time of the study. Neonatal blood AcAc and 3-OHB concentrations averaged 296 ± 112 μm (SEM) and 486 ± 67 μM, respectively, with a 3-OHB/AcAc concentration ratio of 3.0 ± 1.0. Total circulating ketone bodies were 781 ± 172 μM. These values are in the range previously reported for newborns in their first days of life having a similar feeding schedule. Plasma FFA level averaged 810 ± 206 μM, a value in newborns that is similar to that previously reported by us for similar infants.

Infants of group B had blood total ketone body and FFA concentrations averaging 1.250 ± 241 μM and 956 ± 110 μM, respectively, within or near normal physiological values for similarly fasted infants. The 3-OHB/AcAc concentration ratio was 2.70 ± 0.03, a normal value.

Ketone Body Transport and Its Relationship with FFA and Glucose Transport

During the study of group A and B subjects, infused ($^2H_3$) OHB tracer reached an overall average isotope enrichment of 1.50 ± 0.12 atom % excess, whereas ($^2H_3$) AcAc enrichment averaged 1.0 ± 0.09 atom % excess. Thus, although complete isotopic equilibrium between the two ketones was not achieved, the value of the ($^2H_3$)AcAc/($^2H_3$)OHB enrichment ratio (0.67 ± 0.03) indicated extensive interconversion between blood 3-OHB and AcAc, resulting in an average ($^2H_3$) enrichment of 1.34 ± 0.1 atom % excess for blood total ketones in group A and B infants. During the last 30 min of study, the inflow-outflow transport rates of blood total ketone bodies were nearly identical in each subject population and averaged 17.3 ± 1.4 μmol/kg/min in group A infants, and 20.6 ± 0.93 μmol/kg/min in group B infants, values not reached in adults until they have fasted for 3–23 days. There was a direct linear relationship ($r = 0.8$, $p < 0.002$) between blood ketone level and rate of inflow-outflow transport as reported in adults over a similar range of blood ketone concentration. Blood ketone body clearance rate ranged from 12 to 51 ml/kg/min (average, 28.6 ± 6.6 ml/kg/min in group A, and 17.8 ± 2.8 ml/kg/min in group B) and correlated negatively ($r = 0.87$, $p < 0.001$) with blood ketone concentration as previously in fasted adults.

From the infants' FFA values and the regression equation previously defined in a similar group of newborns, the plasma FFA inflow-outflow rate could be estimated for each infant. FFA turnover averaged 14 ± 2 μmol/kg/min in the newborns, and 15 ± 1 μmol/kg/min in group B infants in good agreement with the value of 11.5 ± 1.7 μmol/kg/min previously measured in neonates. Plasma FFA (and therefore FFA outflow rate) were correlated ($r = 0.6$, $p < 0.002$) with ketone body production as anticipated from the precursor-product relationship between FFA and ketone bodies. Because the synthesis of 1 mol of AcAc or 3-OHB requires ~ 0.25 mol of plasma FFA, and assuming that all ketones are derived from FFA oxidation, the amount of FFA utilized for ketogenesis was estimated from ketone body production rate. Thus, 4.2 ± 0.54 μmol/kg/min of FFA was converted to ketone bodies in group A, and 5.2 ± 0.5 μmol/kg/min in group B infants. Therefore, the fraction of FFA flux that served for ketone body synthesis averaged 31 ± 2%, and was nearly constant in group A and B infants.

Discussion

This study shows that ketone body production and utilization are very active processes that occur at accelerated rates in term newborns, even when these neonates are fed every 4 h according to current nursery practices. The observed neonatal ketone body transport rates of 12.8–21.9 μmol/kg/min, and those in older infants fasted for ~ 8 h (17.9–26.0 μmol/kg/min), are achieved by the adults only after several days of starvation. Because the newborn is currently fed on a basis of approximately every 4 h, the total daily ketone body transport can, therefore, be estimated to be on the order of 2–3 g/kg/day. In fasted adults, about 85% of ketone body production is oxidized, mostly in brain, muscle, and kidney. If one assumes the same fractional oxidation rate for the newborn, the neonate would oxidize ~ 2 g of ketone bodies per kilogram body weight daily. This oxidation would yield the equivalent of ~ 10 kcal/kg/day, one-fourth of the minimal, basal energy requirements on the first days of life for an infant in a thermoneutral environment. Most importantly, at a time when glucose production is just sufficient to serve the demand of the newborn brain, ketone bodies can thus serve as alternate substrates for the oxidative requirement of the central nervous system.

The increased capacity for taking up ketone bodies from the blood stream in the neonate is consistent with its large brain size in relation to total body weight, and the fourfold increase in neonatal cerebral ketone body uptake compared with the adult. The close agreement between the regression equation for ketone body production and FFA levels in our patients and the regression calculated from data presented in adult studies is supported by the similar fraction (~ 30%) of the FFA flux, which is converted into ketones. These similar relationships, taken together with the ability of the neonate to produce large amounts of ketones, suggest that ketogenesis is already mature in humans on the first day of life, and that the intrahepatic and extrahepatic regulatory systems controlling the conversion of FFA into KB are well established by this early postnatal age.

References

1 Bougnères, P. F.; Karl, I. E.; Hillman, L. S.; Bier, D. M.: Lipid transport in the human newborn. Palmitate and glycerol turnover and the contribution of glycerol to neonatal hepatic glucose output. J. clin. Invest. *70:* 262–270 (1982).

2 Persson, B.; Settergren, G.; Dahlquist, G.: Cerebral arteriovenous difference of acetoacetate and D-β-hydroxybutyrate in children. Acta paediat. scand. *61:* 273–278 (1972).

3 Kraus, H.; Schlenker, S.; Schwedesky, D.: Developmental changes of cerebral ketone body utilization in human infants. Hoppe-Seyler's Z. physiol. Chem. *355:* 164–170 (1974).

4 Patel, M. S.; Johnson, C. A.; Rajan, R.; Owen, O. E.: The metabolism of ketone bodies in developing human brain: Development of ketone-body-utilizing enzymes and ketone bodies as precursors for lipid synthesis. J. Neurochem. *25:* 903–905 (1975).

5 Bougnères, P. F.; Balasse, E. O.; Ferre, P.; Bier, D. M.: Determination of ketone body kinetics using a D-(−)-3-hydroxy(4,4,4-$^2H_3$) butyrate tracer. Lipid Res. (in press).

6 Bougnères, P. F.; Lemmel, C.; Ferre, P.; Bier, D. M.: Ketone body transport in the human neonate and infant. J. clin. Invest. *77:* 42–48 (1986).

Dr. P. F. Bougnères, U 188 Institut National de la Santé et de la Recherche Médicale,
Unité de Recherches sur la Croissance, Hôpital Saint-Vincent de Paul,
74, Ave. Denfert-Rochereau, F-75014 Paris (France)

Dietze, Grünert, Kleinberger, Wolfram (eds.), Clinical Nutrition and Metabolic Research. Proc. 7th Congr. ESPEN, Munich 1985, pp. 242–246 (Karger, Basel 1986)

Stable Isotope Techniques in Studies of Trace Element Metabolism and Possible Clinical Applications

M. J. Jackson

Dept. of Medicine, University of Liverpool, Liverpool, UK

Introduction

Although stable isotope techniques have been utilised in the study of energy for a considerable period of time [8], they have only been utilised in the field of trace element metabolism relatively recently [4, 7]. The capacity for the development of this field is large since a wide selection of isotopes are commercially available in the enriched form. However, their widespread use is currently limited by the lack of availability of suitable analytical instrumentation in nutritional or metabolic research laboratories. Stable isotope techniques have been used in the study of several trace elements with most work centering on zinc, copper, iron and selenium (for example see [3, 7, 11]). This paper will discuss briefly the factors involved in the use of enriched stable isotopes and possible applications of this technique to nutritional and metabolic research.

Choice of Isotope

For many elements there is a choice of isotope which can be used (e.g. see table I for selenium). The choice between these is dependent upon a variety of factors – these are:

(a) the natural enrichment of isotope;
(b) the availability and cost of enriched products;
(c) limitations on the total amount of isotope which can be used; and
(d) the analytical techniques available.

In general it is better to try to enrich the isotope with the lowest natural enrichment (e.g. 74 selenium in table I), but this may be impossible either because the isotope cannot be measured by the chosen analytical technique, because it is not available in an enriched form, or it is available but the cost of the enriched product is excessively high. The level of enrichment which must be achieved in order to obtain valid results is dependent upon the precision of the analytical technique and the length of time for which the study will proceed. However, the use of large amounts of enriched product to ensure an adequate deviance from the natural abundance must be undertaken with care since this may well influence the results obtained and, in addition, many trace elements are toxic.

Analytical Techniques

The analytical techniques which have been utilised in the study of stable isotopes are shown in table II. Although most early studies in this field utilised neutron activation analysis (e.g. see [4, 7]) there is now a greater reliance on mass spectrometric methods. The highest precision of analysis can be achieved with thermal ionisation mass spectrometry, but the sample applied to this system must be very clean and ideally would consist of a pure salt solution of the element in question. The separation techniques used to overcome this problem have included the use of selective chelators [2, 6] or ion exchange chromatography [11]. Other mass

Table I. Naturally occurring isotopes of selenium

Isotope	74	76	77	78	80	82
Natural abundance (%)	0.9	9.0	7.6	23.5	49.8	9.2

Table II. Techniques used for stable isotope analysis in biological materials

1. Neutron activation analysis	
2. Mass spectrometry (MS):	thermal ionisation MS
	fast atom bombardment MS
	secondary ion MS
	gas chromatography MS
	inductively coupled plasma MS
	laser ionisation MS

spectrometric techniques have not been extensively used although the relatively widespread availability of fast atom bombardment mass spectrometry will probably see further application of this technique in the near future [9].

In principle, inductively coupled plasma mass spectrometry should be ideally suited to this problem, the high temperature of the argon plasma permitting analyses of materials with a high organic content. The disadvantages of this technique are large sample volumes required with conventional nebulisers and the relatively poor precision obtained on certain isotopes. We have recently examined the suitability of this technique in analysis of zinc and selenium isotopes in normal blood plasma. A subject was infused with 4 mg 67 zinc and 50 micrograms 74 selenium and blood samples were removed at intervals over the next 14 days. In a very simple sample preparation procedure 5 ml samples of blood plasma were wet-washed with nitric acid and hydrogen peroxide and reconstituted to 5 ml with deionised, distilled water. The samples were analysed using a VG Isotopes Plasamaquad (VG Isotopes Limited, Winsford, Cheshire, UK) with a nebuliser flow rate of 1 ml/min. The results obtained demonstrate that the technique can provide adequate precision in the analysis of zinc isotopes (0.5–1.5% relative standard deviation) to be useful for nutritional studies, but the precision obtained in the selenium analyses was much larger (1.5–29.5% relative standard deviation). The major factor influencing the precision in this circumstance is the concentration of the element in human blood plasma (i.e. selenium is present at approximately 1 μmol/l which is an order of magnitude less than zinc). Modifications designed to increase the effective concentration seen by the mass spectrometer, such as use of a carbon furnace system or a recirculating nebuliser, may improve this in the future, but this remains to be tested. Laser ionisation mass spectrometry [1] may also possibly become a useful technique in this field since it could be theoretically used to examine isotope ratios in very small tissue samples and may therefore allow stable isotopes to be used in examining tissue uptake of trace elements in man.

Applications of Enriched Stable Isotopes to Clinical Nutrition

Enriched stable isotope preparations can be administered via the oral or the intravenous route during nutritional studies. The major applications have been to assess the gastrointestinal absorption of trace elements, either in the study of normal absorptive processes or to examine bioavailability of nutrients from foodstuffs [10]. Oral administration followed by faecal monitoring has been the major technique used in this work [5, 11]. A useful extension of this has been the growing of specific foodstuffs on nutrients enriched in the isotope to be used in order to obtain intrinsically labelled foods for the study of bioavailability. Intravenous administration of a zinc isotope (67 zinc) followed by concurrent measurement of the plasma and faecal enrichment has been used to follow gastrointestinal excretion of zinc [2]. When used in conjunction with a conventional metabolic balance study, values for the absorption of zinc can also be obtained using this technique.

Stable isotopes can also be utilised to examine the kinetics of trace element movements within the body. Both oral and intravenous administration of the material has been utilised for this purpose.

Conclusion

The potential uses of enriched stable isotopes of trace elements are now recognised but widespread use of these techniques is limited by the availability of suitable analytical instrumentation. However, it is likely that developments in mass spectrometry will alter the situation in the future and will permit more investigators to utilise this extremely powerful tool. However, the extension of this field to the level of sophistication seen in studies examining amino acid and protein metabolism (e.g. see the accompanying papers presented at this Workshop) will require considerable emphasis on precision and accuracy of analysis and may only be possible with a limited number of the analytical techniques listed in table II.

References

1 Chaplin, A. J.; Millard, P. R.; Schmidt, P. F.: The use of a laser microprobe to identify calcium oxalate in histological material. Histochem. *75:* 259 (1982).

2 Jackson, M. J.; Jones, D. A.; Edwards, R. H. T.; Seainbank, I. G.; Coleman, M. L.: Zinc homeostasis in man: Studies using a new stable isotope dilution technique. Br. J. Nutr. *51:* 199 (1984).

3 Janghorbani, M.; Christensen, M. J.; Nahapetin, A.; Young, V. R.: Selenium metabolism in healthy adults: Quantitative aspects using the stable isotope. Am. J. clin. Nutr. *35:* 647 (1982).

4 Janghorbani, M.; Ting, B. T. G.; Young, V. R.: Absorption of iron in young men studied by monitoring excretion of a stable isotope (^{58}F3) in faeces. J. Nutr. *110:* 2190 (1980).

5 Janghorbani, M.; Young, V. R.: Use of stable isotopes to determine bioavailability of minerals in human diets using the method of faecal monitoring. Am. J. clin. Nutr. *33:* 2021 (1980).

6 Johnson, P. E.: A mass spectrometric method for use of stable isotopes as tracers in studies of iron, zinc and copper absorption in human subjects. J. Nutr. *112:* 1414 (1982).

7 King, J. C.; Reynolds, W. L.; Margen, S.: Absorption of stable isotopes of iron, copper and zinc during oral contraceptive use. Am. J. clin. Nutr. *31:* 1198 (1978).

8 Schoenheimer, R.: The dynamic state of body constituents, pp. 3–78 (Harvard University Press, Boston 1942).

9 Smith, D. L.: Determination of stable isotopes of calcium in biological fluids by fast atom bombardment mass spectrometry. Analyt. Chem. *55:* 2391 (1983).

10 Solomons, N. W.: Biological availability of zinc in humans. Am. J. clin. Nutr. *35:* 1048 (1982).

11 Turnland, J. R.; Michel, M. C.; Keyes, W. R.; King, J. C.; Margen, S.: Use of enriched stable isotopes to determine zinc and iron absorption in elderly men. Am. J. clin. Nutr. *35:* 1033 (1982).

M. J. Jackson, Dept. of Medicine, University of Liverpool, P.O. Box 147, Liverpool L69 3BX (UK)

Dietze, Grünert, Kleinberger, Wolfram (eds.), Clinical Nutrition and Metabolic Research. Proc. 7th Congr. ESPEN, Munich 1985, pp. 247–259 (Karger, Basel 1986)

Resting and Postprandial Fuel Utilization in Normal and Diabetic Humans[1]

O. E. Owen, M. A. Mozzoli, S. Caprio, G. Boden

Depts. of Medicine and General Clinical Research Center, Temple University School of Medicine, Philadelphia, Pa., USA

Introduction

Type II (non-insulin dependent) diabetes mellitus is characterized by obesity and disturbed carbohydrate, fat, and protein metabolism. Before the adverse effects of trauma on macronutrient metabolism in type II diabetic patients can be evaluated, the abnormalities related to type II diabetes independent of other stresses must be defined.

Recent refinements and automatization have advanced the technique of indirect calorimetry so that measurements can readily be made to determine the energy requirements and the nature and quantities of macronutrients oxidized in resting postabsorptive and postprandial periods. We used indirect calorimetry to determine the resting metabolic requirements and total body oxidation and storage rates of carbohydrate and fat before and after a standard mixed-meal breakfast in obese volunteers and obese type II diabetic patients.[2]

Methods

Six type II diabetic patients were selected for this study from our hospital and Diabetic Clinic. Their body weights ranged from 130–195% of ideal body weight (table I). None were dependent on insulin for the prevention of ketonuria. Nonetheless, the metabolic control of

[1] This work was supported in part by U.S. Public Health Service Grants AM25386, AM19397, and RR00349, General Clinical Research Centers Branch, NIH.

[2] Part of this data has been previously published [1].

Table I. Clinical characteristics (mean ± SEM)

Subjects	Sex	Age years	% of ideal body weight	Duration of diabetes years	Fasting plasma glucose mg/dl	Insulin dose units/day	Fasting serum C-peptide pmol/ml
Type II	0M/6F	42 ± 4	160 ± 12	7 ± 3.0	184 ± 10	69 ± 23	0.52 ± 0.23
Obese controls	1M/6F	43 ± 3	147 ± 8		94 ± 4		0.38 ± 0.04

all these patients was poor. There was persistent fasting hyperglycemia despite taking oral chlorpropamide 500–750 mg/day and receiving diet and exercise recommendations. Four of these patients (C.C., M.C., S.Mc., and E.U.) received supplementary subcutaneous insulin daily to aid in controlling their symptomatic hyperglycemia. However, all were free of acute illnesses. 7 age and weight matched non-diabetic volunteers served as controls.

Experimental Design

Patients and controls were hospitalized on the General Clinical Research Center at Temple University Hospital. They were placed on a weight-maintaining diet of approximately 22 kcal/kg/day (carbohydrate 48%, fat 33%, protein 18%). Breakfast, lunch, supper, and bedtime snack were served at 8 am, 12 noon, 5 pm and 10 pm, respectively. After an 11 h overnight fast, plasma glucose, free fatty acids (FFA) and serum C-peptide concentrations were measured simultaneously with respiratory exchange rates of O_2 and CO_2, and urinary excretion rates of glucose and nitrogen (indirect calorimetry) [12] at −15 and 0 min before and every 30 min for 4 h after consuming a mixed breakfast (11 kcal/kg; carbohydrate 43%, fat 42%, protein 15%) during a 10-min period. In addition, plasma total lipids were measured at 0 and 240 min. The last chlorpropamide doses were given 24 h before the breakfast tests, and insulin doses were withheld the morning of the studies. During the breakfast studies, physical activity and smoking were prohibited. Immediately after the breakfast studies were completed, insulin and/or chlorpropamide therapy was administered.

Indirect Calorimetry

Respiratory gaseous exchange rates were measured with a Beckman Metabolic Measurement Cart (Beckman, Schiller Park, Illinois). The operational aspects of this machine have been detailed by Foss et al. [2]. Urine was collected to measure glucose and nitrogen excretion before and after breakfast. The non-protein respiratory quotients (npRQ) were determined by subtracting the oxygen consumed and CO_2 produced during protein oxidation which was calculated from the urinary nitrogen excretion. Determinations of carbohydrate and lipid oxidation rates were made using the npRQ tables of Cathcart and Cuthbertson [3]. The amounts of carbohydrate and fat oxidized during the breakfast tests were calculated by determining the areas under the carbohydrate and fat oxidation curves. Glucose intracellular storage was calculated by the following formula:

Glucose intracellular storage (g/4 h) = intake –
(oxidation + excretion + quantity of glucose left in extracellular space).

Glucose volume of distribution in the diabetic patients and normal subjects has been reported as being between 25–30% of body weight. We used 27% of the body weight for the glucose volume of extracellular distribution [4–6]. The amount of the glucose remaining in this space was calculated from the differences between the plasma glucose concentrations at times 0 and 240 min multiplied by the volumes of distribution. All values were corrected to 1.73 m^2 body surface area.

Chemical Analyses

Plasma and urine glucose concentrations were determined using a Beckman Glucose Analyzer (Beckman Instruments, Inc., Fullerton, CA). Plasma FFA were extracted by the Dole and Meinertz technique [7], and concentrations determined by a modification of the colorimetric method of Lorch and Gey [8]. Serum C-peptide concentrations were determined using radioimmunoassay kits (Novo, Copenhagen, Denmark) [9]. The detection limit of C-peptide was 0.01 pmol/ml; the intraassay and interassay variations were 4% and 6%, respectively. Urinary nitrogen was measured by the micro-Kjeldahl method [10].

Statistical Methods

Unless otherwise stated, all values are presented as mean ± SEM. Basal values for the breakfast studies were calculated by averaging −15 min and 0 min time values. Statistical differences among different studies were calculated by using Student's t-test for paired or unpaired samples and analysis of variance for repeated measurements [11].

Results

Circulating Glucose, C-Peptide and FFA Concentrations before and after Breakfast (Fig. 1)

Overnight fasting glucose concentrations in type II diabetic patients were significantly greater than those observed in the obese controls (184 ± 10 vs. 94 ± 4 mg/dl; $p < 0.001$), and all plasma glucose concentrations remained high throughout the breakfast test. Fasting serum C-peptide concentrations in the type II diabetic patients were comparable to those observed in the obese controls (0.52 ± 0.23 pmol/ml vs. 0.38 ± 0.04 pmol/ml; $p > 0.4$). However, postcibal values were lower at 30, 60, 90, 120, and 150 min than obese controls ($p < 0.005$). Further, the peak value of 0.92 ± 0.31 pmol/ml reached at 150 min postcibal was not statistically different ($p < 0.1$) than the basal value in these patients. Overnight fasting and postcibal plasma FFA concentrations in the type II diabetic patients were not significantly different than the obese control values.

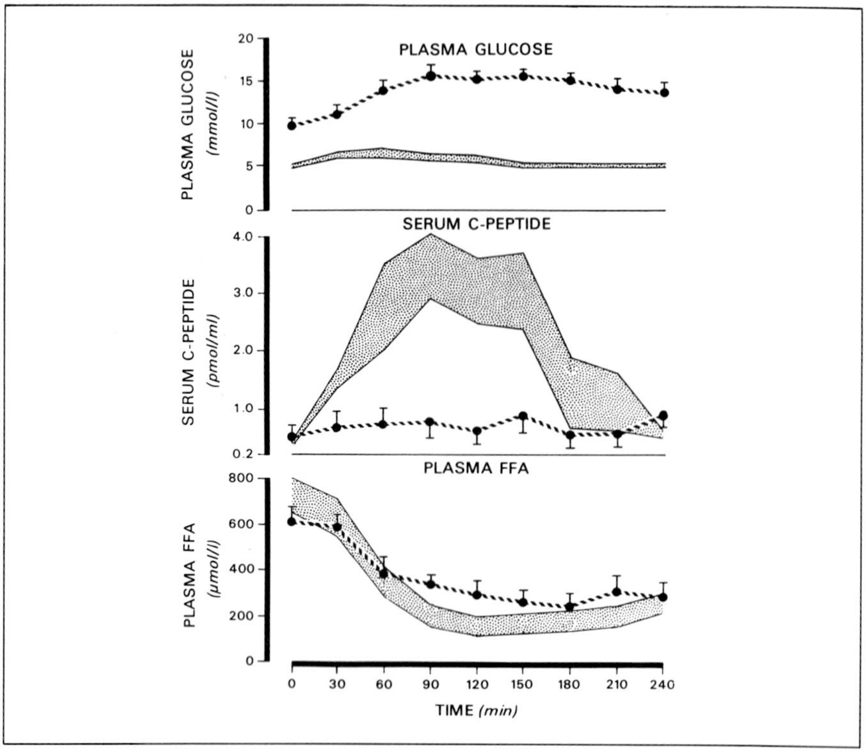

Fig. 1. Circulating concentrations of glucose, C-peptide, and FFA in response to the breakfast in obese controls and type II diabetic patients before breakfast. The shaded area represents one standard error above and below the mean observations in obese controls. Results are expressed as mean ± SEM.

Resting Metabolic Rate (RMR) and Nature and Quantities of Fuels Oxidized (Fig. 2)

The measured RMR of the type II diabetic patients and the obese controls in this study fall within our previously observed 95% confidence limits for lean and obese non-diabetic women after an overnight fast [12]. Since body weight is highly correlated with other measures of active protoplasmic tissue (body surface area, lean body mass, fat-free mass, etc.) [12] and is the most accurately and easily determined variable of body size, we chose to relate RMR to body weight.

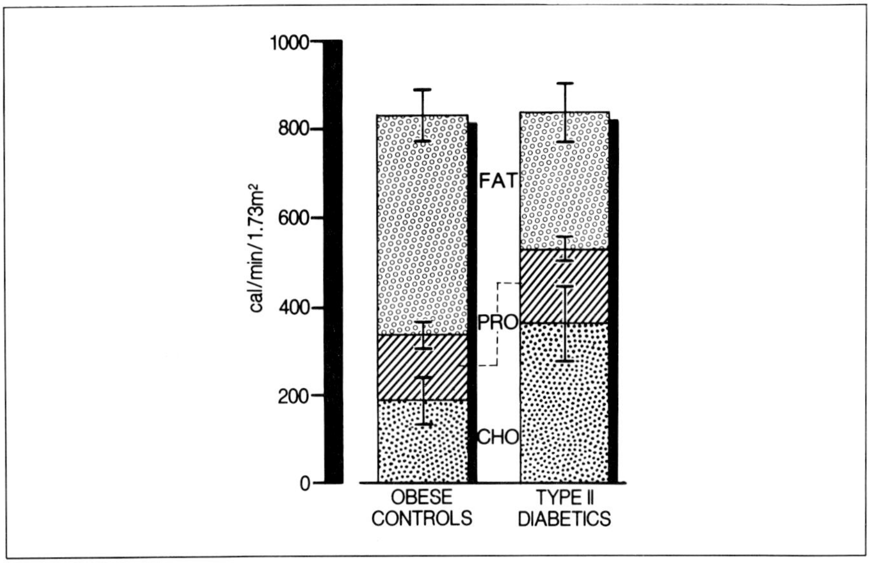

Fig. 2. The resting metabolic rate and the nature and quantity of fuels oxidized in obese controls and type II diabetic patients after an overnight fast.

The quantities of carbohydrate (54 ± 16 vs. 114 ± 69 mg/min), fat (68 ± 9 vs. 63 ± 9 mg/min), and protein (42 ± 9 vs. 54 ± 12 mg/min) oxidized in obese controls and type II diabetic patient were similar.

Non-Protein Respiratory Quotient (npRQ) (Fig. 3)

In obese controls the resting npRQ was 0.77 ± 0.01. It promptly reached a peak value of 0.94 ± 0.03 30 min postcibal and declined slowly thereafter. This change in npRQ was significant ($p < 0.05$). Although there was no statistical numerical difference in the npRQ values between type II diabetic patients and obese controls before and after breakfast, probably because of the limited number of controls and patients studied, there was a physiological difference: the npRQ rose after breakfast in the obese controls, but no significant npRQ changes occurred after breakfast in the type II diabetic patients.

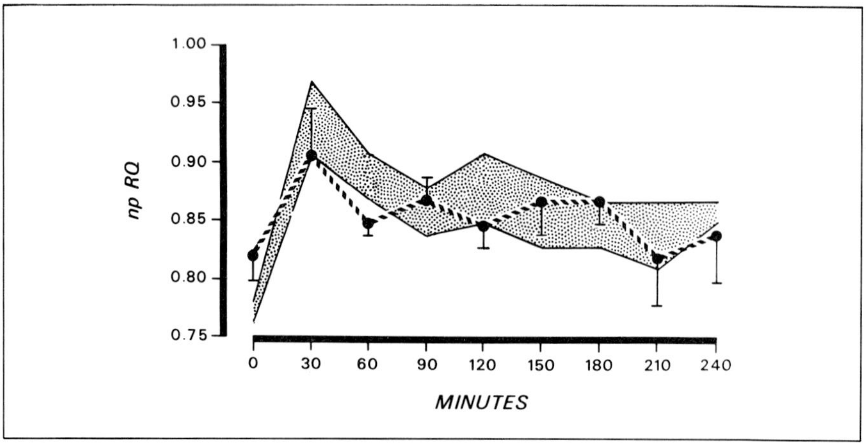

Fig. 3. The npRQ in obese controls and type II diabetic patients after an overnight fast before and after eating breakfast. The faded area represents 1 standard deviation above and below the mean observations for the obese controls. The results are expressed as mean ± SEM.

Postprandial Carbohydrate and Fat Oxidation Rates (Figs. 4 and 5)

From the npRQ data the oxidation rates of carbohydrate and lipid can be calculated. Figure 4 shows a temporal relationship of glucose and fat oxidation in the obese controls and the type II diabetic patients during the study. In the obese controls carbohydrate oxidation was rapidly augmented and fat oxidation was simultaneously suppressed. These acute and reciprocal postcibal changes in the rate and nature of fuels oxidized did not develop in the type II diabetic patients.

The total glucose disposed during the study is shown in figure 5. Before and after breakfast, type II diabetic patients and obese controls oxidized comparable amounts of carbohydrate (30 ± 6 g/4 h vs. 29 ± 2 g/4 h; $p > 0.2$) and fat (9 ± 1 g/4 h vs. 10 ± 1 g/4 h; $p > 0.2$). On the other hand, urinary glucose excretion amounted to 10 ± 4 g/h in the type II diabetic patients whereas the obese controls were free of glycosuria. The amount of glucose left in the extracellular space was also different between the two groups. The type II diabetic patients accumulated 20 ± 4 g/4 h of glucose in the extracellular space. Although the amount of carbohydrate stored in type II diabetic patients (65 ± 10 g/4 h) appeared to be less than the quantity of carbohydrate stored in the obese controls (83 ± 8 g/4 h), these numerical values were not significantly different ($p < 0.2$).

Discussion

We combined measurements of plasma glucose and FFA and C-peptide concentrations with indirect calorimetry before and after a mixed meal breakfast to determine carbohydrate and lipid metabolism in obese controls and type II diabetic patients. These techniques allowed us to estimate the quantities of carbohydrate, protein, and fat oxidized in the basal resting state and to determine the amount of carbohydrate present in the extracellular space, excreted in the urine, and stored in the intracellular space during the postprandial state.

The resting metabolic requirements of type II diabetic patients were normal for their body sizes. Furthermore, the nature and quantity of carbohydrate, protein, and fat oxidized were comparable between obese controls and type II diabetic patients (fig. 2). Specifically basal glucose oxidation after an overnight fast was not curtailed in mild type II diabetic patients with hyperglycemia. Thus, our results agreed with the results of other investigators who showed normal rates of glucose oxidation in obese type II diabetic patients with hyperglycemia [13–15]. Normal resting rates

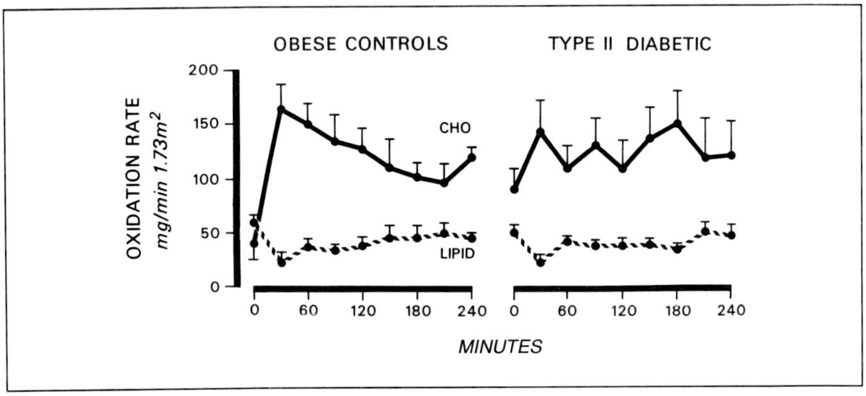

Fig. 4. Carbohydrate and fat oxidation rates in obese controls and type II diabetic patients before and after breakfast.

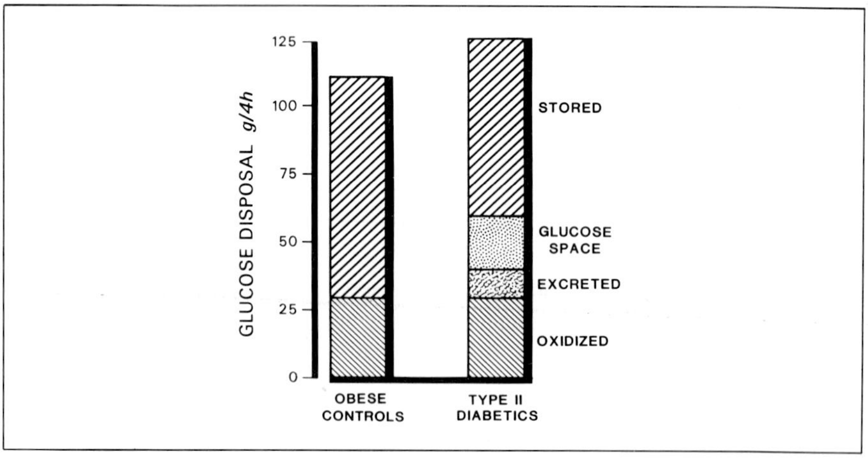

Fig. 5. Total glucose disposal rates (g/4 h) in obese controls and type II diabetic patients following breakfast. Results are not corrected to 1.73 m^2 BSA.

of glucose oxidation after an overnight fast were in part due to persistent consumption of large quantities of glucose by the central nervous system, a tissue that appears to be relatively non-insulin dependent. Another reason for normal rates of glucose oxidation in our patients was their hyperglycemia which is known to compensate for hypoinsulinemia of type II diabetic patients [16, 17]. Although the fasting and postprandial C-peptide concentrations were abnormally low for the plasma glucose concentrations in our type II diabetic patients, plasma FFA before and after breakfast were comparable to those present in the obese controls. Thus, in addition to maintaining normal rates of glucose oxidation in the resting fasted state, hyperglycemia modulates lipolysis. Our data show that the product of circulating high glucose and low insulin (C-peptide) concentrations, with their accompanying transport and receptor expressions [18] maintain normal rates of fuel utilization after an overnight fast in obese type II diabetic patients.

The obese controls rapidly increased glucose oxidation from 26 ± 8 to 70 ± 15 mg/kg/min 30 min postcibal (Δ 269%). The augmented glucose oxidation was transient in the obese controls and rose and fell in parallel with C-peptide concentrations (fig. 4). Concurrently with the increased and decreased glucose oxidation rates, there were reciprocal decreased and increased fat oxidation rates which changed from 33 mg/

kg/min antecibal to 20 mg/kg/min 30 min postcibal and returning toward basal values thereafter. Thus, in obese controls, a tight reciprocal relationship developed postprandially between glucose and fat oxidation. In contrast, the quantities of glucose and fat oxidized by the type II diabetic patients following breakfast were clearly abnormal. The acute and reciprocal changes in glucose and fat oxidation were absent in the diabetic patients. Nonetheless, the slightly increased antecibal glucose oxidation rate persisted throughout the 4 h after breakfast. Therefore, the total quantity of glucose oxidized during the 4 h after breakfast was comparable in the obese controls and type II diabetic patients. Similarly, the fat oxidation over the 4 h postcibal period was also comparable between the two groups.

A large proportion of ingested nutrients are normally disposed by non-oxidative (storage) pathways; specifically, when carbohydrate, protein, and fat intake exceeds energy requirements, these macronutrients are directly or indirectly stored.

In this study, we calculated the amount of glucose stored by assuming that 100% of the ingested carbohydrate was absorbed from the gut during the 4 h after breakfast (fig. 5). The quantities of glucose oxidized, excreted in urine and left in extracellular space were determined. The remaining quantity was considered stored. Although glucose stored in the type II diabetic patients was less than that observed in the obese controls, the difference was not statistically significant. Thus, the quantities of glucose oxidized and stored were roughly comparable in the obese controls and type II diabetic patients. However, hyperglycemia and glycosuria occurred only in the diabetic patients. Based on a retrospective analysis of the glucose disposal data, the type II diabetic patients in this study should be considered as having mild diabetes.

In a previous study [19], we showed that obese type II diabetic patients with more impaired glycemic control (fasting plasma glucose concentration 267 ± 24 mg/dl, glycosuria 29 ± 6 g/24 h but no ketonuria) than those in this report had normal resting glucose oxidation rates after an overnight fast. Following a mixed-meal breakfast, both resting glucose oxidation and storage were impaired. However, the defect in storage had a greater impact than oxidation on impaired glucose disposal in these moderately severe type II diabetic patients [19].

In another report we used indirect calorimetry to study type I diabetic patients during ketoacidosis [20]. In these patients, plasma glucose, FFA, and total ketone body concentrations were 25 ± 6 mM (450 ± 108 mg/

dl), 1.74 ± 0.24 mM, and 20.83 ± 2.93 mM, respectively. These patients were in a florid catabolic state. Body stores were being catabolized, but glucose oxidation to CO_2 and H_2O was nil, and severe glycosuria and ketonuria were depleting the body of carbohydrate, protein, and fat [21].

Figure 6 schematically summarizes postprandial glucose metabolism in a broad spectrum of diabetic patients. In this scheme, glucose delivery from food intake is considered constant [22, 23]. Similarities probably exist among all of the macronutrients (glucose, fat, and protein) metabolized by type I and II diabetic patients.

Glucose oxidation and storage are comparable in obese controls and type II diabetic patients with mild abnormalities in carbohydrate metabolism. However, glucose accumulates in the extracellular space and glycosuria occurs only in the diabetic patients. Thus, hyperglycemia is the first abnormality in carbohydrate metabolism that develops in diabetes mellitus. As the diabetic state deteriorates, the next abnormality detectable in carbohydrate metabolism is impaired glucose storage. Augmented lipolysis and subsequent ketogenesis develop as the diabetic state worsens, and glucose oxidation progressively diminishes. Heightened rates of recycling of lactate and pyruvate develop simultaneously with augmented gluconeogenesis from amino acids and glycerol, and inappropriate rates of

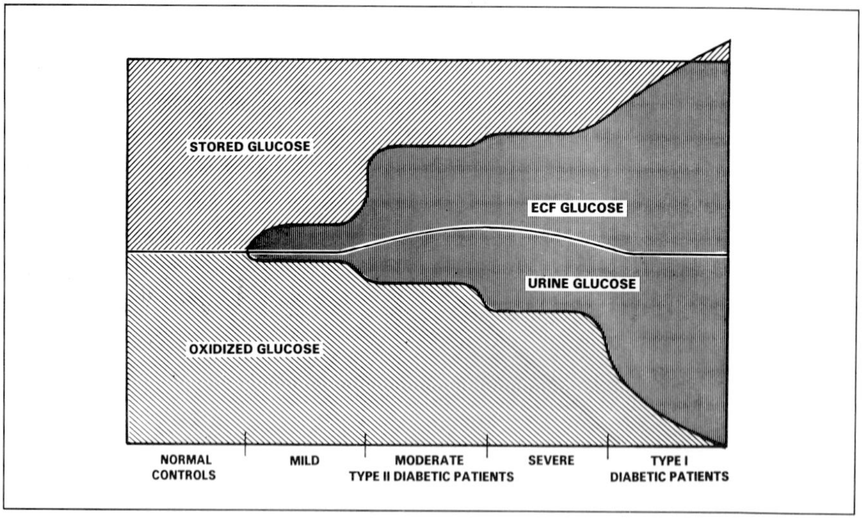

Fig. 6. Schematic presentation of glucose disposal rates in normal controls and patients with various degrees of deterioration.

ketogenesis from FFA occur. Eventually the insulin secretory capacity is 90% or more compromised [24], and food intake can no longer reverse catabolism. Inappropriately elevated hepatic production rates of glucose and ketone bodies coupled with increased FFA mobilization (and concurrent proteolysis) flood the extracellular fluids with an overabundance of fuels that compete as oxidative substrates. The renal capacities to conserve glucose and ketone bodies are exceeded, and progressive glycosuria and ketonuria develop, reflecting loss of carbohydrate, protein, and fat from the body.

Conclusions

Type II and type I diabetes mellitus can be viewed as a spectrum of metabolic disorders progressing from mildly impaired anabolism manifested by postprandial accumulation of metabolites in the extracellular space to grossly augmented catabolism indicated by diabetic ketoacidosis. The stress of trauma and sepsis with its accompanying catabolic hormones combined with the disposal challenges accompanying parenteral or enteral nutrition can convert mild type II diabetes with antecedent hyperglycemia, glycosuria and storage defects into severe hyperglycemia with ketoacidosis.

References

1 Caprio, S.; Ray, T.; Boden, G.; Reichard, Jr., G.; Shuman, C.; Smith, R.; Mozzoli, M.; Dayal, V.; Hoeldtke, R.; Owen, O.: Improvement of metabolic control in diabetic patients during mebendazole administration: Preliminary studies. Diabetologia *27:* 52–55 (1984).
2 Foss, M.; Vlachokosta, F.; Cunningham, L.; Aoki, T.: Restoration of glucose homeostasis in insulin-dependent diabetic subjects. An inducible process. Diabetes *31:* 46–52 (1982).
3 Cathcart, E.; Cuthbertson, D.: The composition and distribution of the fatty substances of the human subject. J. Physiol. *72:* 349–360 (1931).
4 Holdsworth, C.: The gut and oral glucose tolerance. Gut *10:* 442–527 (1969).
5 Shreeve, W.; Baker, N.; Miller, M.; Shipley, R.; Incefy, G.; Craig, J.: C^{14} studies in carbohydrate metabolism. II. The oxidation of glucose in diabetic human subjects. Metabolism *5:* 22–23 (1956).
6 Forbath, N.; Hetenyi, Y.: Glucose dynamics in normal subjects and diabetic patients before and after a glucose load. Diabetes *15:* 778–789 (1966).

7 Dole, V.; Meinertz, H.: Microdetermination of long-chain fatty acids in plasma and tissues. J. biol. Chem. *223:* 2595–2599 (1960).
8 Lorch, E.; Gey, K.: Photometric 'titration' of free fatty acids with Technicon Autoanalyzer. Analyt. Biochem. *16:* 244–252 (1966).
9 Heding, L.: Radioimmunological determination of human C-peptide in serum. Diabetologia *11:* 541–548 (1975).
10 Koch, F.; McMeekim, T.: A new direct nesslerization micro Kjeldahl method and a modification of the Nessler-Folin reagent for ammonia. J. Am. chem. Soc. *46:* 2066–2071 (1924).
11 Snedecor, G.; Cochran, W.: Statistical methods (Iowa State University Press, Ames 1967).
12 Owen, O. E.; Kavle, E.; Owen, R. S.; Polansky, M.; Caprio, S.; Schmidt, M. L.; Mozzoli, M. A.; Kendrick, Z. V.; Bushman, M. C.; Boden, G.: A reappraisal of caloric requirements of healthy women (submitted for publication).
13 Felber, P.; Magnenat, G.; Casthelaz, M.; Geser, C.; Muller-Hess, R.; de Kalbermatten, N.; Ebiner, J.; Curchod, B.; Jequier, E.: Carbohydrate and lipid oxidation in normal and diabetic subjects. Diabetes *26:* 693–699 (1977).
14 Meyer, H.; Curchod, B.; Maeder, E.; Pahud, P.; Jequier, E.; Felber, J.: Modifications of glucose storage and oxidation in nonobese diabetics, measured by continuous indirect calorimetry. Diabetes *29:* 752–756 (1980).
15 Felber, J.; Meyer, H.; Curchod, B.; Iselin, H.; Rousselle, J.; Maeder, E.; Pahud, P.; Jequier, E.: Glucose storage and oxidation in different degrees of human obesity measured by continuous indirect calorimetry. Diabetologia *20:* 39–44 (1981).
16 Jeanrenaud, B.; Renold, A.: Studies on rat adipose tissue in vitro. IV. Metabolic patterns produced in rat adipose tissue by varying insulin and glucose concentrations independently from each other. J. biol. Chem. *234:* 3082–3087 (1959).
17 Thiebaud, D.; Jacot, E.; DeFronzo, R.; Maeder, E.; Jequier, E.; Felber, J.: The effect of graded doses of insulin on total glucose uptake, glucose oxidation, and glucose storage in man. Diabetes *31:* 957–963 (1982).
18 Cryer, P. E.: Does central nervous system adaptation to antecedent glycemia occur in patients with insulin-dependent diabetes mellitus? Ann. intern. Med. *103:* 284–286 (1985).
19 Boden, G.; Ray, T.; Smith, R.; Owen, O.: Carbohydrate oxidation and storage in obese non-insulin-dependent diabetic patients. Effects of improving glycemic control. Diabetes *32:* 982–987 (1983).
20 Owen, O.; Trapp, V.; Reichard, G., Jr.; Mozzoli, M.; Smith, R.; Boden, G.: Effects of therapy on the nature and quantity of fuels oxidized during diabetic ketoacidosis. Diabetes *29:* 365–372 (1980).
21 Owen, O.; Licht, J.; Sapir, D.: Renal function and effects of partial rehydration during diabetic ketoacidosis. Diabetes *30:* 510–518 (1981).
22 Owen, O.; Block, B.; Patel, M.; Boden, G.; McDonough, M.; Kreulen, T.; Shuman, C.; Reichard, G.: Human splanchnic metabolism during diabetic ketoacidosis. Metabolism *26:* 381–398 (1977).
23 Owen, O.; Reichard, G., Jr.; Boden, G.; Patel, M.; Trapp, V.: Interrelationships among key tissues in the utilization of metabolic substrates; in Katzen, Mahler, Diabetes, obesity and vascular disease. Metabolic and molecular interrelationships.

Part 2. Advances in modern nutrition. Chapter 15, pp. 517–550 (John Wiley & Sons, New York 1978).

24 Ward, K.; Beard, J.; Halter, J.; Pfeifer, M.; Porte, D., Jr.: Pathophysiology of insulin secretion in non-insulin-dependent diabetes mellitus. Diabetes Care *7*(5): 491-502 (1984).

Oliver E. Owen, MD, Temple U. Hospital, 3401 N. Broad Street, Philadelphia, PA 19140 (USA)

Dietze, Grünert, Kleinberger, Wolfram (eds.), Clinical Nutrition and Metabolic Research. Proc. 7th Congr. ESPEN, Munich 1985, pp. 260–268 (Karger, Basel 1986)

Glucose versus Sugar Substitutes in Parenteral Nutrition of Diabetics

M. Wicklmayr, G. Dietze, J. Grunst, K. Rett, B. Sauter, H. Mehnert

III. Med. Dept., Schwabing Hospital, and II. Med. Dept., Hospital Red Cross, Munich, FRG

Complete parenteral nutrition of metabolically healthy subjects and diabetics means substitution of carbohydrates, lipids, and protein in a percentage of 45, 35, and 20 of total calories as in normal oral food uptake. The only way to apply carbohydrates intravenously is through monosaccharides, most simply as glucose. However, in diabetics this is not possible without problems since parenteral nutrition in most cases becomes necessary in times of immobilization, acute illness, or postoperative stress. Thereby the impaired diabetic glucose metabolism rather deteriorates: noninsulin-dependent diabetics type II now need exogenous insulin in most cases, insulin-dependent diabetics need more insulin.

It should be emphasized that intermittent insulin therapy at present should be done exclusively with human insulin, because it is less antigenic. Thereby a clinically relevant formation of antibodies can be prevented, which would be a serious disadvantage in the future if the patient should need permanent insulin therapy.

The amount of additional insulin varies from patient to patient and is closely correlated with the actual clinical state: if this is being improved, for instance by an effective therapy of an infection, the additional insulin requirement promptly decreases.

Insulin therapy in parenteral nutrition of diabetics should preferably be managed by continuous intravenous infusion using a pump. In this context it is also important to continuously infuse the glucose for 24 h as well in order to avoid rapid changes of insulin requirement.

However, alterations of blood glucose levels can never be avoided even if insulin therapy is correct and adequate. Hereby hyperglycemia, since not acutely life threatening, should be recognized in time and treated sufficiently in a well-organized clinic. Much more dangerous are intermittent hypoglycemic states, since these can occur without any clinical symptoms in the severely ill patient and since they lead to irreversible cerebral damage within a few hours.

Because of these problems, fructose could be used instead of glucose in parenteral nutrition of diabetics, since fructose increases blood glucose level only by a small amount [1–4]. In figure 1 the course of blood glucose

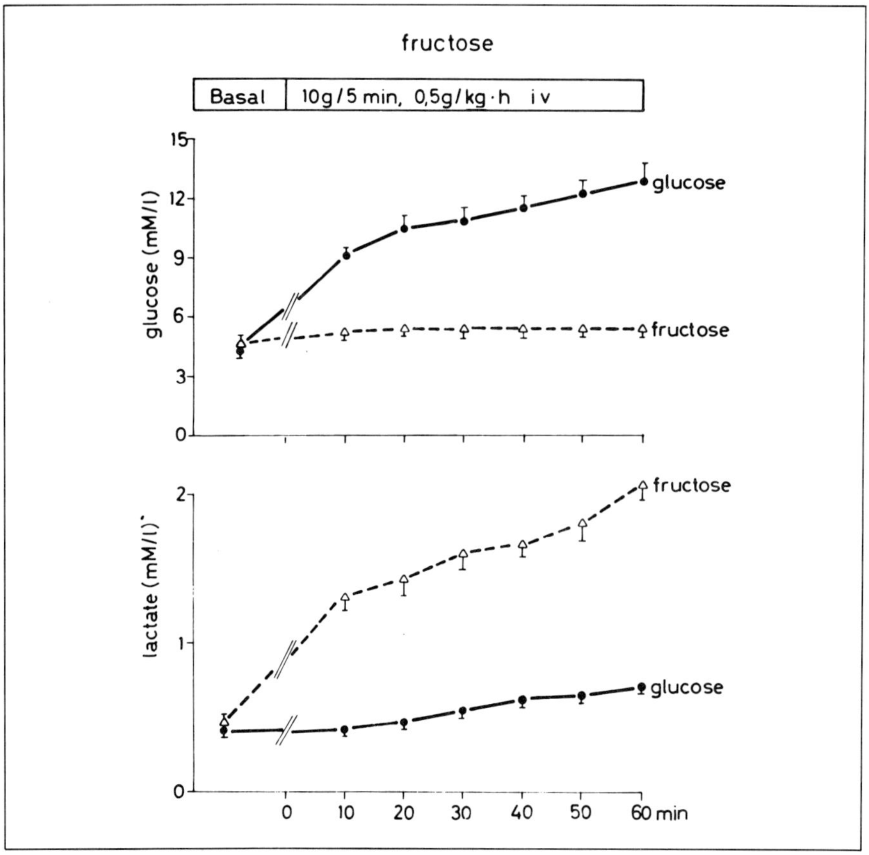

Fig. 1. Arterial concentrations of glucose and lactate in healthy volunteers during an intravenous infusion of equimolar doses of glucose (n = 6) and fructose (n = 6).

during an i.v. infusion of identical amounts of glucose and fructose in healthy volunteers is shown. While glucose leads to a marked increase of blood glucose, there is almost no change during fructose infusion. There are two explanations for this phenomenon: Initially the infused fructose has to be taken up by the liver and will be transformed to glucose in the metabolic pathway of gluconeogenesis with some delay [5–7]. In addition as recent studies have shown, fructose is directly utilized in relevant amounts by skeletal muscle [8]. Fructose concentrations in arterial and deep venous blood of the forearm in one healthy volunteer and one insulin-dependent diabetic are shown in figure 2. As indicated by the constant

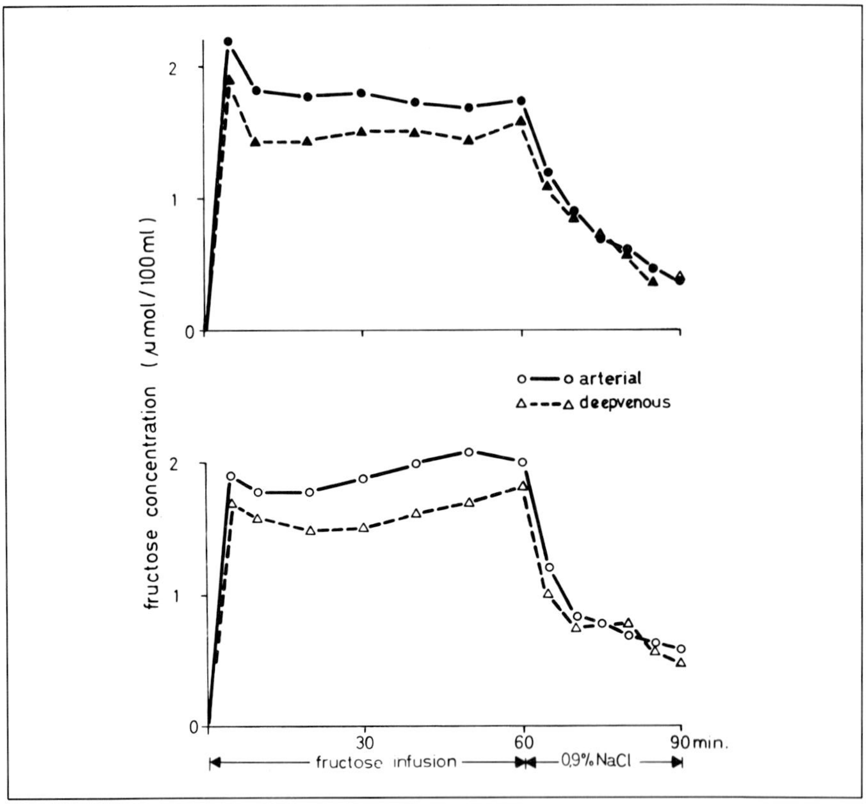

Fig. 2. Arterial and forearm deep venous concentrations of fructose in a healthy volunteer (•) and an insulin-dependent diabetic in acute insulin deficiency (o) before, during and after intravenous infusion of fructose (0.5 g/kg BW × h).

positive arterial deep venous difference, fructose is taken up by the muscle during the 1-h infusion period. That the fructose taken up is really metabolized is shown by the fact that there is no back diffusion after the end of the fructose infusion. Grossly calculated, approximately 10% of the infused fructose is utilized by the muscle. Together with the delayed hepatic transformation of fructose into glucose, this finding of the direct peripheral fructose utilization may explain the comparably weak impact of fructose on blood glucose levels.

Thus with regard to the blood glucose response, fructose would be the ideal alternative carbohydrate in parenteral nutrition of diabetics. However, caused by its rapid hepatic metabolization, the parenteral application of fructose is followed by several metabolic reactions.

Figure 1 shows the behavior of peripheral venous lactate levels under the influence of equimolar amounts of high dose fructose and glucose in healthy volunteers. While glucose causes only a small lactate rise, the application of fructose leads to a considerable increase [5, 9–11] which is secondary to the rapid glycolytic breakdown of fructose in the liver [11, 12]. This hyperlactemia must by no means be taken for lactic acidosis, since fructose application alone does not lead to changes in blood pH. In figure 3 the possible causes of elevated lactate levels are shown schematically. Clinical relevance is given only if hyperlactemia is accompanied by acidosis like in peripheral oxygen deficiency. Other reasons for hyperlactemia are in part physiological like in states of muscular activity, increased fat oxidation, and oral carbohydrate intake. In addition, hyperlactemias

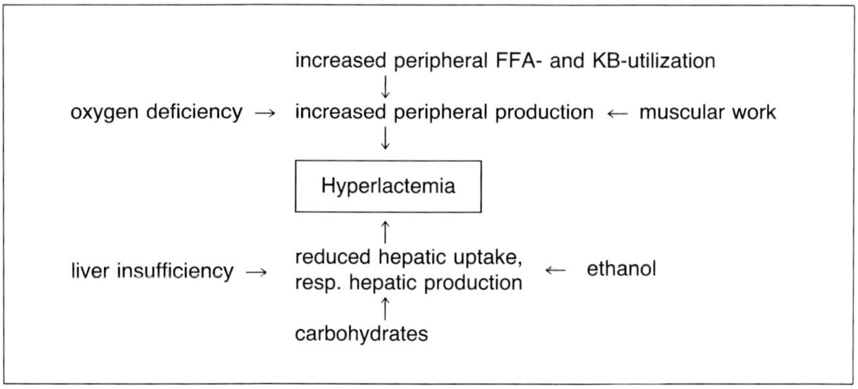

Fig. 3. Possible factors leading to hyperlactemia.

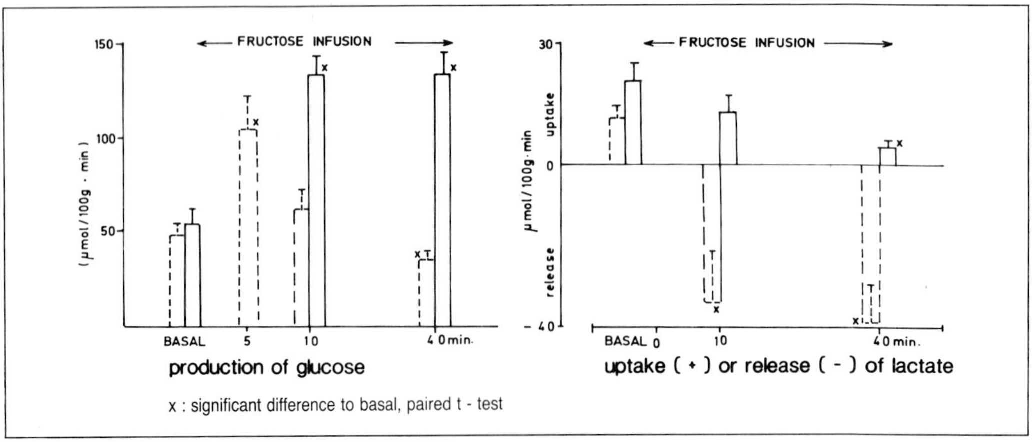

Fig. 4. Hepatic uptake/production of glucose and lactate during an intravenous infusion of fructose (0.5 g/kg BW × h) in healthy volunteers (n = 5) and surgical patients (n = 5).

are seen in disturbed liver function and after alcohol ingestion. In conclusion, the elevated lactate level under the influence of fructose is not primarily negative. However, in states of reduced hepatic lactate clearance or peripheral oxygen deficiency, fructose should not be used.

Since physiological blood fructose levels are near zero, while there is a highly active fructose phosphorylation system in the liver [13, 14], parenteral fructose application leads to a marked dose-dependent decrease of hepatic energy-rich phosphates as was shown in the isolated rat liver by Bode [15]. This phenomenon can also be seen in vivo in man. At arterial fructose levels of about 2 mmol/l which develop during high dose fructose infusion, fructose is rapidly taken up by the liver and transformed to glucose, thus leading to an initially doubled hepatic glucose production in healthy volunteers. Thereby blood glucose level is slightly elevated, which leads to a small insulin secretion. This in turn inhibits hepatic glucose output again and leads to lactate production from glycolytic cleavage of fructose. Basal uptake of lactate by the liver is changed into an increasing lactate release. However, in surgical patients with their known impaired insulin sensitivity, the initially increased hepatic glucose production from fructose persists in spite of the same insulin secretion. Correspondingly less lactate is produced (fig. 4). This different hepatic metabolization of fructose in healthy volunteers and surgical patients is also reflected by different hepatic oxygen consumption, which increases

Table I. Effect of fructose infusion (0.5 g/kg BW × h) on hepatic oxygen uptake (ml/100 g × min) in healthy volunteers (N), diabetics in acute insulin deficiency (D), and surgical patients (OP)

Basal		Fructose infusion	
		10 min	40 min
N	3.9 ± 0.6	6.0 ± 0.9*	3.6 ± 0.5
D	4.8 ± 0.6	6.8 ± 0.9*	7.1 ± 1.1*
OP	4.0 ± 0.8	6.3 ± 1.0*	6.5 ± 1.0*

* $p < 0.05$, paired t-test versus basal

initially in both groups when fructose is transformed into glucose thereby consuming energy. Then in the healthy group increased hepatic oxygen uptake is renormalized, since the fructose taken up is now transformed to lactate, thus glycolytically producing energy. This is not the case in insulin-deprived diabetics and in surgical patients, where increased hepatic oxygen consumption persists (table I).

Increased energy metabolism of the liver can also be seen from the hepatic uric acid production, which is raised in healthy volunteers as well as in diabetics (table II). Elevation of uric acid levels by fructose was described 20 years ago [16–18]. It is due to both increased hepatic production [19, 20] and a decreased renal excretion [21]. However, clinically relevant elevations of uric acid levels are most probably very rare.

Table II. Effect of a fructose infusion (0.5 g/kg BW × h) on hepatic uric acid production (μmol/100 g × min) in healthy volunteers (N, n = 6) and in diabetics in acute insulin deficiency (D, n = 6)

Basal		Fructose infusion	
		10 min	40 min
N	0.4 ± 0.3	2.1 ± 0.2*	1.1 ± 0.5*
D	0.1 ± 0.3	1.5 ± 0.3*	1.3 ± 0.2*

* $p < 0.05$ versus basal, paired t-test

In summary: At a high fructose dosage, producing fructose levels of 2 mmol/l, hyperlactemia, increased hepatic energy turnover, and uric acid production develop. For xylitol in general the same side effects are known [22]. These effects are strictly dose-dependent. That means that they are negligible when fructose or xylitol are applied in limited amounts.

This became possible in the last years. The first reason is that in parenteral nutrition of diabetics, lipids can be used [23], which allows a reduction of the part of carbohydrates in total calories. Secondly, we have learned that parenteral nutrition should be given around the clock to reduce the acute carbohydrate load. A further step was the use of a combination of glucose, fructose, and xylitol, which produces a reduction in the dose-dependent side effects of the individual monosaccharides despite of full caloric supply. It was shown that the glucose, fructose, xylitol mixture leads to lower blood glucose levels in diabetics – although less insulin substitution was required [24]. In severely ill patients, total parenteral nutrition including lipids and fructose, glucose, xylitol infusions had no relevant impact on lactate and glucose levels in the blood (table III). The fact of only minimally increased lactate concentration is explained by the low fructose level of about 0.3 mmol/l. This is made possible because of the continuous 24-h infusion, the use of lipids covering 35 % of total calories, and because of the use of the glucose, fructose, xylitol mixture.

Thus, it can be suggested that parenteral nutrition of diabetics should be done using fructose, glucose, xylitol mixtures, because full caloric substitution of the carbohydrate demand is possible without greater alterations of blood glucose level. Because of the known side effects of fructose and xylitol, they should not be used in states of disturbed lactate homeostasis, when peripheral oxygen supply is impaired or in the case of relevant liver disease. In favor of the use of xylitol are some recent findings indicating that it per se has a positive anabolic effect on protein metabolism [25].

Table III. Arterial concentrations of glucose, fructose, and lactate (mmol/l) in severely ill patients during parenteral nutrition (30 kcal/kg BW × day; F : CH : P = 35 : 45 : 20; CH : FGX)

	1st	3rd	5th	7th day
Glucose	6.2 ± 0.6	7.1 ± 0.8	7.1 ± 0.7	6.8 ± 0.6
Fructose	0	0.35 ± 0.02	0.36 ± 0.7	0.40 ± 0.04
Lactate	0.63 ± 0.01	0.93 ± 0.06	0.77 ± 0.02	0.89 ± 0.001

The question, whether to use glucose or sugar substitutes, cannot be answered in general for all patients. The problem requires a more differentiated approach. If the management of blood glucose concentrations seems difficult, fructose should be preferred; if liver metabolism or lactate homeostasis are disturbed, glucose should be used instead.

References

1 Altwell, M. E.; Waterhouse, C.: Glucose production from fructose. Diabetes *20:* 193 (1971).

2 Bergström, J.; Fürst, P.; Gallays, F.; Hultmann, E.: Aspects of fructose metabolism in normal man. Symp. Clin. Metab. Asp. Fructose, p. 57 (1972).

3 Bünger, R.; Sommer, O.; Walter, G.; Scholz, R.: Fructose, a substrate for energy-yielding metabolism in the heart? Hoppe-Seyler's Z. physiol. Chem. *359:* 819 (1978).

4 Weichselbaum, T. E.; Markgraf, H. W.; Elman, R.: Metabolism of intravenously infused fructose in man. Metabolism *2:* 434 (1953).

5 Dietze, G.; Wicklmayr, M.; Grunst, J.; Mehnert, H.: Die Verwertung von Glukose und Fruktose in Leber und Muskel beim Menschen. Int. J. Vitam. Nutr. Res. *15:* 31–43 (1976).

6 Atwell, M. E.; Waterhouse, C.: Glucose production from fructose. Diabetes *20:* 193 (1971).

7 Öckermann, P. A.; Lundberg, H.: Conversion of fructose to glucose by human jejunum. Absence of galactose to glucose conversion. Biochim. biophys. Acta *105:* 34 (1956).

8 Wicklmayr, M.; Dietze, G.; Günther, B.; Schöps, H.; Hartl, W.; Mehnert, H.: Untersuchungen zur Verwertung von Fruktose durch die menschliche Skelettmuskulatur. Akt. Ernähr. *8:* 192–199 (1983).

9 Andersson, G.; Brohult, J.; Sterner, G.: Increasing metabolic acidosis following fructose infusion in two children. Acta paediat., Stockh. *58:* 301 (1968).

10 Bergström, J.; Hultman, E.; Roch-Norlund, A. E.: Lactic acid accumulation in connection with fructose infusion. Acta med. scand. *184:* 359 (1968).

11 Sestoft, L.; Tenneson, K.; Hansen, F. V.; Damgaard, S. E.: Fructose and glyceraldehyde metabolism in the isolated perfused pig liver. Eur. J. Biochem. *30:* 542 (1972).

12 Dietze, G.: Untersuchungen über den Stoffwechsel der menschlichen Leber mit Hilfe der Kathetertechnik sowie einer neuen Methodik zur Messung der Leberdurchblutung; Habschr. München (1974).

13 Adelman, R. C.; Ballard, F. J.; Weinhouse, S.: Purification and properties of rat liver fructokinase. J. biol. Chem. *242:* 3360 (1967).

14 Heinz, F.; Lamprecht, W.; Kirsch, J.: Enzymes of fructose metabolism in human liver. J. clin. Invest. *47:* 1826 (1968).

15 Bode, C.; Schumacher, H.; Goedell, H.; Zelder, O.; Pelzel, H.: Fructose induced depletion of liver adenine nucleotides in man. Hormone metabol. Res. *3:* 289 (1971).

16 Förster, H.; Mehnert, H.; Alhough, I.: Anstieg der Serumharnsäure nach Verabreichung von Fruktose. Klin. Wschr. *45:* 436 (1967).

17 Heuckenkamp, P. U.; Zöllner, N.: Fructose-induced hyperuricaemin in man. Lancet *i:* 808 (1971).

18 Perheentupa, J.; Raivio, K.: Fructose-induced hyperuricaemia. Lancet *ii:* 9–11 (1967).

19 Grunst, J.; Dietze, G.; Wicklmayr, M.; Holz, S.; Eisenburg, J.; Mehnert, H.; Hepp, K. D.: Die Harnsäureproduktion der menschlichen Leber während parenteraler Fruktosezufuhr. Verh. dt. Ges. inn. Med. *80:* 487 (1974).

20 Grunst, J.; Dietze, G.; Wicklmayr, M.; Hoppe, F.; Mehnert, H.: Einfluß parenteraler Fruktose- bzw. Glukosezufuhr auf die Harnsäurebildung und Phosphataufnahme der menschlichen Leber. Z. ErnährWiss. *14:* 259 (1975).

21 Lieber, C. S.; Jones, D. P.; Losowsky, M. S.; Davidson, C. S.: Interrelation of uric acid and ethanol metabolism in man. J. clin. Invest. *41:* 1863 (1962).

22 Förster, H.; Zagel, D.: Stoffwechseluntersuchungen während und im Anschluß an Dauerinfusionen von Glucose und Zuckeraustauschstoffen. Dt. med. Wschr. *99:* 1300–1304 (1974).

23 Kleinberger, G.: Parenterale Fettzufuhr bei Diabetes mellitus; in Eckart, Wolfgram, Fett in der parenteralen Ernährung, pp. 155–165 (Zuckschwerdt, München 1981).

24 Leutenegger, A. F.; Göschke, H.; Stutz, K.; Mannhart, H.; Werdenberg, D.; Wolff, G.; Allgöwer, M.: Comparison between glucose and a combination of glucose, fructose and xylitol as carbohydrates for total parenteral nutrition of surgical intensive care patients. Am. J. Surg. *133:* 199–208 (1977).

25 Georgieff, M.; Moldawer, L. L.; Bistrian, B. R.; Blackburn, G.: Xylitol, an energy source for intravenous nutrition after trauma. J. parent. ent. Nutr. *9,* 2: 199–209 (1985).

Priv.-Doz. Dr. M. Wicklmayr, III. Med. Abteilung, Krankenhaus Schwabing, Kölner Platz 1, D-8000 München 40 (FRG)

Dietze, Grünert, Kleinberger, Wolfram (eds.), Clinical Nutrition and Metabolic Research. Proc. 7th Congr. ESPEN, Munich 1985, pp. 269–279 (Karger, Basel 1986)

Use of Insulin Infusion Pumps during Hyperalimentation of the Stressed Diabetic Patient

M. Bergman[a], *S. RaviKumar*[a], *C. Auerhahn*[a], *N. Del Savio*[a], *J. Savino*[a], *R. Hendler*[b], *R. Jacob*[b], *P. Felig*[b]

[a] New York Medical College, Dept. of Medicine, Rachmiel Levine Diabetes Center, Valhalla, New York, USA
[b] Yale University School of Medicine, Dept. of Internal Medicine, Div. of Endocrinology and Metabolism, New Haven, Connecticut, USA

Parenteral and enteral hyperalimentation are frequently complicated by hyperglycemia. In as many as 15% of patients receiving total parenteral hyperalimentation, at least one blood glucose concentration may exceed 400 mg/dl on at least one occasion [1]. The impairment in glucose disposal in these circumstances has been attributed to overt or latent diabetes mellitus, reduced insulin secretion in response to the glycemic stimulus because of 'stress' (pain, trauma, infection, shock), or prior starvation [1]. Hyperglycemia may also be attributed to insulin resistance seen in sepsis and stress during which levels of counterregulatory hormones (e.g. catecholamines and glucocorticoids) are elevated [1, 2]. Furthermore, it has also been shown that infused glucose is less able to suppress glucose production, thereby sparing amino-acid precursors, in sepsis [3]. Hyperglycemia is generally treated by the periodic subcutaneous administration of intermediate and short-acting insulins, by adding regular insulin to the parenteral infusion, or, in severe cases, by the continuous intravenous administration of insulin.

Continuous subcutaneous insulin infusion (CSII) has been demonstrated to be effective in the outpatient management of diabetes [4]. Whether CSII can improve blood glucose control in a setting of a marked increase in carbohydrate intake (e.g. hyperalimentation) and intercurrent stress has not been established. The present study was therefore conducted to evaluate the effectiveness of CSII in the treatment of hyperglycemia occurring during enteral feedings in patients with postoperative sepsis or extensive burns. Since the enteral feedings were administered continuously, it was postulated that CSII administered solely as a continuous basal infusion without intermittent bolus doses of insulin would be effective. In a second part of this study, the impact of improved glucose control on metabolic and hormonal substrate concentrations was evaluated.

Material and Methods

Four patients treated with enteral hyperalimentation at the Westchester County Medical Center were studied. A consent form, approved by the institutional committee on human research, was signed by each patient. One patient (pt. 1) was treated on two separate occasions. Characteristics of these patients are shown in table I. All of the patients received enteral feedings via a naso-gastric tube consisting of 3,000 kcal/day containing 390 g of simple carbohydrate. During the pre-CSII period, blood glucose levels were measured approximately 3–5 times daily for 3–6 days without making any significant attempt at achieving tight control with conventional insulin therapy.

CSII was administered using a portable infusion pump (Autosyringe, model AS 6C, Hooksett, New Hampshire). Blood glucose monitoring and insulin pump adjustments were based on written guidelines (table II) and were made by the nursing staff in each intensive

Table I. Patient characteristics

Patient	Sex	Age	Height/ Weight	Diagnosis	History of Diabetes	Duration	Therapy
1	f	60	5′2″/204 lbs	toxic epidermonecrolysis	yes	3 years	oral agent
2	m	51	N/A	Whipple's procedure for pancreatic carcinoma	no	–	–
3	f	58	5′6″/134 lbs	coronary artery bypass, graft + endarterectomy	yes	16 years	oral agent
4	f	60	5′7″/140 lbs	coronary artery bypass, graft and sepsis	yes	6 years	insulin

care unit to which the patients were admitted. Treatment was initiated using the basal mode of infusion at 12–15 mU/kg/h [5]. Bolus doses of insulin were only administered for the rapid lowering of blood glucose levels in the event of marked hyperglycemia. Adjustments in the basal rate were made depending on the results obtained from capillary blood glucose monitoring using the Glucometer (Ames, Elkhart, Indiana). Fingerstick monitoring of blood glucose was performed every 2–4 h when blood glucose results were demonstrated to be stable. A target blood glucose in the range of 150 mg/dl was considered to constitute desirable control. More frequent capillary blood glucose monitoring was performed when values fell below or exceeded this range. On the average 14 determinations were obtained daily from every patient (range 11–19 per day). 24-h coverage was provided by the 'pump team' which included two physicians, a diabetes nurse practitioner, and a dietitian.

A metabolic profile in 3 additional patients [5–7] and patient 2 in the initial group was performed including measurements of serum cholesterol, triglyceride, free fatty acid, and

Table II. Guidelines for use of the insulin pump

Goal: Maintain blood glucose values in physiologic range (approximately 150 mg/dl).
Modalities: Portable insulin pump, reflectance meter with strips.
Technique:

(1) Capillary blood glucose values are performed q2h until stable and then q4h.
(2) Capillary glucose determinations need to be made more frequently if glucose values are rising or falling rapidly (i.e. q½h–q1h).
(3) Insulin concentrations are usually prepared to provide either a basal rate of 1 U/h at 24% (100 U/cc) or 2 U/h at 24% with (200 U/cc).
(4) The basal rate is increased at 0.5 to 1.0 unit increments each 1–2 h until the capillary blood glucose approximates 150 mg/dl.
(5) The basal rate is increased at 1.0 U/h if the capillary blood glucose is rising at a rate of about 30–50 mg/h.
(6) Additional bolus doses of insulin may be necessary at times if basal rate adjustment is inadequate. This decision will be made in conjunction with M.D. contact.
(7) The basal rate is decreased by 1.0 U/h if blood glucose reading falls at 30–50 mg/h and is decreased by 0.5 U/h if glucose levels fall at a lower rate until an optimal range is achieved.
(8) If the capillary blood glucose falls below 100 mg/dl but above 80 mg/dl, the pump should be turned off and a glucose determination repeated within ½ h.
(9) The pump should be restarted when glucose values climb above 100 mg/dl at a rate of 0.5–1.0 U/h *less* than the previous setting. Capillary blood glucose need to be repeated within ½–1 h and appropriate adjustments made again.
(10) If capillary blood glucose values fall $<$ 70 mg/dl, the pump should be turned off and either p.o. or i.v. 50% dextrose administered in accordance with the level.
i.e. 6–8 oz OJ or ½ AMP D50 for values 60–70 mg/dl
10–12 oz OJ or 1 AMP D50 for values $<$ 50–60 mg/dl.
Capillary blood glucose values need to be repeated q 15 min until values stabilize $>$ 80 mg/dl $\times$ 2 or 3.

growth hormone concentrations. All specimens were drawn at 8 a.m. at least 12 h after the infusion of lipids.

Data in the text are presented as the mean ± S.E. Student's t-test was used for all statistical analysis.

Results

The results of 5 separate trials of treatment with CSII are shown in table III. The mean duration of treatment with CSII was 16.8 days (range from 7 to 32 days). The mean capillary blood glucose concentration fell to 61% of pre-treatment levels with CSII ($p < 0.001$). Table IV demonstrates that only 1.3% of the 1,254 capillary blood glucose determinations performed were less than 60 mg/dl. Most of the values (61.6%) were between 61 and 200 mg/dl. Only 5.6% of all determinations were excessively hyperglycemic (greater than 350 mg/dl). The insulin infusion rate during CSII (table III) varied from 1.1–5.4 U/h, averaging 2.5 U/h. Bolus insulin doses via CSII were only administered in approximately 5 instances during the study for severe hyperglycemia. Small, pea-size, nontender, subcutaneous nodules occurred occasionally in areas where the needle had been inserted. Cellulitis or abscess formation was not observed. Table V demonstrates that the improvement in blood glucose control was associ-

Table III. Response of capillary blood glucose (CBG) to CSII in patients receiving enteral hyperalimentation*

Patient	Duration of CSII (days)	Mean CBG+ (mg/dl)		Mean insulin infusion rate (U/h)
		Pre-CSII	Post-CSII	
1 (1st course)	19	326 ± 67	172 ± 40	1.8 ± 0.7
1 (2nd course)	13	233 ± 70	187 ± 47	1.7 ± 0.6
2	13	319 ± 18	162 ± 27	1.1 ± 0.4
3	32	399 ± 102	199 ± 34	2.3 ± 0.6
4	7	331 ± 30	256 ± 21	5.4 ± 1.8
Mean ± SE	17 ± 8.5	322 ± 52	195 ± 33	2.5 ± 1.5

* Mean values ± SE are shown ($p < 0.001$)
+ Capillary blood glucose

Table IV. % of capillary blood glucose values (mg/dl) by range

	0–60	61–75	76–100	101–150	151–200	201–250	251–300	301–350	> 350
1 (1st course)	3%	4.3%	10.6%	25.1%	28.1%	14.9%	10.2%	2.6%	1.3%
1 (2nd course)	0.7%	2.1%	10.3%	21.2%	36.3%	13.0%	8.2%	3.4%	4.8%
2	1.4%	1.4%	3.4%	46.9%	29.3%	10.9%	4.1%	2.0%	0.7%
3	1.2%	1.5%	6.1%	24.3%	23.8%	16.5%	12.9%	8.3%	5.6%
4	–	–	3.4%	12.9%	16.4%	17.0%	19.0%	15.5%	15.5%
Mean	1.3 ± 1.0	1.9 ± 1.4	6.8 ± 3.2	26.1 ± 11.3	26.8 ± 6.6	14.5 ± 2.3	10.9 ± 5.0	6.4 ± 5.1	5.6 ± 5.3

Table V. Metabolic profile

Patient		Pre-CSII	Normal range	Post-CSII
2	chol	135 ± 10.2	145–250 mg/dl	114.8 ± 30
	tg	95 ± 19	46–236 mg/dl	74 ± 13
	cortisol	21.5 ± 0.7	7–25 μg/dl	15.2 ± 3.1
	GH	2.65 ± 0.78	5 ng/ml	4.08 ± 2.27
	FFA	398 ± 170	300–700 μmol	266 ± 14
	mean CBG	319 ± 18	75–125 mg/dl	162 ± 27
5*	chol	136 ± 19		117 ± 16
	tg	197 ± 121		114 ± 57
	cortisol	25 ± 8.9		14 ± 4
	GH	8.1 ± 1.9		5.3 ± 2.1
	FFA	1009 ± 383		307 ± 214
	mean CBG	265 ± 162		142 ± 78
6	chol	161 ± 36		139
	tg	369 ± 45		179
	cortisol	35.3 ± 11.9		9.6 ± 3.1
	GH	4.05 ± 4.5		2.85 ± 2.6
	FFA	970 ± 492		539 ± 190
	mean CBG	270 ± 38		209 ± 51
7	chol	132 ± 12		102
	tg	192		90 ± 2.8
	cortisol	14.6 ± 2.5		13.4 ± 1.5
	GH	1.8 ± 0.6		1.56 ± 0.07
	FFA	915 ± 124		484 ± 115
	mean CBG	272 ± 15		159 ± 35

* Patient received parenteral hyperalimentation

ated with a reduction in serum cholesterol, triglyceride, cortisol, and free fatty acid levels without any consistent change noted in growth hormone concentrations.

Discussion

Normally, glucose is metabolized at a rate varying between 0.4 and 1.2 g/kg/h [6]. When the glucose infusion rate exceeds this range, hyperglycemia may occur. The tendency for hyperalimentation feedings to provoke hyperglycemia or even hyperglycemic hyperosmolar nonketotic coma is compounded by the stress already evident in these patients in whom such feedings are administered. Patients experiencing severe burns, sepsis, or trauma are exposed to elevated levels of counter-regulatory hormones resulting in an insulin-resistant state and/or insulin deficiency. The development of hyperglycemia during hyperalimentation may be counterproductive to the nutritional process as the catabolic state already present in these patients may become exacerbated. Therefore, the goal of treatment should be to preserve as close to a euglycemic state as possible.

Hyperglycemia complicating hyperalimentation can be treated in various ways. If the metabolic disturbance is mild, then a combination of intermediate-acting and short-acting insulins can be administered as multiple injections. However, when hyperglycemia becomes more severe, intravenous administration of insulin may be necessary. With prolonged use, the intravenous route may be complicated by phlebitis, thrombosis, or infection. Furthermore, to minimize the risk of developing these complications, the i.v. site needs to be changed frequently. As hyperalimentation is generally prescribed for extended periods, intravenous access may become limited, making an alternate modality of insulin administration desirable. This is particularly true in patients receiving hyperalimentation via the enteral route in whom a central venous catheter is not required for feeding purposes.

CSII has been demonstrated to be successful in the ambulatory treatment of type I diabetes [4]. In this setting, the insulin infusion pump is designed to mimic two physiological functions of the pancreas. One function, termed the basal mode, provides a constant insulin infusion between meals which generally approximates 0.8 U/h [5]. The other function is the provision of a preprandial bolus of insulin which simulates meal-induced secretion of insulin and prevents an excessive blood glucose excursion following a meal. This function is referred to as the bolus mode.

The use of CSII in the treatment of patients receiving hyperalimentation has not previously been reported. This system has the advantage of not requiring i.v. access in order to regulate blood glucose concentrations. Furthermore, the rate of insulin administration can be adjusted to need, based on frequent blood glucose determinations by using capillary blood glucose monitoring. CSII therapy would be particularly useful if it can be demonstrated that successful application is feasible by a clinical nursing staff even in the absence of a specialized research unit.

Since the patients in this study received continuous enteral feedings, it was theorized that only the basal mode of CSII would be necessary to regulate hyperglycemia. The basal mode could be rapidly adjusted to reflect changes in ambient blood glucose levels. Blood glucose concentrations may fluctuate markedly during hyperalimentation resulting from variation in the flow rates of solutions, from the variability of carbohydrate concentration of the solution infused, and the amount absorbed from the intestine. As a result of the osmotic load, diarrhea occurs frequently during enteral feedings which may also contribute to the variability of glucose absorption.

In the present study, we found that the mean capillary blood glucose fell significantly as a result of pump treatment. It should be noted that an attempt was not made to optimize blood glucose control by using more conventional treatment regimens as this study purported to study the feasibility of CSII in the setting of hyperglycemia complicating hyperalimentation. The overall improvement in glucose control following the initiation of CSII would have been even more impressive were it not for one patient (pt. 4). This patient also demonstrated a greater degree of insulin resistance based on basal rate requirements than did the other study patients. Even with the increased insulin requirement (5.4 ± 1.8 U/h), optimal regulation became difficult and ultimately the patient required intravenous insulin infusion as the insulin requirements exceeded the maximum amount of insulin that can be provided with the AS 6C pump (approximately 11 U/h). The increased insulin requirement in this patient most likely resulted from the postoperative fever due to sepsis.

CSII was well tolerated regardless of the duration of infusion. One patient (pt. 3) was treated with the pump for 32 days without developing any local complications. The infusion site was changed in each patient every 2–3 days, minimizing the likelihood that an abscess or cellulitis would develop. Areas of subcutaneous induration were, however, occasionally noted in sites where the needle had been inserted. These areas were nontender, pea-size, and noninflamed, frequently only recognizable by palpation.

Hypoglycemia occurred rarely in this study. Only 1.3% of the 1,254 capillary blood glucose determinations were below 60 mg/dl. The infrequent occurrence of hypoglycemia is related to the frequency with which capillary glucose monitoring was performed. When hypoglycemia did occur, it resulted primarily from the inadvertent failure to adequately decrease the basal rate infusion setting, either when a delay resulted in obtaining the hyperalimentation solution from the pharmacy, or at a time when blood glucose levels were declining. Hypoglycemia was also rarely seen when the basal rate setting was inadequately lowered after a prescribed change in the concentration or flow rate of the enteral solution had occurred.

An average of 14 finger-sticks were obtained daily from each patient by the nursing staff. Despite the frequency with which finger-sticks were performed, patients did not complain of undue discomfort, and inflammation or infection were not observed at the puncture sites.

The mean capillary blood glucose achieved with CSII (195 ± 33 mg/dl) was acceptable although not optimal. The reason for this stemmed largely from the desire of the nursing staff to maintain blood glucose levels above 150 mg/dl, fearing that sudden drops below this level could potentially result in hypoglycemia. Furthermore, despite supervision and availability of frequent contact with the 'pump team' the nursing staff was responsible for regulating CSII following an initial training period. The fluctuation and variability in blood glucose levels (table III) may therefore be partially attributed to the experience, interest, and ability of a very large clinical nursing staff. Nevertheless, these results showed a clear-cut improvement as compared to the pre-pump control period. In addition, the exact blood glucose value, below which the catabolic process associated with hyperglycemia is impeded, has not been ascertained.

Since the purpose of this study was to evaluate the feasibility of CSII in this particular setting, it cannot be concluded that intensified conventional management with multiple insulin injections in conjunction with more frequent blood glucose monitoring could not achieve similar results observed with CSII therapy. A prospective study comparing these two therapeutic modalities would therefore be needed to clarify this issue. This present study does, however, demonstrate the effectiveness and feasibility of basal rate CSII in the management of patients undergoing enteral hyperalimentation.

Since previous studies have demonstrated abnormalities in a variety of metabolic substrates and hormones in the uncontrolled diabetic state and restoration to normal with improved control [7, 8], we were interested in assessing the metabolic profile in patients treated with hyperalimentation while under severe stress. Although a study of a larger number of patients and intermediary metabolites is required to confirm the present findings, our preliminary data would seem to indicate that improved diabetes control in this setting is accompanied by a reduction in several substrates. FFA levels were restored to normal while cholesterol and triglyceride concentrations were further reduced although they had not been elevated in most patients prior to CSII therapy. Cortisol levels were also lowered in most patients with improved metabolic control while GH levels remained essentially unchanged.

In conclusion, basal CSII is a safe and effective means of improving blood glucose control in patients receiving enteral hyperalimentation, despite the markedly elevated intake of carbohydrate and the presence of insulin resistance. CSII can enhance the metabolic response to hyperalimentation without requiring an intravenous access route. CSII may improve abnormal substrate metabolism associated with poor metabolic control. Finally, CSII can be safely applied by a clinical nursing staff in an intensive care setting for prolonged periods without the development of significant complications including frequent hypoglycemia or skin infections. Adequate training and supervision of the nursing team with 24-h access to an experienced 'pump team' are vital for a successful outcome of such a program.

Acknowledgments

Partial funding for this study was made available through a contribution from Autosyringe Inc., Hooksett, New Hampshire.

We thank Mrs. Nina Cascello for her secretarial assistance in the preparation of this manuscript. The assistance of Ms. Susan Trepel and the technical expertise of Ms. Miriam Levitt are greatly appreciated.

References

1 Ryan, J. A., Jr.: Complications of total parenteral nutrition; in Fischer, Total Parenteral Nutrition, pp. 55–100 (Little, Brown and Co., Boston 1976).

2 Sanderson, I.; Deitel, M.: Insulin response in patients receiving concentrated infusions of glucose and casein hydrolysate for complete parenteral nutrition. Ann. Surg. *179:* 387–394 (1974).

3 Shaw, J. H. F.; Wolfe, R. R.: Response to Glucose and Lipid Infusions in Sepsis: A Kinetic Analysis. Metabolism *34:* 442–449 (1985).

4 Tamborlane, W. V.; Sherwin, R. S.; Genel, M.; Felig, P.: Outpatient treatment of juvenile-onset diabetes with a programmed portable subcutaneous insulin infusion system. Am. J. Med. *68:* 190–196 (1980).

5 Tamborlane, W. V.; Sherwin, R. S.; Genel, M.; Felig, P.: Reduction to normal of plasma glucose in juvenile diabetes by subcutaneous administration of insulin with portable infusion pump. New Engl. J. Med. *300:* 573–578 (1979).

6 Geyer, R. P.: Parenteral Nutrition. Physiol. Rev. *40:* 150–186 (1960).
7 Tamborlane, W. V.; Sherwin, R. S.; Koivisto, V.; Genel, M.; Felig, P.: Normalization of the growth hormone response to exercise in juvenile-onset diabetic subjects treated with a portable insulin pump. Diabetes *28:* 785–788 (1979).
8 Tamborlane, W. V.; Sherwin, R. S.; Genel, M.; Felig, P.: Restoration of normal lipid and amino-acid metabolism in diabetic patients with a portable insulin-infusion pump. Lancet *i:* 1258–1261 (1979).

Michael Bergman, MD, New York Medical College, Dept. of Medicine, Rachmiel Levine Diabetes Center, Valhalla, NY 10595 (USA)

Dietze, Grünert, Kleinberger, Wolfram (eds.), Clinical Nutrition and Metabolic Research. Proc. 7th Congr. ESPEN, Munich 1985, pp. 280–290 (Karger, Basel 1986)

Perioperative Management of Diabetes Mellitus

R. Gunnarsson

Dept. of Medicine, Karolinska Institute, Huddinge Hospital, Stockholm, Sweden

It has been estimated that about one half of all diabetics will undergo surgery some time during their life, in many cases for late vascular complications of the disease. The commonest reasons for surgical intervention that are associated with diabetes have recently been discussed by Reynolds [24]. Diabetes mellitus occurs in approximately 2–3% of the population in the Western countries. The disease often becomes manifest during surgery; as many as 23% of the series of 487 diabetic patients reported by Galloway and Shuman [12] were discovered in this way. As the disease can influence the outcome of the operation, it is important for both surgeons and anesthesists to be aware both of its presence and its late complications. Furthermore, surgical stress can seriously interfere with glucose metabolism, and the diabetes therapy therefore often requires postoperative adjustment.

This review discusses aspects of the management of diabetes before, during and after elective surgery. For more detailed information the reader is referred to reviews of the work in this field [11, 16, 22].

Goals for the Perioperative Management of Diabetes Mellitus

The overall goal is to ensure that the morbidity or mortality among diabetic patients undergoing surgery do not exceed the figures for the non-diabetic population. The primary objectives for the management during the various perioperative stages are presented in table I.

Table I. Aims of perioperative management of the diabetic patient

	Primary objective (s)
Preoperative management	assessment of current metabolic control, correction of metabolic imbalance if necessary, evaluation of secondary late vascular complications
Perioperative management	avoidance of hypoglycemia and marked hyperglycemia
Postoperative management	minimizing catabolism

Preoperative Management

Before operation the metabolic control should be checked and an examination for the presence and severity of late complications should be conducted. It is usually considered advisable to admit the patient to hospital 2–3 days prior to a planned operation.

Glycemic control can be assessed by repeated measurements of the blood glucose concentration. In addition, an impression of the control during the previous weeks can be obtained from a measurement of glycosylated hemoglobin. Determination of urinary glucose excretion is of limited value since the renal threshold for glucose displays a large inter-subject and intra-subject variability. A routine check for the presence of ketonuria should be made.

Well-controlled insulin-dependent diabetic patients can continue with their insulin regimen. Unsatisfactory glycemic control may be improved by giving, twice, daily, an injection of a mixture of short- and intermediate-acting insulin or, alternatively, multiple injections of a short-acting insulin. In the case of poor control, correction is achieved most rapidly by intravenous infusion or intramuscular injections.

For well-controlled non-insulin-dependent diabetic patients where diet alone or sulfonylurea drugs are the forms of treatment, the only special precaution required is withdrawal of long-acting sulfonylureas at least 36 h prior to operation. (The most commonly used long-acting sulfonylurea compound is chlorpropamide.) Biguanides should also always be withdrawn prior to surgery because of the increased risk for lactic acidosis associated with their use. If control is poor in the non-insulin-dependent diabetic patient or if major surgery is planned, it is advisable to begin with insulin therapy following one of the above regimens. If the insulin treatment is supposed to be intermittent, it is essential to use insulins of the modern human type and with highest purity grade in order to reduce the risk of sensibilization.

While there are no controlled studies in which the results of surgery in patients with different degrees of glycemic control have been compared, there are at least theoretical advantages of a good control. It is generally held that effective glycemic control improves the conditions for wound healing and lowers the risk for postoperative bacterial infections. Furthermore, hemostatic regulation, which can be impaired in diabetics, seems to be dependent on glycemic control.

Prior to surgery, a check for late vascular complications of the disease should be made and, if such are found, their severity should be assessed. Diabetic microangiopathy includes lesions in the eyes, the kidneys, and the peripheral nerves. Proliferative retinopathy should, if possible, be treated with photocoagulation before surgery in order to reduce the risk of perioperative retinal hemorrhages. As regards the kidneys, the glomerular filtration rate should be assessed; usually a serum creatinine determination suffices. A reduced filtration rate will predispose fluid retention and electrolyte disturbances, and may impair drug metabolism or excretion – for example, of some antibiotics. One dominant feature of nephropathy can be nephrosis, with hypoalbuminemia and edema, which may call for treatment with high doses of furosemide. Certain neuropathic lesions call for special consideration. Sensory neuropathy can not only lower the pain threshold but also elicit severe burning pain, usually in the calves. Another common manifestation is the loss of some tendon reflexes. Of especial interest are those neuropathic lesions affecting the autonomic nervous system. Such lesions can give rise to a wide variety of symptoms; those of interest in relation to surgery include abnormal pupillary reactions with, for example, loss of the reaction to light; postural hypotension, which can complicate the postoperative mobilization, and abnormalities in gastrointestinal motility, with constipation, diarrhea, and gastroparesis. In the latter case, gastric emptying can be extremely slow, with undigested food remaining in the stomach after an overnight fast. Patients with gastroparesis usually complain of nausea and vomiting. One objective method of evaluating autonomic neuropathy is to measure the heart beat-to-beat variation during rest and hyperventilation; the normal variability in heart rate is considerably reduced if not absent. It has been suggested that disturbance of the cardiac innervation may lead to an increased risk of cardiac arrythmias. For this reason, it may be advisable to keep patients with evidence of autonomic neuropathy under close observation.

In addition to microangiopathy, diabetic patients may also suffer from atherosclerotic vascular lesions similar to those seen in non-diabetics. In fact it is the cardiovascular status that largerly determines the surgical risk; the supposed increased perioperative morbidity and mortality of diabetic patients can probably be ascribed to their higher prevalence of atherosclerosis. If corrected for this, there should, however, be no increased perioperative morbidity or mortality in diabetic patients [28].

Perioperative Management

The primary aim of perioperative management of the diabetic patient is to ensure his or her maximum safety; both hypoglycemia – with the potential risk for brain damage – as well as marked hyperglycemia and ketosis must be avoided. Several protocols for the management of diabetes during surgery have been described and reviewed [2].

In most diabetic patients, the blood glucose level does not change greatly during surgery. In general, any variation tends to be related to the severity and duration of the operation [9, 17].

For well-controlled non-insulin-dependent diabetic subjects treated with diet alone, no special perioperative treatment is required; blood glucose is followed repeatedly and corrected with short-acting insulin if necessary. If the patient is treated with a modern sulfonylurea drug as glibenclamide or glipizide, the treatment is stopped on the operation day. Blood glucose is determined regularly and insulin given if the control deteriorates. An earlier suggestion by Fähndrich et al. [10], to give intravenous therapy with sulfonylurea during operation, has not been widely accepted.

Many protocols for perioperative insulin administration in insulin-dependent diabetics have been reported. Insulin can be given by the subcutaneous or the intravenous route, in the former case either by injection or as a continuous infusion. For injection therapy, an intermediate-acting insulin (NPH or lente insulin) has usually been chosen, supplemented when necessary by intermittent doses of regular insulin. Simultaneously with the injection of the intermediate-acting insulin, a constant intravenous glucose infusion is started, using, for example, a 5% solution delivered at a rate of 100 ml/h. There is no consensus on the insulin dose to be given bevore operation. Some authors prefer to give from 50 to 75% of the usual daily dose as intermediate-acting insulin in the morning, the rest being by some authors supplied after the operation; others give the full dose beforehand.

The use of a portable pump for continuous subcutaneous insulin infusion can improve the glycemic control in many insulin-dependent diabetics but the technique has not gained wide acceptance for perioperative use although Barnett et al. [3] achieved satisfactory control with it in minor surgery (0.5 U/h; no intravenous glucose). There seems to be no controlled study in which the outcome of the various subcutaneous techniques, injection or infusion, have been compared but the available data indicate that injection is a safe and easy mode of delivery.

According to most modern protocols, however, the intravenous route is the better route for perioperative insulin delivery. Usually, the infusion rate is adjusted manually on the basis of regular blood glucose measurements (open loop system) but automatic adjustment of the insulin supply can be effected through an 'artificial pancreas' (closed loop system). The use of continuous intravenous infusion during surgery was encouraged by its successful introduction for the treatment of diabetic ketoacidosis during the early seventies. Taitelman et al. [26] compared a subcutaneous injection of NPH insulin (⅔ of the ordinary dose) with an intravenous insulin infusion (1 or 2 U/h); the higher insulin infusion rate being given if the preoperative daily insulin requirement had exceeded 20 U. A parallel infusion of glucose was given 5% solution; 500 ml 1st h, then 125 ml/h for 4 h). The rate of 2 U/h was found to yield the better result but in 2 of their 6 patients a tendency for hypoglycemia necessitated a reduction of the rate of supply and increase in the dextrose infusion rate. Hypoglycemia did not, however, present any problem in the series of 20 patients receiving 2 U/h reported by Bowen et al. [6] who, however, used a higher glucose infusion rate during the operation (100 ml/h of a 10% glucose solution). In a comparison of perioperative intravenous and subcutaneous administration, Goldberg et al. [15] found no statistically significant difference in the degree of control achieved with 1 U/h given as intravenous infusion and that provided by the subcutaneous injection of one half of the conventional daily dose, but recommended the former route on grounds of its greater flexibility.

Perioperative adjustment of the insulin infusion rate based on the blood glucose is probably necessary to achieve optimal blood glucose control. In a technique to this end, proposed by Alberti and Thomas [2] and, later Alberti et al. [1], insulin-glucose mixtures were prepared that had an insulin concentration related to the prevailing blood glucose level.

They recommended insulin in a 10% glucose solution which they infused at a rate of 100 ml/h. Although the method seems to reliably avoid hypoglycemia, it is inconvenient to have to make new solutions following a change in the blood glucose level. To circumvent this drawback, a 'piggy back' system entailing a separate and variable insulin infusion has been used (Meyer et al. [20]). In a system for adjusting the infusion rate, Edouard and coworkers [7] used an initial rate of 2 U/h, which they subsequently modified in steps of 0.5 U/h according to the blood glucose level.

In earlier studies, a 2–3 h interval between the blood glucose measurements was recommended but more recently the frequency has increased. Woodruff and coworkers [29] used a 15-min interval, which enabled a fairly tight control of blood glucose to be maintained; a range of

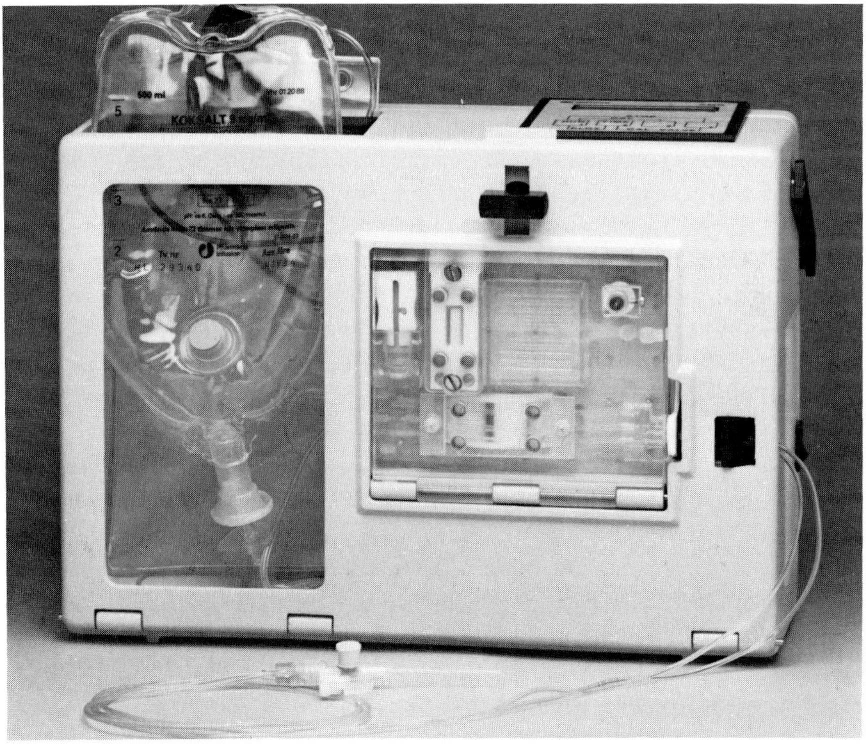

Fig. 1. Portable apparatus for continuous measurement of blood glucose concentration (photograph kindly provided by Gambro, Lund, Sweden).

4.4–11.1 mmol/l was aimed at. Within this range, insulin was infused at a rate of 1 U/h but when the upper limit was passed, the rate was raised to as much as 20 U/h; this would seem to be too high, however, since in the treatment of diabetic ketoacidosis a rate of 4–6 U/h is commonly used to achieve the maximum lowering of blood glucose. In fact, Woodruff and coworkers observed a tendency for hypoglycemia to develop in 2 of their 8 patients on this high-dose insulin regimen.

With modern measurement techniques, frequent checking of the blood glucose concentration during surgery presents little difficulty. Small, portable, and cheap glucose meters are eminently suitable for this purpose. If not available, visual reading from strips seems to provide satisfactory guidance [19]. The ease with which the blood glucose level can be monitored should enable us to dispense with arbitrary management regimens and to individualize the perioperative insulin treatment [5]. The need for an individualized approach is underlined by evidence that the insulin requirement varies according to the type of operation [14].

As for the future, continuous perioperative blood glucose monitoring will probably be more commonly available. A recently developed small and portable apparatus (fig. 1) would seem to be ideal in this context. If combined with a computer regulating the insulin infusion rate, an artificial pancreas is at hand. The only commercially available today is the Biostator® (Miles-Ames Co, Elkhart, Indiana); this system for glucose controlled insulin delivery has been used successfully for the perioperative management of diabetes mellitus [18, 21, 25]. However, the fact that an open-loop system with frequent blood glucose measurements can offer the same degree of control as the Biostator has recently been demonstrated in a controlled study on patients undergoing coronary bypass surgery [8].

To summarize: For perioperative control of diabetes, a constant glucose and variable insulin infusion by the intravenous route would seem to be the optimal system provided that the blood glucose concentration is measured at frequent intervals and that the insulin infusion rate is adjusted so as to keep the blood glucose level within a range of about 5–10 mmol/l.

Postoperative Management

In healthy subjects, the postoperative depression of glucose tolerance is due mainly to the development of an insulin resistance [13]. The duration of the reduced glucose tolerance is then dependent on the extent of the operation and to the occurrence of postoperative complications, it usually lasts for about a week [31]. The difficulty attending the management of diabetes after an operation is illustrated by the fact that only 8% of the postoperative blood glucose measurements obtained in 100 patients by Belcaro and coworkers [4] fell within the normal range. In non-insulin-dependent diabetic patients, a deterioration in glycemic control was observed to last for about a week [10]. The insulin-dependent diabetic patient will usually need greater amounts of insulin, but the actual requirement is difficult to predict. An intravenous infusion started during the operation may be continued for as long as the patient is receiving parenteral nutrition, but then the blood glucose level should be measured at frequent intervals. If glucose is included in the nutrition – as is to be recommended – it should preferably be given around the clock so as to facilitate adjustment of the insulin infusion rate. A 2–4 h monitoring interval is usually short enough to ensure satisfactory control. Algorithms for adjustment of the insulin infusion rate have been published by, among others, Woolfson [30]. If for some reason the intravenous route is not used, multiple subcutaneous injections may be resorted to; the optimal frequency is then 4–6 times a day. For injection of short-acting insulin every 4 h, proposed sliding scales based on bedside glucose measurements are given in table II. Higher doses should be used if the preoperative daily requirement has been in excess of, say, 60 U/d, or if corticosteroids are given postoperatively. If a schedule tends to result in too low blood glucose values, a slower delivery rate should be used, but if the hyperglycemia persists, a schedule with higher doses is used or should be designed. For the subcutaneous injections, the modern human insulin preparations

Table II. Proposed sliding scales for subcutaneous injection of regular insulin (preferably of human type) every 4 h based on bedside glucose measurements. If the preoperative insulin requirement has been normal, the regimen may be introduced with schedule B or C

Blood glucose concentration mmol/l		< 4	4.0 – 4.9	5.0 – 5.9	6.0 – 7.9	8.0 – 9.9	10.0 – 14.9	15.0 – 19.9	> 20.0
Insulin dose, U	A	0	4	6	6	8	10	12	14
	B	0	4	6	8	10	12	14	16
	C	0	6	8	10	12	14	16	18
	D	0	6	8	12	14	16	18	20

should be used since they have the advantage of being more rapidly absorbed from subcutaneous depots than the corresponding porcine insulins [23]. The blood glucose concentration should be frequently monitored so that the insulin supply rate can be reduced when the postoperative insulin requirement diminishes.

Concluding Remarks

The perioperative management of diabetic patients presents a challenge for both the surgeon and the anesthesist. While it must be based on local convention, the inclusion of a diabetologist in the team has been strongly recommended [1, 27]. The modern techniques for rapid bedside measurement of blood glucose has greatly improved our prospects of attaining the goals for the various perioperative stages, and they may afford an opportunity for adopting a more individualized approach. Further development in the field should include development of a reliable system for continuous monitoring of the blood glucose level, perhaps coupled with computerized adjustment of the insulin delivery.

Acknowledgments

This study has been supported in part by the Hagbergs Foundation, the Swedish Diabetes Association, and the Karolinska Institute.

References

1 Alberti, K. G. M. M.; Gill, G. V.; Elliott, M. J.: Insulin delivery during surgery in the diabetic patient. Diabetes Care *5:* suppl. 1, pp. 65–77 (1982).
2 Alberti, K. G. M. M.; Thomas, D. J. B.: The management of diabetes during surgery. Br. J. Anaesth. *51:* 693–710 (1979).
3 Barnett, A. H.; Robinson, M. H.; Harrison, J. H.; Watkins, P. J.: Minipump: Method of diabetic control during minor surgery under general anaesthesia. Br. med. J. *280:* 78–79 (1980).
4 Belcaro, G.; Cotellese, R.; Gargano, E.; Filippini, A.; Magri, M.: Diabetes and surgery. Acta chir. belg. *82:* 133–138 (1982).
5 Biddle, C. J.; Hernandez, S.: Perioperative control of diabetes mellitus – revisited. AANA J. *51:* 138–141 (1983).
6 Bowen, D. J.; Nancekievill, M. L.; Proctor, E. A.; Norman, J.: Perioperative manage-

ment of insulin-dependent diabetic patients. Use of continuous intravenous infusion of insulin-glucose-potassium solution. Anaesthesia *37:* 852–855 (1982).

7 Edouard, D.; Francois, P.; Langlois, B.: Anesthésie et réanimation des diabétiques. Nouv. Presse méd. *13:* 943–946 (1980).

8 Elliott, M. J.; Gill, G. V.; Home, P. D.; Noy, G. A.; Holden, M. P.; Alberti, K. G. M. M.: A comparison of two regimens for the management of diabetes during open-heart surgery. Anesthesiology *60:* 364–368 (1984).

9 Fletcher, J.; Langman, M. J. S.; Kellock, T. D.: Effect of surgery on blood-sugar levels in diabetes mellitus. Lancet *ii:* 52–55 (1965).

10 Fähndrich, W.; Liebermeister, H.; Schmitt, H.; Daweke, H.: Die Einstellung von Altersdiabetikern mit intravenösen Tolbutamidgaben während und nach der Operation im Vergleich zu herkömmlichen Behandlungsverfahren. Dt. med. Wschr. *99:* 121–127 (1974).

11 Gallina, D. L.; Mordes, J. P.; Rossini, A. A.: Surgery in the diabetic patient. Compr. Ther. *9:* 8–16 (1983).

12 Galloway, J. A.; Shuman, C. R.: Diabetes and surgery. Am. J. Med. *34:* 177–191 (1963).

13 Giddings, A. E. B.; Rowlands, B. J.; Mangnall, D.; Clark, R. G.: Plasma insulin and surgery. II. Later changes and the effect of intravenous carbohydrates. Ann. Surg. *186:* 687–693 (1977).

14 Gill, G. V.; Sherif, I. H.; Alberti, K. G. M. M.: Management of diabetes during open heart surgery. Br. J. Surg. *68:* 171–172 (1981).

15 Goldberg, N. J.; Wingert, T. D.; Levin, S. R.; Wilson, S. E.; Viljoen, J. F.: Insulin therapy in the diabetic surgical patient: Metabolic and hormone response to low dose insulin infusion. Diabetes Care *4:* 279–284 (1981).

16 Johnston, D. G.; Alberti, K. G. M. M.: Diabetic emergencies. Practical aspects of the management of diabetic ketoacidosis and diabetes during surgery. Clin. Endocrinol. Metab. *9:* 437–460 (1980).

17 Knick, B.: Besonderheiten der Diabetesbehandlung während operativer Eingriffe. Anaesthesist *9:* 303–308 (1966).

18 Kuntschen, F. R.; Taillens, C.; Galletti, P. M.; Hauf, E.; Hahn, C.: Coronary surgery in diabetics: Metabolic aspects of glycemia control by an artificial pancreas. Trans. Am. Soc. artif. internal Organs *28:* 236–239 (1982).

19 Madsbad, S.; Adelhoj, B.; Bigler, D.; Hilsted, J.: Evaluation of two methods of rapid blood-glucose monitoring by unskilled personnel during surgery. Acta anaesth. scand. *28:* 649–651 (1984).

20 Meyer, E. J.; Lorenzi, M.; Bohannon, N. V.; Amend, W.; Feduska, N. J.; Salvatierra, O.; Forsham, P. H.: Diabetic management by insulin infusion during major surgery. Am. J. Surg. *137:* 323–327 (1979).

21 Moulin, J. P.; Vialettes, B.; Lassmann, V.; Vague, P.: Le pancréas artificiel en chirurgie. Nouv. Presse méd. *11:* 3627–3630 (1982).

22 Podolsky, S.: Management of diabetes in the surgical patient. Med. Clins N. Am. *66:* 1361–1372 (1982).

23 Pramming, S.; Lauritzen, T.; Thorsteinsson, B.; Johansen, K.; Binder, C.: Absorption of soluble and isophane semi-synthetic human and porcine insulin in insulin-dependent diabetic subjects. Acta endocr. Copenh. *105:* 215–220 (1984).

24 Reynolds, C.: Management of the diabetic surgical patient. A systematic but flexible plan is the key. Postgrad. Med. *77:* 265–279 (1985).

25 Schwartz, S. S.; Horwitz, D. L.; Zehfus, B.; Langer, B.; Moossa, A. R.; Ribeiro, G.; Kaplan, E.; Rubenstein, A. H.: Use of a glucose controlled insulin infusion system (artificial beta cell) to control diabetes during surgery. Diabetologia *16:* 157–164 (1979).

26 Taitelman, U.; Reece, E. A.; Bessman, A. N.: Insulin in the management of the diabetic surgical patient. J. Am. med. Ass. *237:* 658–660 (1977).

27 Thai, A. C.; Husband, D. J.; Gill, G. V.; Alberti, K. G. M. M.: Management of diabetes during surgery. A retrospective study of 112 cases. Diabète Métab. *10:* 65–70 (1984).

28 Walsh, D. B.; Eckhauser, F. E.; Ramsburgh, S. R.; Burney, R. B.: Risk associated with diabetes mellitus in patients undergoing gallbladder surgery. Surgery *91:* 254–257 (1982).

29 Woodruff, R. E.; Lewis, S. B.; McLeskey, C. H.; Graney, W. F.: Avoidance of surgical hyperglycemia in diabetic patients. J. Am. med. Ass. *244:* 166–168 (1980).

30 Woolfson, A. M. J.: An improved method for blood glucose control during nutritional support. J. parent. ent. Nutr. *5:* 436–440 (1981).

31 Wright, P. D.; Henderson, K.; Johnston, I. D. A.: Glucose utilization and insulin secretion during surgery in man. Br. J. Surg. *61:* 5–8 (1974).

Rolf Gunnarsson, MD, Department of Medicine, Huddinge Hospital,
S-141 86 Huddinge (Sweden)

Dietze, Grünert, Kleinberger, Wolfram (eds.), Clinical Nutrition and Metabolic Research. Proc. 7th Congr. ESPEN, Munich 1985, pp. 291–299 (Karger, Basel 1986)

All-in-One Solutions for TPN of Diabetic Patients

G. Kleinberger

1st Medical Department, LKH Steyr, Austria

Introduction

The indication of nutritional support to traumatized patients [1, 2] and the effectiveness of metabolic care of diabetics [3, 4] have been published in numerous papers and are not the topics of the following paper. A nutrition regime for traumatized diabetic patients with an all-in-one (AIO) solution which is based on recommendations for a diabetic diet should be presented.

AIO solutions were recommended first by Sollasol and Joyeux [5] who mixed all nutrients necessary for complete parenteral nutrition in a glass bottle or silastic bag. In my own unit, mixing of AIO solutions has been done since 1972 [6].

Objections were raised to this system due to the possibility of Maillard reaction and the instability of some vitamins and electrolytes [7]. From previous studies it is known that fat emulsions are sensitive to electrolytes and carbohydrates [7]. Therefore, the stability of fat emulsions in AIO solutions is an important factor.

In electron microscopic studies we were able to demonstrate that our AIO solution for traumatized diabetic patients shows only insignificant morphological changes within 2 months of storage at 4 °C or within two weeks of storage at room temperature [8]. After mixing, the lipid particles of Intralipid 20% show a spherical shape with a homogenous center which carries highly osmiophilic inclusion bodies configurated as granules or globules [8]. High magnification demonstrated that these granules and the borderline of the globules were built up by osmiophilic spots of about 30 Å. The coarse rim of the lipid particles is thought to be built up by phospholipids of the emulsifier which bind osmium tetroxide to its double bonds. The granules and globules should be an effect of certain amino acids (AA) or additives in AA solutions necessary for stability [8].

Nutrition Regime for Traumatized Diabetic Patients

The AIO solution for traumatized diabetic patients consists of 250 ml of 30% glucose, 500 ml of a 10% L-AA-mixture and 250 ml of a 20% fat emulsion. The solution contains all electrolytes, trace elements, and vitamins recommended for complete parenteral nutrition (table I).

The diabetes solution consists of 1090 ml with 131 g carbohydrates, 50 g fat and 50 g amino acids. The carbohydrates are a mixture of glucose, sorbitol, xylitol and glycerol. Sorbitol and xylitol come from the amino acid solution and glycerol from the fat emulsion (table II). The total energy amounts to 1200 kcal. 44% are derived from carbohydrates, 39% from fat and 17% from amino acids. The nitrogen comes to 8.1 g and the energy nitrogen ratio to 150 kcal/g nitrogen. The osmolality of the solution is 1470 mosm/kg H_2O.

According to the pioneering work of Cuthbertson, the metabolic response to injury can be separated to the early 'ebb' shock phase with a low metabolic rate, followed by the 'flow' or catabolic phase, with an increased metabolic expenditure [9]. In the transition of these two phases, when nutrition should be started, the endogenous production rate of most substrates is above and the total utilization rate is below normal. In this situation normal nutritional supply of traumatized diabetic patients may cause severe metabolic disturbances.

Table I. Composition of the fat-containing all-in-one (AIO) solution for traumatized diabetic patients

Glucose 30%	250 ml
Amino Mel Optimal 10%	500 ml
Intralipid 20%	250 ml
Potassium malate	20–40 mmol
Glucose-1-phosphate	10–20 mmol
Trace elements Leopold	1 Amp
Solu vit	1 Amp
Vitalipid	1 Amp
Heparin	5000 IU

Table II. Content of substrates of the fat-containing all-in-one (AIO) solution for traumatized diabetic patients

Fluid	1090 ml
Carbohydrates	131 g
Glucose	75 g
Sorbitol	25 g
Xylitol	25 g
Glycerol	6.3 g
Fat	50 g
L-amino acids	50 g
Total energy supply	1200 kcal
Carbohydrates	44 %
Fat	39 %
L-amino acids	17 %
Nitrogen	8.1 g
kcal/g N	150

Therefore, after stabilization of circulation we can start intravenous nutrition below basal requirements with an infusion rate of 30–40 ml/h and increase it by 5 ml every 8 h during the first 2 days [6]. At the end of this adaptation phase, the maintenance dose amounts to 1 ml nutrition solution/kg B.W./h. This infusion rate provides 26 kcal (0.11 MJ), 2.9 g carbohydrates, 1.1 g fat, and 1.1 g amino acids/kg B.W./day. In the late phase of injury we increase the infusion rate by 1/3 to 1.3 ml/kg B.W./h which provides 36 kcal (0.15 MJ), 3.9 g carbohydrates, 1.5 g fat, and 1.5 g amino acids per kg B.W./day.

In addition to the adaptation of the patients to i.v. nutrition, certain adjustments of the composition of the AIO solution to the metabolic need of the individual patients have to be made during the course of the post-traumatic period. These adjustments are facilitated by the continuous infusion of the nutrition solution with a fixed formula (table III).

By changing the content of glucose or the amount of insulin in the bottle, we try to stabilize the blood glucose level between 5 and 10 mmol/l. The amino acid content is decreased from a 10% to a 5% solution if the blood urea nitrogen exceeds 80 mg/100 ml or the increase of the production rate of urea nitrogen indicates that the infused amino acids are mainly oxidized. The fat content of the solution is decreased from a 20% to a 10% emulsion if the triglyceride level exceeds 4.5 mmol/l (400 mg/100 ml). In the same way the electrolyte content is adjusted to the serum levels of the patients.

Table III. Variation of the composition of the all-in-one (AIO) solution according to the serum concentration of the infused substrates

Substrate	Variation	Serum level
Glucose	30–60%	5–10 mM/l
AA-mixture	5–10%	PUN 20 g/d
Fat	10–20%	TG 4 mM/l
Potassium	0–40 mM	4–5 mM/l
Chloride	0–40 mM	95–100 mM/l
Phosphate	0–20 mM	1.0–2.0 mM/l
Insulin	0–80 IU	BG 5–10 mM/l

Evaluation of the Diabetic Nutrition Regimes

A reliable evaluation of a nutrition regime in traumatized diabetic patients is difficult. The individual variations in the duration and severity of the ebb and flow phase and the unpredictability of complications prevent the realization of a controlled trial with comparable patients. Therefore, we selected 7 patients who just came out of a severe, but uncomplicated diabetic ketoacidosis for examination of our diabetes solution [10, 11]. These patients were selected because of their diabetes with a well defined stress, a metabolic situation comparable to traumatized diabetic patients.

We started our nutritional protocol after the blood glucose level decreased to 10 mmol/l and the pH exceeded 7.3, with an infusion of 0.12 g glucose/kg B.W./h to avoid hypoglycemia and to diminish diabetic ketosis further.

After an 8-h glucose infusion, we changed to our diabetes solution with an infusion rate of 1 ml/kg B.W./h, which supplies the same amount of carbohydrates as was given before. Figure 1 shows that the blood glucose increases during the glucose phase and decreases during the period of complete parenteral nutrition. This decrease occurs despite a reduction of the insulin dosis from 5 to 2 U/h. Later experience with our diabetes nutrition solution confirms that 4 U of insulin/h are too much and 2 U/h are generally insufficient. No significant changes in serum osmolality or lactate were noticed.

Because some authors claim that in diabetic patients fat emulsions should not be used, we were interested in the change of the triglycerides

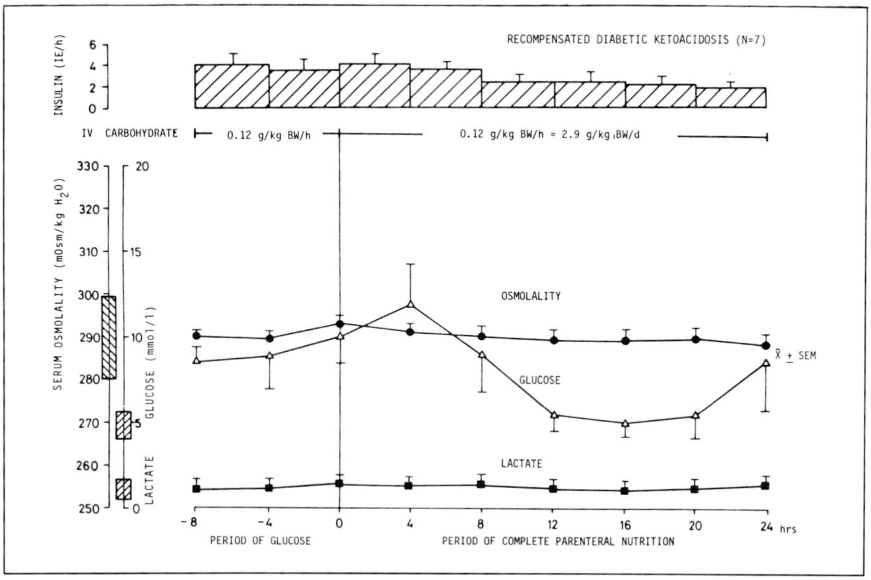

Fig. 1. Mean value of plasma glucose, osmolality, and lactate of 7 patients who just came out of severe diabetic ketoacidosis during continuous administration of 0.12 g glucose/kg B.W./h and diabetic nutrition solution, respectively.

and beta-OH-butyrate concentrations in serum. In our patients who just came out of a diabetic ketoacidosis, 1.1 g fat/kg B.W./day produced only a small increase in the triglyceride levels (fig. 2). The initial mean value was 0.8 mmol/l and reached a steady state after an 8-h period of 1.3 mmol/l. The serum beta-OH-butyrate concentration showed a decrease during the glucose period. After starting complete parenteral nutrition, beta-OH-butyrate increased during the first 4 h from 0.6 to 0.9 mmol/l and afterwards decreased to normal range. These data show that fat amounting to 1.1 g/kg B.W./day is eliminated from serum sufficiently in patients with still evident diabetic ketosis.

In an insulin deficient state, characteristic disturbances of the amino acid metabolism can be detected which cause changes in the plasma amino acid concentrations. Figure 3 shows the mean plasma amino acid concentrations of 9 patients with severe diabetic ketoacidosis prior to therapy. These disturbances raise the question whether or not a special amino acid mixture is necessary for adequate nutrition of diabetic patients.

First I want to emphasize that the disturbance in the amino acid

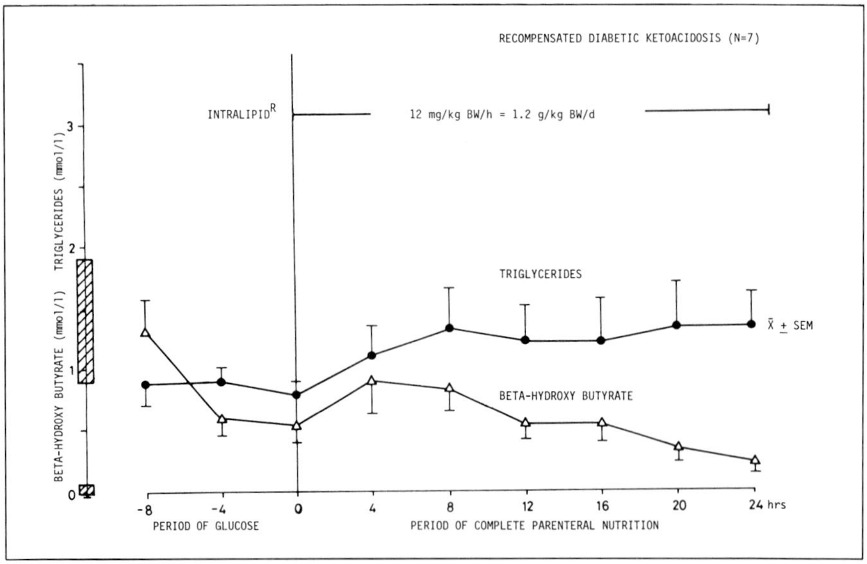

Fig. 2. Mean value of plasma concentration of triglycerides and beta-hydroxy-butyrate of 7 patients who just came out of severe diabetic ketoacidosis during continuous administration of 0.12 g glucose/kg B.W./h (glucose phase) and complete parenteral nutrition, respectively.

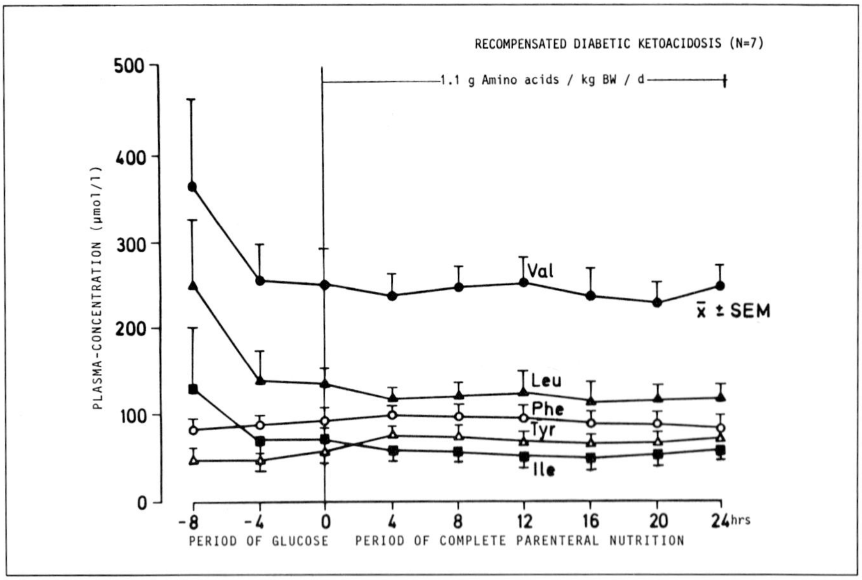

3

Table IV. Electrolyte solution for rehydration of severely metabolic deranged diabetic patients

Fluid	1000 ml
Sodium	90 mM
Chloride	65 mM
Potassium	25 mM
Calcium	1 mM
Phosphate	10 mM
Magnesium	1.5 mM
Malate	43 mM
Osmolality	236 mosm/kg H_2O

metabolism of uncontrolled diabetes is not only the consequence of insulin deficiency and the overproduction of the contraregulatory hormones, it is also the consequence of dehydration [12]. The BCAA valine, leucine, and isoleucine decreased in severe diabetic ketoacidosis by plain rehydration without exogenous administration of insulin with our diabetes electrolyte solution (table IV) [13].

During the above mentioned study, we measured the plasma concentration of the amino acids and got the following results. The BCAA valine, leucine, and isoleucine which were elevated in the insulin deficient state, decreased during insulin therapy and reached the normal range during the glucose phase. No change was detectable during complete parenteral nutrition in which the patients got 1.1 g L-amino-acids/kg B.W./day of a conventional AA mixture. The aromatic amino acids showed no significant change during all periods investigated (fig. 3).

It is of some interest that the gluconeogenic amino acids glycin, alanin, threonine, and serin increased during the intravenous administration of the diabetes nutrition solution (fig. 4). This increase of the gluconeogenic AA cannot be explained by the exogenous administration of these AA. We have not been able to find a significant correlation between the increase of the PAA concentrations and the AA dosage administered [11]. Thus, it can be assumed that the increase of these

Fig. 3. Mean value of plasma concentration of Val, Leu, Phe, Tyr, and Ile of 7 patients who just came out of severe diabetic ketoacidosis during continuous administration of 0.12 g glucose/kg B.W./h (glucose phase) and complete parenteral nutrition, respectively.

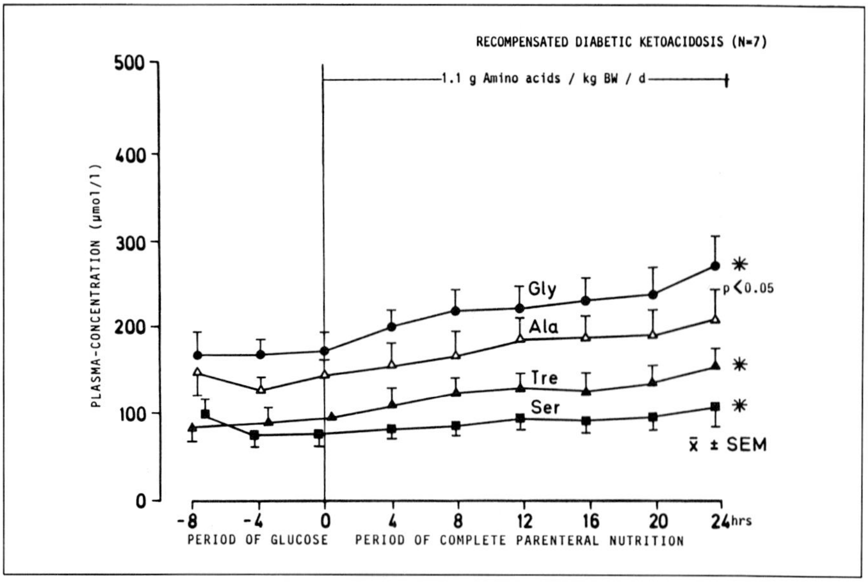

Fig. 4. Mean value of plasma concentration of Gly, Ala, Tre, and Ser of 7 patients who just came out of severe diabetic ketoacidosis during continuous administration of 0.12 g glucose/kg B.W./h (glucose phase) and complete parenteral nutrition, respectively.

gluconeogenic amino acids is due to an insulin-induced inhibition of the hepatic gluconeogenesis. The individual values of these amino acids remained within the normal range or exceeded insignificantly the upper limit of normal range. Therefore, in diabetic patients with sufficient insulin supply no special amino acid mixture is necessary.

Conclusion

Diabetes is the most frequent metabolic disease in traumatized patients and influences the metabolic response to injury. The nutritional support of the patients is often complicated by severe metabolic complications. An all-in-one solution with a decreased content of carbohydrates, compared to a normal solution, and a sufficient amount of lipids facilitates the metabolic treatment of these patients. There is some evidence that no special amino acid mixture is necessary for diabetic patients if insulin is sufficiently supplied. During the first 2 days of intravenous nutrition, a gradual adaptation of the patients and a constant rate of intravenous infusion are recommended to avoid unexpected metabolic complications.

References

1 Elwyn, D. H.: Nutritional requirements of adult surgical patients. Crit. Care Med. *8:* 9–20 (1980).

2 Schmitz, J. E.; Ahnefeld, F. W.; Burri, C.: Nutritional support of multiple trauma patient. World J. Surg. *7:* 132–142 (1983).

3 Mehnert, H.; Dehmel, K. H.: Stoffwechselkrankheiten: Diät bei Diabetes mellitus; in Kühn, Zöllner, Allgemeine und spezielle klinische Ernährungslehre, vol. II/1, pp. 48–75 (Thieme, Stuttgart 1978).

4 Liebermeister, H.: Diätetische Therapie; in Oberdisse, Diabetes mellitus; Hdb. inn. Med., vol. VII/2, pp. 757–786 (Springer, Berlin, Heidelberg, New York 1977).

5 Solassol, C.; Joyeux, H.; Serrou, B.; Pujol, H.; Romiau, C.: New techniques of long-term parenteral feeding for intestinal replacement. Report of 54 cases. J. Chir., Paris *105:* 15–24 (1973).

6 Kleinberger, G.; Durml, W.; Lochs, H.; Pamperl, H.; Widhalm, K.: Fetthaltige Gesamtnährlösungen für die parenterale Ernährung. Ernährung *8:* 143–153 (1984).

7 Kleinberger, G.; Pamperl, H.: Allgemeine Charakteristika und Fragen zur Galenik von Fettemulsionen. Infusionstherapie *10:* 108–117 (1983).

8 Pamperl, H.; Kleinberger, G.: Morphological changes of Intralipid 20% liposomes in all-in-one solutions during prolonged storage. Infusionstherapie *9:* 86–91 (1982).

9 Cuthbertson, D. P.: Disturbances of metabolism produced by bony and bony injury, with notes on certain abnormal conditions of bone. Biochem. J. *24:* 1244–1263 (1930).

10 Kleinberger, G.: Parenterale Ernährung bei Diabetes mellitus. Intensivmed. *18:* 91–96 (1981).

11 Kleinberger, G.: Infusionstherapie und parenterale Ernährung bei Patienten mit diabetischer Stoffwechselstörung. Ernährung *8:* 547-558 (1984).

12 Waldhäusl, W.; Kleinberger, G.: Acute treatment of diabetic coma; in Podolsky, Viswanathan, Secondary diabetes. The spectrum of diabetic syndromes, pp. 215–240 (Raven Press, New York 1980).

13 Kleinberger, G.; Bauer, K.; Gaßner, A.; Pichler, M.; Waldhäusl, W.; Westphal, G.: Treatment of electrolyte derangement in uncontrolled diabetes; in Waldhäusl, Diabetes 1979, International Congress Series 500, pp. 693–699 (Excerpta Medica, Amsterdam 1980).

Doz. Dr. G. Kleinberger, 1. Med. Abteilung, LKH Steyr, Sierningerstraße 170, A-4400 Steyr (Austria)

Dietze, Grünert, Kleinberger, Wolfram (eds.), Clinical Nutrition and Metabolic Research. Proc. 7th Congr. ESPEN, Munich 1985, pp. 300–310 (Karger, Basel 1986)

Parenteral versus Tube Feeding in the Diabetic Patient

S. P. Allison

University Hospital, Nottingham, UK

The diabetic and non-diabetic patient differ in only one respect: the former suffers from a permanent state of insulin deficiency or insulin resistance, whereas the latter may suffer a transitory state of altered insulin secretion and activity, associated with the metabolic response to acute illness and injury. The type I or insulin deficient diabetic requires insulin treatment at all times and knows that with the insulin resistance associated with acute illness he needs to increase his insulin dose. Without insulin treatment, such patients develop ketoacidosis and the severe illness which goes with it. The type-II diabetics on the other hand are often obese and suffer insulin resistance with a degree of insulin deficiency. They are normally treated by dietary restriction and, in some instances, with tablets. Although they do not become ketotic in the face of acute illness, they may develop very high blood sugars necessitating temporary insulin treatment until the illness is over.

The therapeutic problem caused by intolerance to carbohydrate in enteral or parenteral nutrition, in both the diabetic and the non-diabetic, is a fairly straightforward one. The aim is:

(1) to avoid overwhelming the patient with an excessive rate of administration of carbohydrate;

(2) to provide insulin at a rate which maintains the blood glucose between 5 and 15 mmol concentration, avoiding persistent hyperglycaemia and its associated fluid problems or hypoglycaemia which the patient and the staff find alarming.

I would like to review briefly the changes in carbohydrate metabolism associated with injury in the non-diabetic patient, and then discuss the technique of insulin administration in the diabetic and non-diabetic. Glucose intolerance, associated with acute illness and injury, has been known for many years, e.g., the 'pseudo diabetes' associated with burns. We [1] and others have described the suppression of insulin secretion in the acute phase of injury giving way to insulin resistance with persistent glucose intolerance and high insulin levels. In figure 1 are shown the insulin responses to a 50 g intravenous glucose tolerance test in the acute phase of burn injury compared with those seen a week later. Insulin response is suppressed in the acute phase, due to alpha adrenergic stimuli. A week later there is persistent glucose intolerance with high insulin levels. Other workers have described the increase in corticosteroid [2, 3], glucagon [4], growth hormone, and catecholamine secretion [3], all of which have an insulin antagonistic effect. These changes are summarised in figure 2

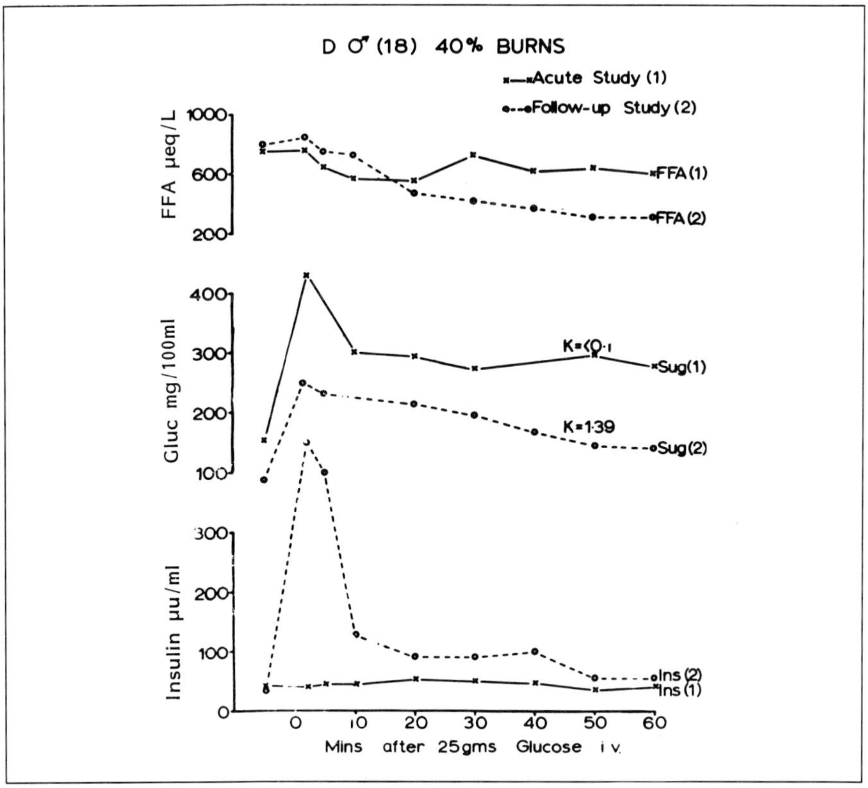

Fig. 1. Insulin responses to a 50 g intravenous glucose tolerance test in the acute phase of burn injury (1) and in follow-up study (2), 1 week later.

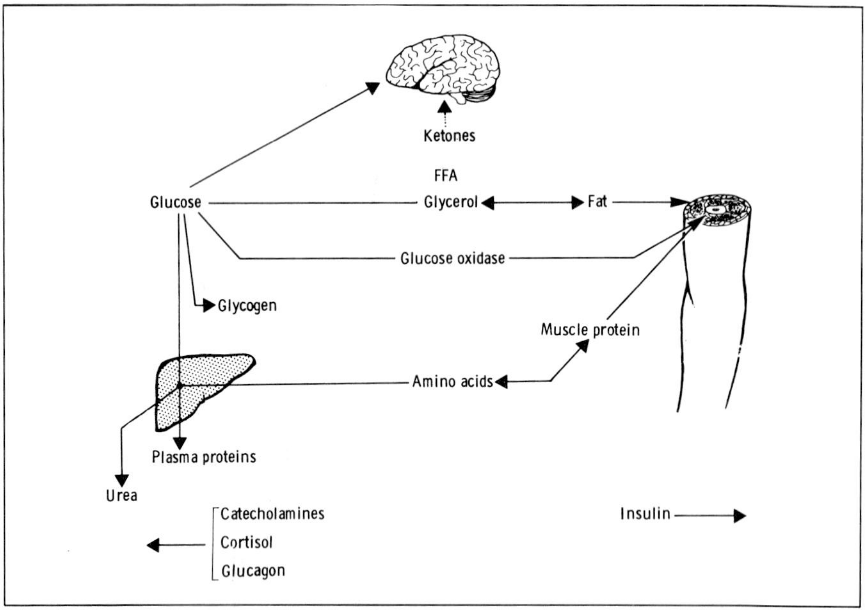

Fig. 2. The role of the balance between the anabolic or storage hormone, insulin, and the catabolic hormones in respect of glucose, fat and protein metabolism in injury.

which emphasises the role of the balance between the anabolic or storage hormone, insulin, and the catabolic hormones, not only in respect of glucose metabolism, but also of fat and protein metabolism. Injury therefore leads to protein breakdown, the resulting amino acids being used for gluconeogenesis in the liver.

We have described how insulin infusion not only controls hyperglycaemia during parenteral nutrition, but also diminishes protein catabolism in the more severely ill patients such as major burns [5].

A constant nitrogen infusion of 10 g daily was given and different but isocaloric energy sources compared in 3-day cross-over periods. The infusion of glucose alone was compared with that of glucose and insulin; the resulting glucose and insulin levels are shown in table I, and the changes in protein catabolism, as measured by urea production rate, are shown in figure 3. The non-catabolic patients with urea production rates between 12 and 20 g/24 h show no effect of insulin, whereas those with major burns, and urea production rates of 40 to 50 g/24 h, showed a 30–40% reduction of in urea production rate when insulin was added to the glu-

Table I. Infusion of glucose alone compared with that of glucose and insulin

Regimen	Blood glucose mmol/l	Serum insulin mU/l
Insulin/Glucose	7.5 ± 4.3	223 ± 219
Glucose alone	11.0 ± 3.3	81 ± 47
P value	< 0.001	< 0.005

cose. In further studies [6], Dr. Woolfson measured insulin resistance, i.e., the rate of insulin infusion required to maintain normoglycaemia in the face of a constant rate of glucose infusion; he showed that this correlated positively with urea production rate, i.e., glucose intolerance and protein catabolism were increased in proportion to each other in the severely ill patient. Similar problems are encountered in patients receiving enteral nutrition. In an early study [7] using peptides as the nitrogen source and 600 g/day of the glucose polymer, Caloreen, as the energy source, we treated a number of patients by nasogastric tube feeding for periods up to 4 weeks. Blood glucose was measured routinely and insulin was given when the blood glucose exceeded a level of 12 mmol. The insulin requirements of these patients are shown in table II. It can be seen that those with

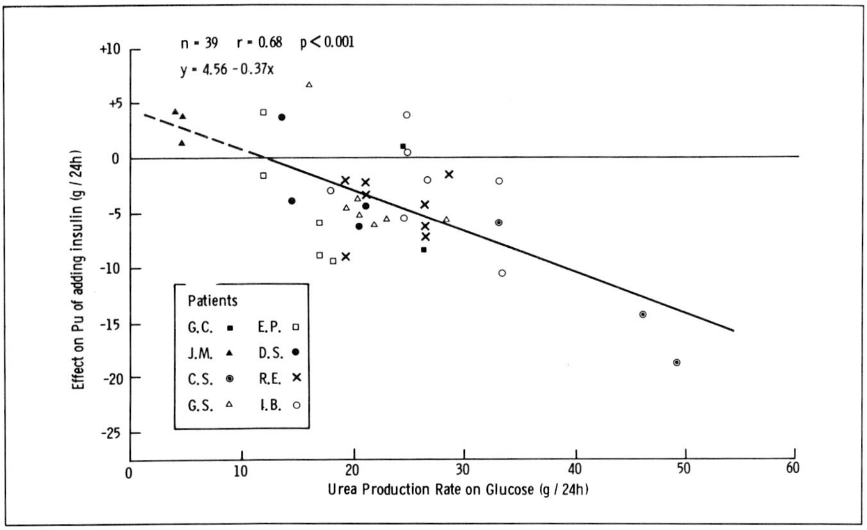

Fig. 3. Changes in protein catabolism as measured by urea production rate.

Table II. Insulin requirements to maintain blood glucose at 100–180 mg/100 ml

Diagnosis	Insulin units
1 Postoperative collapse	60–120
2 Crushed chest	40–120
1 Head injury + Crushed chest	40–80
1 Ca mouth	< 20 u. for 3 days only
3 Head injury	0
1 Respiratory failure	0
6 Ca mouth	0*

minor injury did not require insulin and the more severely ill patients required insulin in proportion to the severity of their injury. The control of blood glucose in enteral and parenteral nutrition has been revolutionised by the introduction of simple, rapid and accurate methods of measuring blood glucose by the bedside, using capillary blood obtained by finger prick [8]. The enzyme sticks made by Boehringer or Ames are excellent for this purpose and can be read either by eye against a colour chart, or more accurately using a small machine. In an unstable situation, the blood glucose may be measured hourly and changes made in insulin or glucose infusion rate. When the patient is stable, a blood glucose measurement every 6 h is perfectly adequate.

In health, the insulin requiring diabetic is taking food in the form of meals every 4 to 6 h. He is also taking intermittent injections of insulin timed to coincide with maximum food absorption. A few patients use portable pumps which maintain a constant fasting infusion rate of approximately 1 U/h to control hepatic glucose output. The rate is turned up at mealtimes to an appropriate level. With enteral and parenteral as opposed to oral nutrition, carbohydrate is given by constant infusion, and the pattern of insulin administration must match this. For the diabetic receiving parenteral nutrition for more than a few weeks, either in hospital or at home, one of the portable insulin pumps giving insulin subcutaneously may be ideal. However, in patients, whether diabetic or non-diabetic, receiving enteral or parenteral nutrition during a period of acute illness, we use a Vickers variable speed pump to give glucose intravenously. This is usually administered via a peripheral vein and not through the central venous line, in order to avoid contamination and infection. All patients should receive a non-immunogenic insulin in the form of short acting,

Table III. Glucose infusion rate – *a*g/h. Start at *b*U/ml at *c*ml/h i.e. *bc*U/h. Test 1 hourly

Blood glucose		Action
< 4.0 mM		Reduce rate by 1.0 ml/h
4.0–6.9 mM		Reduce rate by 0.5 ml/h
7.0–10.9 mM		Same rate
11.0–15.0 mM	If lower than last test	Same rate
	If higher than last test	Increase rate by 0.5 ml/h
> 15.0 mM	If lower than last test	Same rate
	If higher than last test	Increase rate by 1.0 ml/h
If rate becomes 0.5 ml/h or zero – half concentration and restart at 0.5 ml/h		
If rate becomes 4.5 or 5 ml/h – double concentration and restart at 2.5 ml/h		

purified porcine or human insulin. Old fashioned, unpurified or beef insulin should be avoided, since immunisation to insulin may cause problems in the future. My colleague, Dr. Woolfson [9], has devised an excellent algorithm (table III) for controlling insulin infusion rate which takes into account not only the prevailing blood sugar, but the direction of change since the previous measurement. The administration of substrate and of insulin separately risks hypoglycaemia if the glucose infusion stops, either through pump failure or blockage of the central venous line, while the insulin infusion continues. This risk is avoided with modern infusion pumps with their alarm systems. If there is any risk that the glucose infusion rate may vary, as with gravity feeding, or where separate bottle reservoirs are used instead of the single big bag, then it can be quite safe and effective to add the insulin to the glucose solution, making some allowance for loss of insulin on to glassware and tubing. I usually find that in the non-insulin resistant patient, a ratio of 1 unit of insulin to 4 g of glucose is safe and adequate. Indeed, in the early days of the use of insulin and glucose in parenteral nutrition, we invariably used this technique. It has the great disadvantage that it is difficult to change the insulin to glucose ratio at frequent intervals in the unstable patient. The intermittent injection of subcutaneous insulin (fig. 4) does not give the same degree of control as constant infusion although we have used this technique for its convenience in some patients receiving enteral nutrition. It has been our practice to meet half to three-quarters of the patient's energy intake from carbohydrate. In parenteral nutrition, this means a glucose infusion rate of between 25–35 g/h. With enteral nutrition we use either a ready made proprietary feed containing whole protein, oligosaccharides and fat, or a

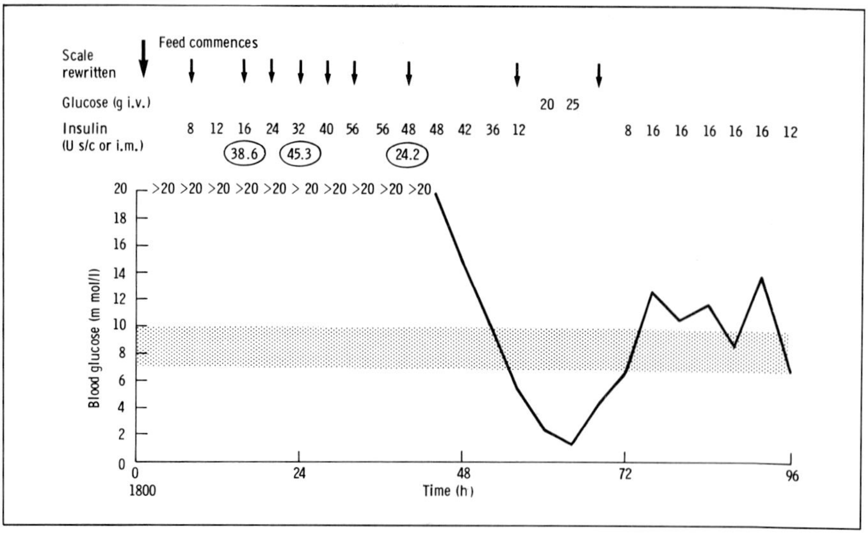

Fig. 4. Intermittent injection of subcutaneous insulin.

more concentrated feed consisting of a high protein preparation with the addition of oligosaccharides or glucose polymer in liquid form, as in Fortical, or powdered form, as in Caloreen. We do not use alternative forms of carbohydrate such as fructose or sorbitol which have been suggested in the glucose intolerant patient. A diagrammatic representation of the glycolytic pathway is shown in figure 5. Although both fructose and sorbitol are independent in terms of their initial phosphorylation, nevertheless, as soon as they enter the intermediary pathways of carbohydrate metabolism, they are influenced by the action of insulin and counter regulatory hormones. In a diabetic or post-injury state where gluconeogenesis is accelerated, they are both converted to glucose and may give rise to hyperglycaemia. Secondly, none of these alternative carbohydrates are easily measured in the peripheral circulation and their effects cannot, therefore, be easily judged. Thirdly, they may be toxic in some patients causing lactic acidosis, hypophosphataemia and hyperuricaemia.

With enteral nutrition, we do not use a dilute starter regimen strength feed, but on the first day use full strength feed administered by pump at half the normal rate. In enteral feeding, it is not the concentration of osmoles or substrates per unit volume which matters, but the administration per unit time [10]. In parenteral nutrition we do not use a starter

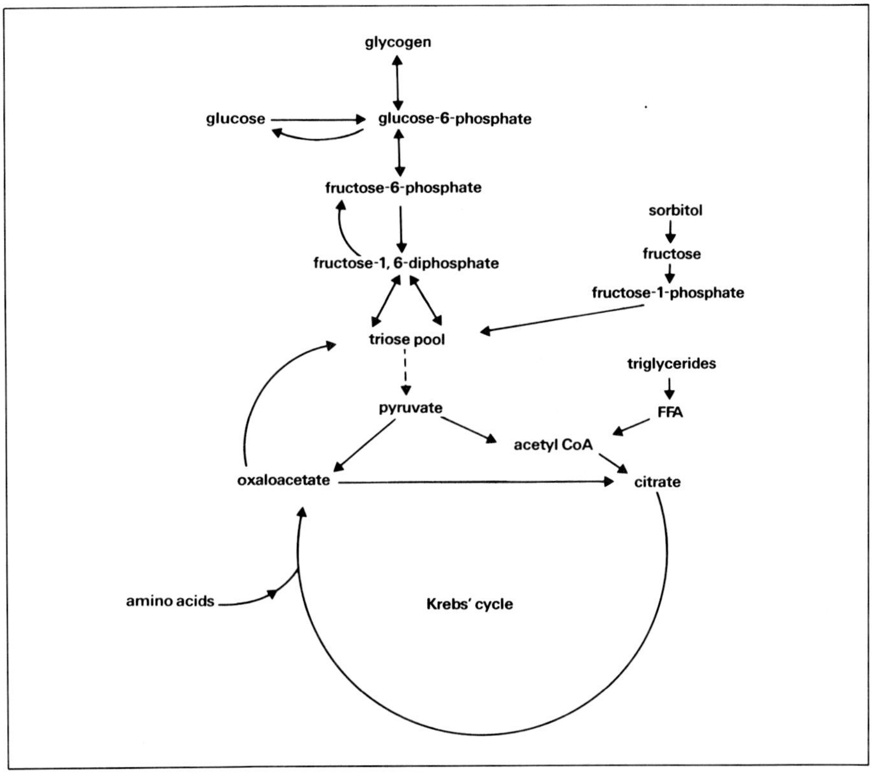

Fig. 5. Glycolytic pathway.

regimen either, prefering to control blood glucose using the insulin infusion algorithm which I have already mentioned. The effects of doing this in a non-diabetic, but glucose intolerant patient are shown in figure 6. Initial hyperglycaemia in excess of 20 mmol is rapidly and smoothly brought under control without any hypoglycaemic overshoot. As soon as stabilisation is achieved, an infusion rate of 4–6 U/h is quite sufficient to maintain normoglycaemia in the face of a glucose infusion rate of 30 g/h. Should there be a worsening in the patient's condition caused, for example, by an infection, there is an immediate increase in insulin resistance. Regular measuring of the blood glucose by the bedside allows this to be observed early and the insulin infusion rate adjusted. In figure 7 are shown the data from a totally insulin deficient diabetic patient with mesenteric artery thrombosis and gangrene of the bowel. Total parenteral nutrition was commenced with a glucose infusion rate of 25 g/h. In the absence of fever and infection, the degree of insulin resistance was small and over three days the insulin infusion rate could be gradually reduced from 6 to 2 U/h.

Conclusions

I have tried to show that the control of glycaemia in the diabetic patient requiring enteral or parenteral nutrition is simple and little different from that in the non-diabetic. The same nutritional regimens can be used in both situations and are determined by the nutritional requirements and not by whether diabetes is present or not. As in the non-diabetic, enteral and parenteral nutrition are complementary, not competitive.

The control of glycaemia is facilitated by frequent bedside measurements of capillary blood using enzyme sticks. Using the appropriate algorithm, the insulin infusion rate can be adjusted and normoglycaemia maintained without any risk of hypoglycaemia. Insulin may also diminish protein catabolism in catabolic patients. For parenteral or enteral nutrition in diabetes, continuous intravenous or subcutaneous insulin infusion is the treatment of choice. In parenteral nutrition it may, in some cases, be

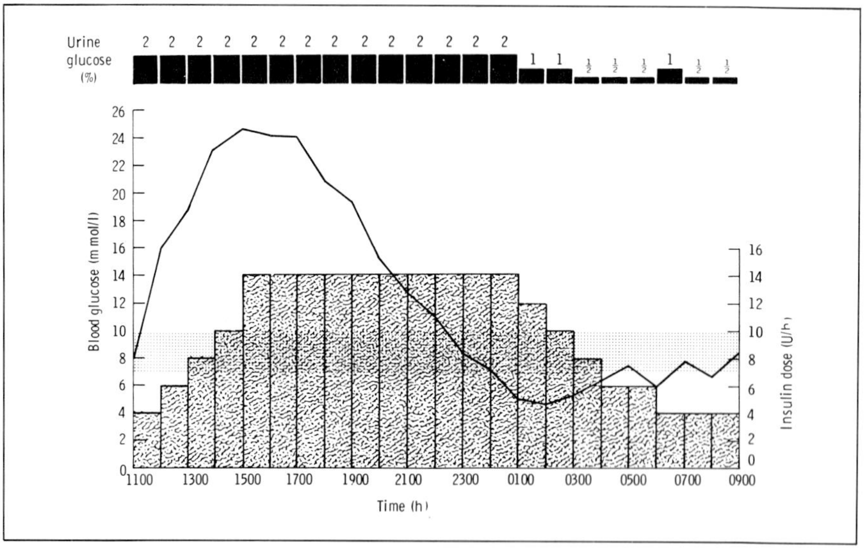

Fig. 6. Control of blood glucose in a non-diabetic, but glucose intolerant patient.

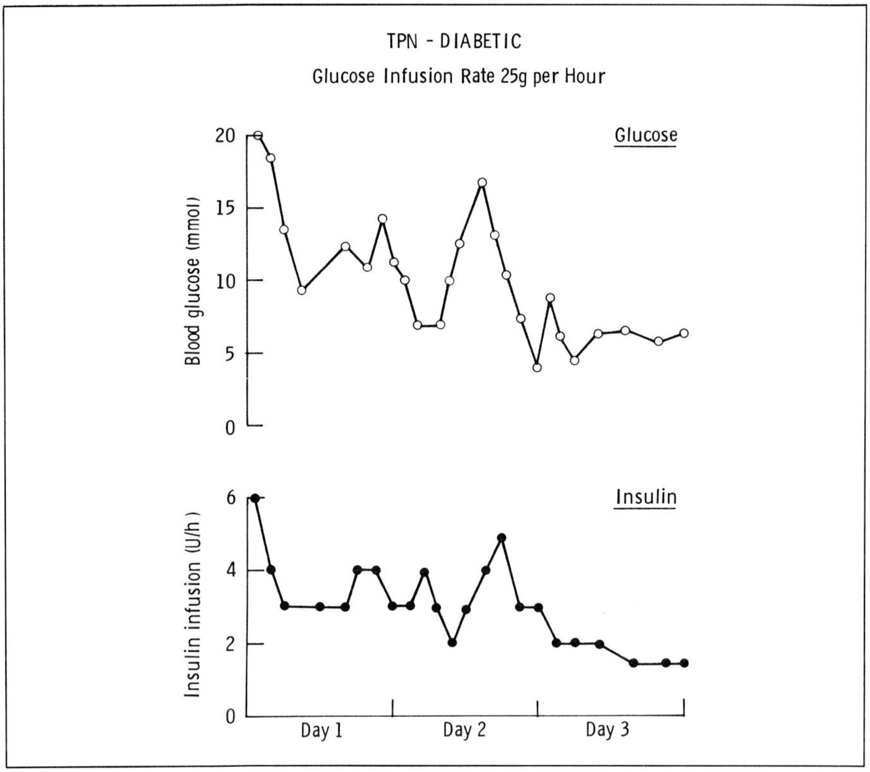

Fig. 7. Data from a totally insulin deficient diabetic patient with mesenteric artery thrombosis and gangrene of the bowel.

satisfactory to add insulin to the glucose reservoir, making allowance for losses on glass or plastic. In enteral nutrition subcutaneous insulin twice or three times daily may be more convenient.

There is no case for using alternative forms of carbohydrate. Glucose polymers and oligosaccharides should be used for enteral, and glucose solutions for parenteral nutrition.

References

1 Allison, S. P.; Hinton, P.; Chamberlain, M. J.: Intravenous glucose tolerance, insulin and free fatty acid levels in burned patients. Lancet *ii:* 1113–1116 (1968).

2 Cope, O.; Nathanson, I. T.; Rourke, G. M. et al.: Metabolic observations on shock. Ann. Surg. *117:* 937 (1943).

3 Birke, G.; Duner, H.; Liljedahl, S. O. et al.: Histamine, catecholamines and adrenocortical steroids in burns. Acta clin. scand. *114:* 87 (1957).

4 Wilmore, D. W.; Moylan, J. A.; Pruitt, B. A. et al.: Hyperglucagonaemia after burns. Lancet *i:* 73 (1974).

5 Woolfson, A. M. J.; Heatley, R. V.; Allison, S. P.: Insulin to inhibit protein catabolism after injury. New Engl. J. Med. *300:* 14 (1979).

6 Woolfson, A. M. J.: Insulin, nutrition and injury; thesis Nottingham University (1979).

7 Woolfson, A. M. J.; Ricketts, C. R.; Hardy, S. M.; Saour, J. N.; Pollard, B. J.; Allison, S. P.: Prolonged nasogastric tube feeding in critically ill and surgical patients. Postgrad. med. J. *52:* 678–682 (1976).

8 Walford, S.; Allison, S. P.; Gale, E. A. M.; Tattersall, R. B.: Self-monitoring of blood glucose. Lancet *i:* 732–735 (1978).

9 Woolfson, A. M. J.: An improved method for blood glucose control during nutritional support. J. parent. ent. Nutr. *5:* 436–440 (1981).

10 Bastow, D.; Rawlings, J.; Allison, S. P.: Overnight nasogastric tube feeding. Clin. Nutr. *4:* 7–11 (1985).

Dr. S. P. Allison, MD, FRCP, Dept. of Medicine, University Hospital, Queen's Medical Centre, GB-Nottingham NG7 2UH (UK)

Dietze, Grünert, Kleinberger, Wolfram (eds.), Clinical Nutrition and Metabolic Research. Proc. 7th Congr. ESPEN, Munich 1985, pp. 311–328 (Karger, Basel 1986)

Species Differences Relevant to Nutrition and Metabolism Research

D. Giesecke

Institute for Physiology, Physiological Chemistry, and Nutrition Physiology, University of Munich, FRG

All animals are equal but some animals are more equal than others. (George Orwell: Animal Farm, 1945)

Mammals have many features in common. However, the gross classification of species into carnivores, herbivores, and omnivores indicates definite differences in nutrition. In fact, nutritional adaptation to ecological niches, the driving force of evolution, has coined the patterns of perception and selection of food, of ingestion and digestion, of metabolism and excretion, i.e. of functions which are more or less typical of individual species. Man in this context has emerged from evolution as a carnivore, but has started to harvest crops and become more of an omnivore about 8000 years ago.

Fortunately, the researcher in the field of experimental biology and medicine has not necessarily to be concerned with the overwhelming diversity of nutritional patterns in animals which evolution has propagated. He can restrict himself to those features which, after domestication, standardization and adaptation, finally have persisted and proved suitable for comparative research. Thus, the present paper is not intended as a catalogue of differences between species which have occasionally been described. Instead, only a limited number of examples have been selected to discuss specific features of digestion, intermediary metabolism, and disposal of catabolites in view of the central question: Which species, including man, 'are more equal than others'?

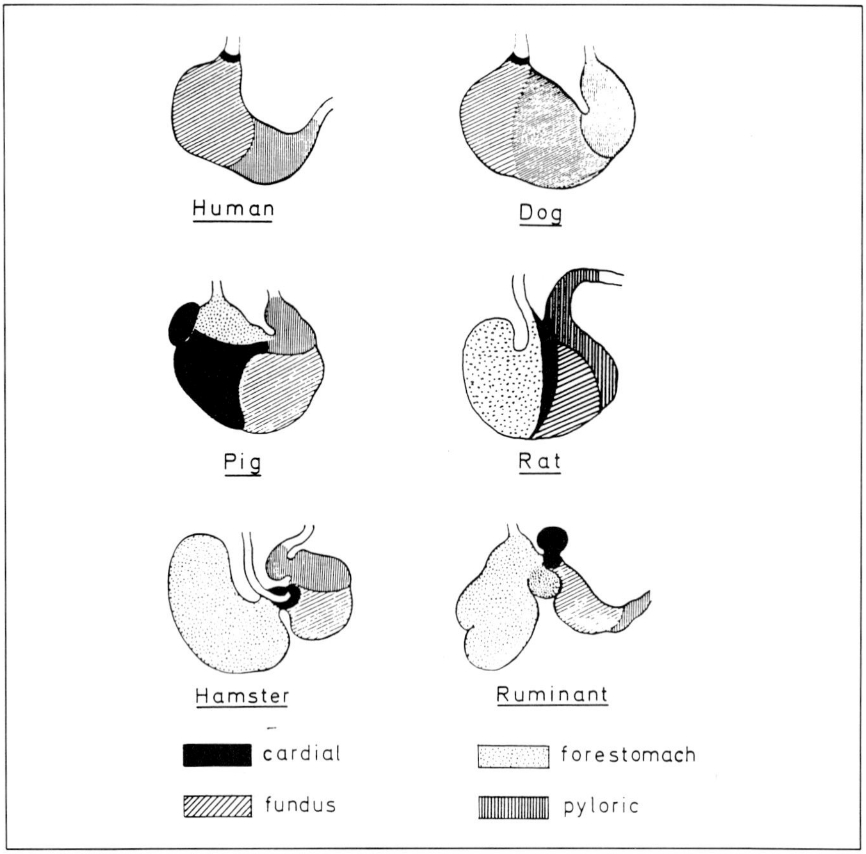

Fig. 1. Stomach in various species [34].

Differences in Digestive Functions

In experimental models based on conventional or enteral nutrition, certain anatomical and functional differences of the gastrointestinal tract gain considerable importance. In fact, the general descriptive term 'monogastric' is frequently used to suggest a similarity of digestive functions between animals and man, which is rarely justified. Except for man, dog, cat, and certain primates, monogastric mammals have more or less extended forestomach areas (fig. 1), enabling microbial fermentation of ingested (or infused) nutrients. Further anatomical differences are the length of the intestine and the extension of the large intestine. The former has been expressed as the proportion of body length: intestinal length [14] again showing a reasonable agreement between dog and man:

cat	dog	man	rabbit	horse	pig	sheep
1 : 4	1 : 6	1 : 6	1 : 10	1 : 12	1 : 14	1 : 28

The extent of gastrointestinal conversion of nutrients into microbial fermentation products is reflected by the concentrations of lactic acid and/ or volatile fatty acids (VFA) in the stomach and hindgut (table I). In rabbits and pigs [38] as well as in rats [43] α-amylase in saliva supports the breakdown of starch for fermentation. Both D(−) and L(+) lactic acid are produced as end products if the stomach environment is not anaerobic enough to allow for microbial transformation into VFA. Particularly high lactate levels in piglets of about 100 mmol l^{-1} [15] as compared to pigs suggest that age may play a role. It is worth noting that in folivorous colobid monkeys the stomach fermentation is comparable to rumen fermentation in sheep.

More recently the similarity of microbes and their metabolic products in the human large intestine and the rumen has been emphasized [16, 52], pointing out at the same time 'that we each have more microbial than human cells' [16]. The molar proportions (mol%) of acetic, propionic, and butyric acids in the colobid stomach of 62, 22, and 8 [18], in the sheep

Table I. Microbial fermention in the gastrointestinal tract

Species	(Fore)-stomach		Large intestine
	DL-lactate mmol l^{-1}	VFA [20] mmol	VFA [20] (100 g dry matter)$^{-1}$
Human	not done		134*
Dog	not done	1	57 [44]
Rat	111 [29]	3	63
Pig	53 [36]	25	57
Horse	14 [1]	8	87
Rabbit	4 [2]	5	29
Colobid monkeys	not done	103–219 [18]	not done
Sheep	0.3 [13]	128	56

* Fecal VFA [19]

Table II. Content of pancreatic ribonuclease in mammals [9]

Species	Ribonuclease* μg/g
Dog, cat	0.5
Human	1
Monkey (Macaca mulatta)	2
Horse	25
Pig	80
Guinea pig	240
Rat, hamster	260
Mouse	395
Cow, goat, sheep	1000–1200

* μg ribonuclease per g of pancreatic tissue

rumen of 64, 22, and 11 [23] and in human feces of 75, 17, and 8 [52] are in reasonable agreement. However, quantitative differences in monogastric hindgut fermentation are apparent; the contribution of VFA to the energy requirements for maintenance have been estimated up to 30% in pigs [22] and rabbits [42] but only 7–10% in man [49].

In a different comparison of species the relative importance of microbial productivity in the foregut has been associated with pancreatic ribonuclease activity (table II), which is needed for the recycling of nucleic acid phosphate [9]. These observations result in a similar sequence of species as anatomical features and fermentation activities had suggested.

Species-Related Patterns in Intermediary Metabolism

Differences between species in metabolism are abundant. The examples selected for this section refer to the metabolism of carbohydrates, lipids, amino acids, and vitamins.

Carbohydrate Metabolism

Microbial carbohydrate breakdown in the GI-tract affects metabolism. One example is D(−)lactic acid, a specific microbial product, the oxidation rate of which after absorption (fig. 2) is related to gastric pro-

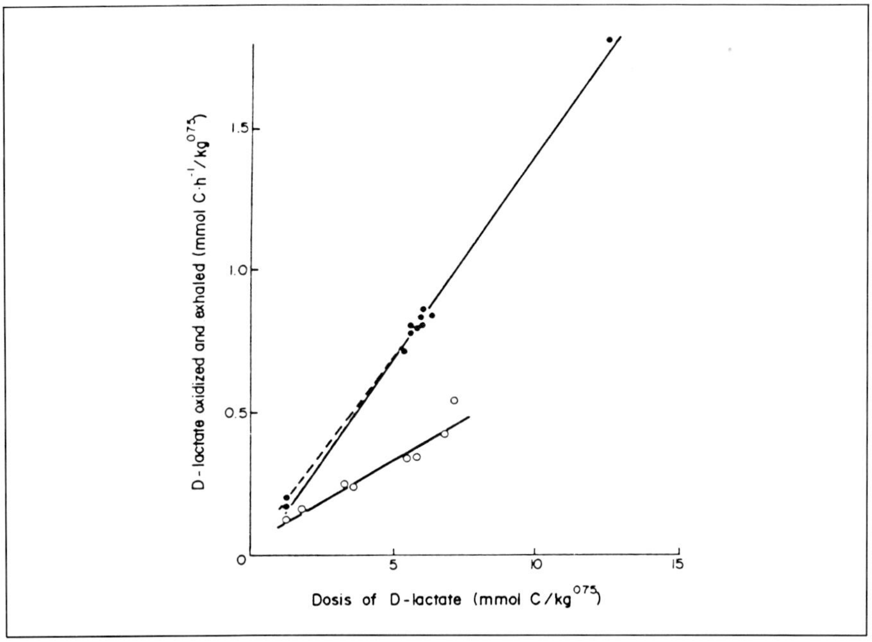

Fig. 2. Oxidation of D(−)lactic acid in the rat -●- and the rabbit -○- [25]; rat: $y = 0.146x - 0.032$; $r = 0.997$; $p < 0.001$; rabbit: $y = 0.062x + 0.030$; $r = 0.963$; $p < 0.001$.

duction (see table I). Obviously the rat handles (D(−)lactate oxidation considerably faster than the rabbit. The adaptive effect of D(−)lactate from the stomach on D-2-hydroxy acid dehydrogenase (EC 1.1.99.6), the rate limiting enzyme, is supported by the observation [27] that D(−) lactate oxidation in the liver is considerably lower in germ-free than in conventional rats. These results and an observed inhibition of D(−)lactate oxidation by L(+)lactate may have a bearing on parenteral nutrition of patients with small bowel surgery who can suffer from D(−)lactic acidosis [26, 27].

The central role of glucose metabolism is well established. Quantitation by metabolic kinetics (^{14}C or ^{3}H-glucose) has revealed that glucose entry rates and body weights of species are connected by a log-log relationship (fig. 3). Even though animals are equal in this respect, biochemical functions necessary for maintaining glucostasis are likely to differ, because of species-related peculiarities in dietary carbohydrate intake and digestion, circadian activity, and glucose recycling. Thus the activity of

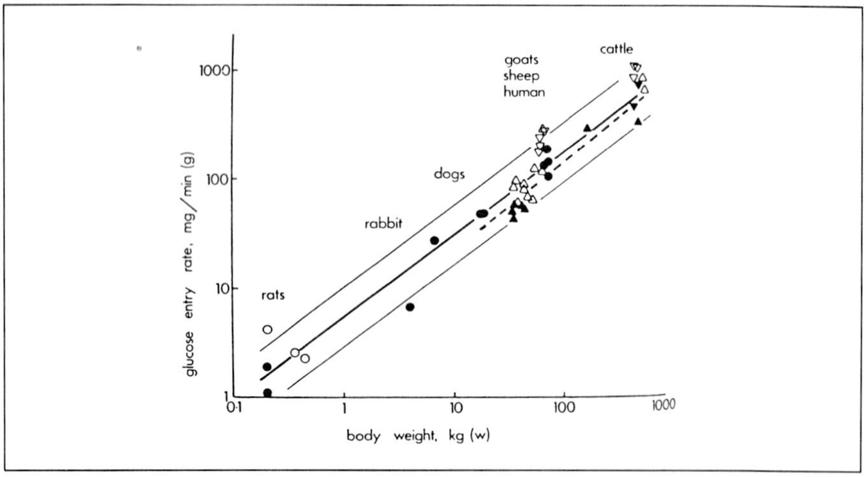

Fig. 3. Relationship between glucose entry rates (post absorptive) and body weights of various species [4]; regression for nonruminants ± SD. (fasted 0–4 h ○ and 12–24 h ●); the regression for 12-24 h after feeding is $G = 2.86\ W^{0.807}$; regression for non-lactating sheep and cattle (fasted 0–16 h △ and 24–96 h ▲); the regression for 24–96 h after feeding is $G = 4.60\ W^{0.804}$; lactating sheep, goat, and cows fasted 0–16 h ▽ or 24–96 h ▼ not included in the calculation.

hepatic glucokinase, the specific enzyme responsible for channelling the portal flux of absorbed glucose into hepatic glucose uptake and glycogen storage, has been shown to vary between 3.8 and 0.03 U per g liver of respective species according to the following sequence [49]:

rat > mouse > pig > dog > rabbit > guinea pig > man > cat, sheep.

It shows starch-feeding omnivores (granivores) at the top, species absorbing very little glucose at the end and intermediate feeding types in between. In an earlier study [37] glucokinase activity in the human liver had been given a similarily low position close to carnivorous felids. This would suggest that the capacity of the human liver to convert high portal glucose fluxes into glycogen is lower than in most of the other experimental animals.

Differences between species are particularly obvious in the classical case of PEP-CK compartmentation. This key enzyme for the regulation of gluconeogenesis transforms mitochondrial oxaloacetate (from glucogenic amino acids, propionate, etc.) into phosphoenolpyruvate for further upgrading to glucose by cytosolic enzymes. PEP-CK is distributed in both cytosol and mitochondria of hepatocytes, however, the activities vary widely: e.g. in rat liver total PEP-CK activity is only about 10% of that in pigeon liver, but more than 90% of it are localized in the cytosol, whereas the pigeon harbors 95% in mitochondria [47].

The compartmentation of the enzyme as given by Hanson and Garber [32] and Söling [47] for a variety of species is shown in table III. The former authors have pointed out that under conditions of hunger or diabetes only the activity of cytosolic PEP-CK is increased (except for ruminants showing no response), not the mitochondrial enzyme, which regulates a more autonomous type of gluconeogenesis. The predominance of cytosolic PEP-CK appears to be a special requirement of the nocturnal granivores (bottom of table), which have also high hepatic glucokinase activity (see above). In species with high activity of mitochondrial PEP-CK (top of table) a more constant supply of glucose is maintained by more frequent diurnal feeding (pigeon, rabbit) or by constant gluconeogenesis in carnivores (cat, dog), feeding infrequently on diets poor in carbohydrates. In the latter species the insulin system appears to be weaker as indicated by more frequent occurrence of diabetes as compared to other animal species.

Even though only of relevance in the early phase of life, fructogenic species should be mentioned, including mainly the ungulates i.e. pig,

Table III. Compartmentation of PEP-CK* in the livers of various species [32]

Species	% of total	
	cytosol	mitochondria
Pigeon	5	95
Rabbit	5	95
Cat	35	65
Dog [47]	35	65
Human	40	60
Guinea pig	40	60
Cattle	50	50
Sheep	65	35
Pig [47]	71	29
Rat	90	10
Mouse	90	10
Hamster	95	5

* Phosphoenolpyruvate carboxykinase (EC 4.1.1.32)

sheep, goat, cattle, horse, and others. In the fetus and neonate of these species, fructose is the main blood sugar, which is replaced by glucose soon after birth.

Lipogenesis

In lipid metabolism differences between species are shown by dietary lipid tolerance, which is high in chicken and rat, but low in sheep and pig, and by the distribution of lipogenic activity between liver and adipose tissue. These two are quantitatively the most important organs even though others are capable of synthesizing fatty acids de novo. Published rates of lipogenesis, as given in table IV, will not allow a strictly quantitative inter-species comparison because of variation in the methods used such as age and nutrition of individuals, sampling of tissues, conditions of sample incubation in vitro (kind and level of substrate, level of insulin), and biological reference used. However, the ratio of adipose tissue to liver of lipogenic activity demonstrates the main difference between species; in

Table IV. Lipogenic activity in adipose tissue and liver

Species	Method substrate	Rate of incorporation (nmol/g/h)*		Ratio	References
		adipose tissue	liver	A :L	
Human	^3H from ^3H_2O glucose	0.74 ± 0.32	6.3 ± 3.5	0.12	[3]
Rat	glucose-^{14}C	186 ± 33	517 ± 90	0.36	[31]
	acetate-^{14}C	10 ± 3	490 ± 120	0.02	
Mouse	^3H from ^3H_2O glucose	3600 ± 1700	2900 ± 200	1.24	[33]
Sheep	glucose-^{14}C	110 ± 40	1 ± 0.1	110	[35]
	acetate-^{14}C	640 ± 140	6 ± 2	107	
Pig	glucose-^{14}C	2480 ± 310	10 ± 3	248	[39]
	acetate-^{14}C	2430 ± 270	17 ± 3	143	
Dog	glucose-^{14}C	1240 ± 270	1 ± 0.3	1240	Giesecke et al. (unpubl.)**

* inter-species comparison of quantitative data appears difficult because of variation in methods (age and feeding of individuals, levels of substrate, of insulin, etc.)
** data from 16 dogs (Beagle and Dalmatian) referred to mg DNA in respective tissue

fact, the ratios of 0.12 in the human, which is indicative of high hepatic lipogenesis, and of 1240 in the dog differ by 4 orders of magnitude. It is important to emphasize that the ratios are calculated from the respective rates per g of tissue. This means that the lipogenic activity of the whole organs may by relatively higher in adipose tissue (the mass of which is difficult to estimate but is much higher than for liver) than the values of the table would suggest. Only few results have been obtained with lactate as a substrate, but observations in porcine [39] and in ovine [45] adipose tissues have demonstrated that lactic acid is a suitable precursor for fatty acids. In metabolism this transformation is favored by high plasma insulin levels (e.g. post-feeding) suppressing gluconeogenesis from lactate.

Metabolism of Amino Acids

Are animals equal in amino acid metabolism? There appears to exist general agreement on whole body protein turnover being connected to body weight by a log-log relationship with the same exponent of 0.73 as basal energy metabolism, some 20% of which are needed to cover the energy costs of protein turnover [50]. This general rule neither excludes deviations of certain species nor of special demands for one or the other amino acid. Indeed, under conditions of conventional or enteral nutrition, the remarkable differences in length of the intestine, but even more so the tremendous volume of the hindgut in some species associated with high microbial activities, should create differences in amino acid requirements [21]. Such special expenses have not yet been quantified, however, the well-known increase in weight gain and feed efficiency of animals fed nutritive amounts of certain antibiotics is an indirect proof of such an effect.

Based on more recent observations [8] felids have higher amino acid requirements than other monogastric species including an essential demand for arginine (see below). Rabbits and avians require a dietary source of glycin and a high level of arginine to achieve maximum growth, and dogs do very poorly on arginine deficient diets. Unique is the high sensitivity of feline species to arginine deficiency and to high dietary levels of glutamic acid [40]. Both result in hyperammonemia at a very early stage which can, however, be prevented by supplementing ornithine. Limitations of enzymes for ornithine synthesis from glutamate in the intestinal mucosa [46] provide an explanation for this peculiarity and cast some light

Table V. Bioefficacy of D-tryptophan

Species	% of L-tryptophan	Reference
Rat	100	[41]
Pig	60	[6]
Dog	36	[17]
Chicken	21*	[41]
Mouse	limited	[5]
Man	capacity	[5]

* 40% after injection

Table VI. Bioefficacy of certain D-amino acids in rat and chicken

Amino Acid	% of L-isomer		Reference
	rat	chicken	
D-Arg	0	0	[7]
D-His	0	19	[7]
D-Ile	16	70	[12]
D-Leu	48	100	[12]
D-Met	100*	100**	* [53], ** [48]
D-Phe	68	75	[11]
D-Thr	0	0	[48]
D-Trp	100	21	[41]
D-Val	–	43	[48]

Table VII. Bioefficacy of L-isoleucin analogues in rat and chicken [11, 12]

Analogues	% of L-isoleucin*	
	rat	chicken
2-DL-amino-3-methylvaleric acid	58	85
2-keto-3-methylvaleric acid	38	60
2-L-hydroxy-3-methylvaleric acid	65	54
2-DL-hydroxy-3-methylvaleric acid	45	49
2-D-hydroxy-3-methylvaleric acid	– 2	– 10

* 2-L-amino-3-methylvaleric acid

on the contribution of the intestine to urea cycle metabolism. The arginine deficient cat offers an interesting model for studying urea cycle functions in view of patients with dysfunction of the liver.

In amino acid nutrition the bioefficacy of D-isomers and L-amino acid analogues is of considerable interest. In this respect species can vary widely as indicated for D-Trp (table V) being utilized as efficiently as L-Trp by the rat but very poorly by mouse and human. The bioefficacy of some other D-amino acids was compared in rat and chicken (table VI). Both are equal in the utilization of D-Met and D-Phe, but differ with regard to other amino acids. The bioefficacy of branched-chain amino acid analogues has also been evaluated in rat and chicken as shown for L-Ile in table VII. In general, the chicken appears to be superior to the rat except for D-Trp (see table V), but it is clear that no generalizations can be made and the bioefficacy of any compound of interest must be evaluated for every species in question.

Vitamins

Observations on species-related patterns of vitamin requirements and effects are rare; the ascorbic acid demands by man, primates, and guinea pig being well-known exceptions. The example selected here is concerned with the relationship between liver storage and plasma levels of vitamin A (table VIII). The relationship is of a lin-log type, i.e. the $\log_{10}$ of total liver vitamin A is correlated with plasma vitamin A concentrations. The regressions for individual species are characterized by the intercept (depending in some way on the varying success of liver vitamin A depletion prior to supplementation) and the slope. The latter indicates definite differences between species, the highest response being observed in rats and the lowest in goats. Apart from indicating interesting differences between species, the relationship enables the researcher to estimate within known limits the total vitamin A storage in the liver by determining the plasma level. This is a potentially helpful tool also in parenteral nutrition once the relationship is established for the species investigated.

One further interesting case is a non-vitamin effect of the vitamin niacin: the hypolipemic and hypocholesterolemic effects of this compound in the human are only achieved with nicotinic acid, whereas in rats, rabbits, and guinea pigs nicotinamide is also effective [24]. This observation indicates differences both between species and between vitamers.

Table VIII. Relationship between plasma vitamin A levels and vitamin A storage in the liver* [54]

Species (n)	Intercept ± SE	Slope ± SE	Correlation coefficient
Rat (138)	– 1.22 0.04	0.1301 0.0057	0.92
Pig (39)	2.24 0.56	0.0800 0.0235	0.60
Calf (48)	2.32 0.21	0.0785 0.0064	0.92
Rabbit (86)	1.17 0.04	0.0319 0.0021	0.93
Goat (40)	4.31 0.21	0.0243 0.0054	0.75

* Regression of $\log_{10}$ (total liver vitamin a in μg) (y) on plasma vitamin A concentration in μg/dl (x)

Differentiation in Disposal of Catabolites

The mechanisms and efficiency by which catabolites are finally disposed can effect metabolism. The first example refers to D(−)lactic acid produced by intestinal microbes (table I) and oxidized in part after absorption (fig. 2). The two compared species, rat and rabbit, differ considerably in renal excretion (fig. 4), indicating reabsorption in the rat at a dosage below 5 mmol $kg^{0.75}$, but not in the rabbit.

An impressive example demonstrating that some animals are more equal than others is urate metabolism and excretion. The human and anthropoid primates have lost uricase, the enzyme of liver peroxisomes which in other mammals oxidizes urate to the easily soluble allantoin. Only the Dalmatian dog excretes urate [10] as discussed below. Urate transport in the kidney (table IX) is now divided into 2 classes (column 1 + 2, column 3 + 4), each with 2 sub-classes. The term 'proved' indicates that some activity of the mechanism in question (tubular reabsorption or tubular net secretion) has been demonstrated, but the quantitative role is still unknown. It is worth noting, that primates are distributed over all 4 sub-classes, and the position of the Dalmatian dog is different from

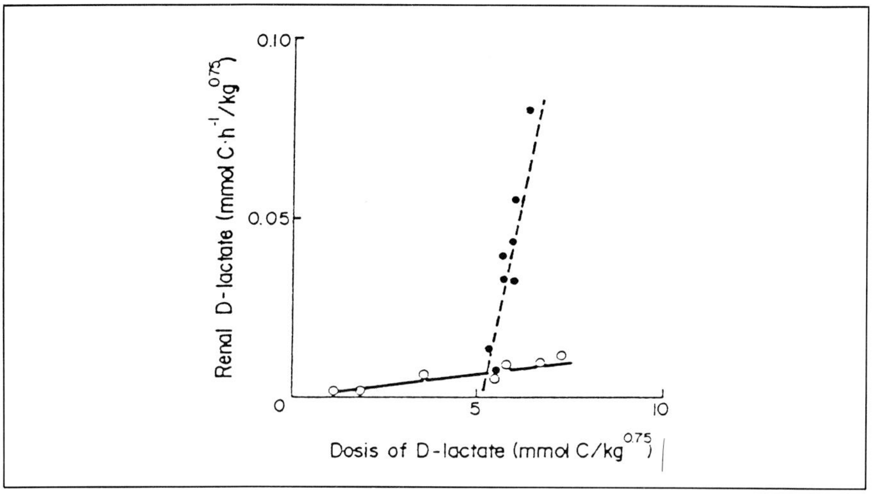

Fig. 4. Renal excretion of D(−)lactic acid in the rat –●– and the rabbit –○– [25]; rat: $y = 0.049x - 0.250$; $r = 0.713$; $p < 0.05$; rabbit: $y = 0.00016x - 0.0014$; $r = 0.929$; $p < 0.01$.

Table IX. Urate transport in the kidney [51]

	Reabsorption	Net secretion
Chicken	−	+
Pig	−	+
Calf	−	+
Rhesus	−	+
Guinea pig	proved	+
Rabbit	proved	+
Goat	proved	+
Dalmatian	proved	+
Olive baboon	proved	+
Rat	+	proved
Dog	+	proved
Cebus	+	proved
Chimpanzee	+	proved
Man	+	proved
Cat	+	−
Gibbon	+	−

dog as a species. In the human renal reabsorption of urate causes the well-known problems of hyperuricemia and gout. The conditions of urate elimination have a bearing on the use of non-glucose carbohydrates in parenteral nutrition [55].

Last but not least, differences between breeds of experimental animals can occur as exemplified above by the Dalmatian dog. Animals of this breed show normal hepatic uricase activity but suffer from the 'Dalmatian dog syndrome,' which has also been observed in man [30], i.e. loss of the carrier system for tubular reabsorption of urate. If this were the reason for urate excretion the pig would also eliminate urate, but this is not the case (see table IX). More recent experiments with Dalmatian and Beagle dogs [26–28] have shown definite difference in urate transport through the hepatic cell membrane (fig. 5). Apparently, the Dalmatian dog has lost the specific high affinity urate carrier (which is present in the liver of the Beagle) and therefore achieves only a limited urate uptake into the liver by the unspecific low affinity carrier occurring also in erythrocyte membranes. It is not unlikely that the specific carrier missing in hepatocyte membranes is genetically identical with that missing in kidney tubuli.

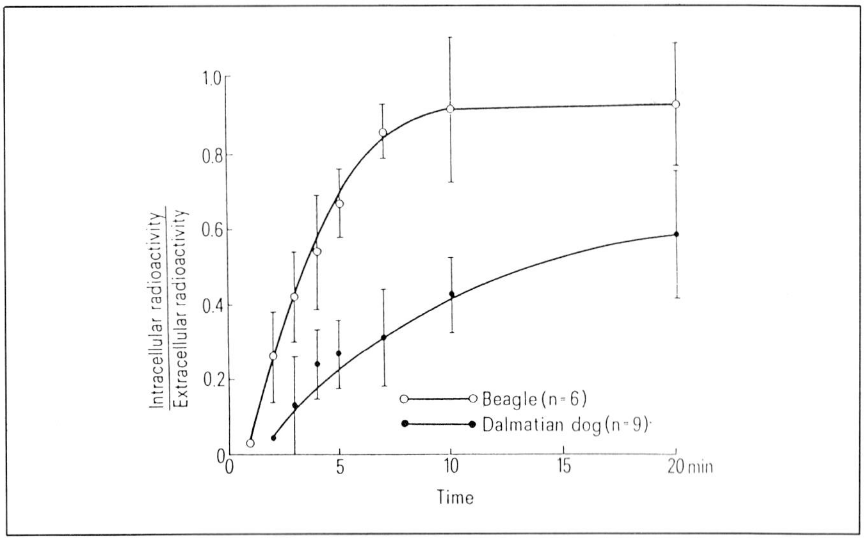

Fig. 5. ^{14}C-uric acid uptake in liver slices from Beagle and Dalmatian dog [28]. Liver slices were transferred at zero time to the incubation medium containing uric acid (0.1 mmol/l) and (^{14}C)uric acid. The uptake was determined by measuring radioactivity. Values shown are means of similar experiments. Vertical bars represent ± SD.

Concluding Remarks

Which species are more equal than others? The data presented in this frame may not lend themselves for a comprehensive evaluation, because of limitations in the numbers of animals, of experimental conditions, and of laboratories involved. Therefore, any comparison can only be tentative. For 8 of the more prominent criteria almost complete data are available for human, dog, pig, and rat. If these are evaluated by a rank system with increasing numbers indicating the degree of difference of the respective species relative to man (= 0), the dog with an average figure of 2.0 is the most similar species, followed by pig (4.1) and rat (4.3). As for the cat, the available data suggest a position reasonably close to the dog, however, some important criteria have not yet been measured. It must be considered, however, that the criteria are unweighed, but may be given quite different priorities depending on the model used, e.g. in conventional, enteral, or parenteral nutrition.

References

1 Alexander, F.; Davies, M. E.: Production and fermentation of lactate by bacteria in the alimentary canal of the horse and pig. J. Comp. Path. Ther. *73:* 1–8 (1963).

2 Alexander, F.; Chowdhury, A. K.: Digestion in the rabbit's stomach. Br. J. Nutr. *12:* 65–73 (1958).

3 Angel, A.; Bray, G. A.: Synthesis of fatty acids and cholesterol by liver, adipose tissue and intestinal mucosa from obese and control patients. Eur. J. clin. Invest. *9:* 355–362 (1979).

4 Ballard, F. J.; Hanson, R. W.; Kronfeld, D. S.: Gluconeogenesis and lipogenesis in tissue from ruminant and nonruminant animals. Fed. Proc. *28:* 218–231 (1969).

5 Baker, D. H.: Equalized versus ad libitum feeding. Nutr. Rev. *42:* 269–273 (1984).

6 Baker, D. H.; Allen, N. K.; Boomgardt, J.; Graber, G.; Norton, H. W.: Quantitative aspects of D- and L-tryptophan utilization by the young pig. J. Anim. Sci. *33:* 42–46 (1971).

7 Baker, D. H.; Boebel, K. P.: Utilization of the D-isomers of arginine and histidine by chicks and rats. J. Anim. Sci. *53:* 125–129 (1981).

8 Baker, D. H.; Speer, V. C.: Protein-amino nutrition of nonruminant animals with emphasis on the pig: Past, present and future. J. Anim. Sci. *57:* 284–299 (1983).

9 Barnard, E. A.: Biological function of pancreatic ribonuclease. Nature *221:* 340–344 (1969).

10 Benedict, S. R.: Uric acid and its relations to metabolism. Harvey Lect. *11:* 346–365 (1916).

11 Boebel, K. P.; Baker, D. H.: Comparative utilization of the isomers of phenylalanine and phenyllactic acid by chicks and rats. J. Nutr. *112:* 367–376 (1982a).

12 Boebel, K. P.; Baker, D. H.: Comparative utilization of the α-keto and D- and L-α-hydroxy analogs of leucine, isoleucine and valine by chicks and rats. J. Nutr. *112:* 1929–1939 (1982b).
13 Brüggemann, J.; Giesecke, D.: Milchsäuregehalt im Pansen und mikrobieller Abbau in vitro. Zentbl. Vet. Med. *A15:* 470–476 (1968).
14 Colin, G. (1871) cited by Hill, K. J.: Prehension, mastication, deglutination, and the esophagus; in Swenson, Duke's physiology of domestic animals; 8th ed., pp. 351–362 (Cornell University Press, Ithaca 1970).
15 Cranwell, P. D.; Noakes, D. E.; Hill, K. J.: Gastric secretion and fermentation in the suckling pig. Br. J. Nutr. *36:* 71–86 (1976).
16 Cummings, J. H.: Fermentation in the human large intestine: Evidence and implications for health. Lancet *i:* 1206–1209 (1983).
17 Czarnecki, G. L.; Baker, D. H.: Utilization of D- and L-tryptophan by the growing dog. J. Anim. Sci. *55:* 1405–1410 (1982).
18 Drawert, F.; Kuhn, H.-J.; Rapp, A.: Gaschromatographische Bestimmung der niederflüchtigen Fettsäuren im Magen von Schlankaffen (Colobinae). Hoppe-Seyler's Z. physiol. Chem. *329:* 84–89 (1962).
19 Ehle, F. R.; Robertson, J. B.; van Soest, P. J.: Influence of dietary fibres on fermentation in the human large intestine. J. Nutr. *112:* 158–166 (1982).
20 Elsden, S. R.; Hitchock, M. W. S.; Marshall, R. A.; Phillipson, A. T.: Volatile acid in the digesta of ruminants and other animals. J. exp. Biol. *23:* 191–202 (1946).
21 Erbersdobler, H.: Zur Übertragbarkeit ernährungsphysiologischer Daten aus Tierversuchen auf den Menschen. Ernährungs-Umschau *28:* 15–19 (1981).
22 Friend, D. W.; Nicholson, J. W. G.; Cunningham, H. M.: Volatile fatty acid and lactic acid content of pig blood. Can. J. Anim. Sci. *44:* 303–308 (1964).
23 Giesecke, D.: Gaschromatographische Bestimmung flüchtiger Fettsäuren und ihre Produktion im Pansen. Z. Tierphysiol., Tierernährg. u. Futtermittelkde. *22:* 354–364 (1967).
24 Giesecke, D.: Nicotinsäure oder Nicotinamid? Biochemische Bedeutung der Vitamere und Wirkungsunterschiede im Stoffwechsel. Übers. Tierernährg. *11:* 133–154 (1983).
25 Giesecke, D.; Fabritius, A.; von Wallenberg, P.: A quantitative study on the metabolism of D(−)lactic acid in the rat and the rabbit. Compar. Biochem. Physiol. *69B:* 85–89 (1981).
26 Giesecke, D.; Kraft, W.; Tiemeyer, W.: Warum Dalmatiner Harnsäure ausscheiden: Ursachen und Folgen einer klassischen Stoffwechselanomalie. Tierärztl. Praxis *13* (in press).
27 Giesecke, D.; Stangassinger, M.; Henle, K.: D(−)Milchsäure – ein Stoffwechselproblem. Z. ErnährWiss. (in press).
28 Giesecke, D.; Tiemeyer, W.: Defect of uric acid uptake in Dalmatian dog liver. Experientia *40:* 1415–1416 (1984).
29 Giesecke, D.; von Wallenberg, P.; Fabritius, A.: D(−)lactic acid – a physiological isomer in the rat. Experientia *36:* 571 (1981).
30 Green, M. L.; Marcus, R.; Aurbach, G. D.; Kazam, E. S.; Seegmüller, J. E.: Hypouricemia due to isolated renal tubular defect: Dalmatian dog mutation in man. Am. J. Med. *53:* 361–367 (1972).

31 Hanson, R. W.; Ballard, F. J.: The relative significance of acetate and glucose as precursors for lipid synthesis in ewes and adipose tissue from ruminants. Biochem. J. *105:* 529–536 (1967).

32 Hanson, R. W.; Garber, A. J.: Phosphoenolpyruvate carboxykinase. Its role in gluconeogenesis. Am. J. clin. Nutr. *25:* 1010–1021 (1972).

33 Hems, D. A.; Rath, E. A.; Verrinder, T. R.: Fatty acid synthesis in liver and adipose tissue of normal and genetically obese (ob/ob) mice during the 24-hour cycle. Biochem. J. *150:* 167–173 (1975).

34 Hill, H.: Die Verdauung; in Scheunert, Trautmann, Lehrbuch der Veterinär-Physiologie; 6th ed., pp. 93–187 (Paul Parey, Berlin 1976).

35 Ingle, D. L.; Baumann, D. E.; Carrigus, U. S.: Lipogenesis in the ruminant: In vivo site of fatty acid synthesis in sheep. J. Nutr. *102:* 617–623 (1972).

36 Koch, G.; Ledinek, M.; Giesecke, D.: Untersuchungen über die Beteiligung von Mikroorganismen am Verdauungsstoffwechsel des Schweines: Untersuchungen an Schlachtschweinen. Z. Tierphysiol. Tierernährg. u. Futtermittelkde. *30:* 222–231 (1972).

37 Lauris, V.; Cahill, G. F.: Hepatic glucose phosphotransferase. Variation among species. Diabetes *15:* 475–479 (1966).

38 Mangold, E.: Die Verdauung bei den Nutztieren (Akademie-Verlag, Berlin 1950).

39 Mersmann, H. J.; Allen, C. D.; Steffen, D. G.; Brown, L. G.; Danielson, D. M.: Effect of age, weaning and diet on swine adipose tissue and liver lipogenesis. J. Anim. Sci. *43:* 140–150 (1976).

40 Morris, J. G.; Rogers, Q. R.: Arginine: An essential amino acid for the cat. J. Nutr. *108:* 1944–1953 (1978).

41 Ohara, I.; Otsuka, S.-I.; Yugari, Y.; Ariyoshi, S.: Comparison of the nutritive values of L-, DL- and D-tryptophan in the rat and chick. J. Nutr. *110:* 634–640 (1980).

42 Parker, D. S.: The measurement of production rates of volatile fatty acids in the caecum of the conscious rabbit. Br. J. Nutr. *36:* 61–70 (1976).

43 Peters, K.; Gärtner, K.: Untersuchungen zur Funktion des Vormagens der Muriden. Passage fester und flüssiger Futterbestandteile, pH-Wert und α-Amylaseaktivität im Vormagen der Ratte. Zentbl. Vet. Med. *A20:* 233–243 (1973).

44 Phillipson, A. T.: The production of fatty acids in the alimentary tract of the dog. J. exp. Biol. *23:* 346–349 (1947).

45 Prior, R. L.: Effect of level of feed intake on lactate and acetate metabolism and lipogenesis in vivo in sheep. J. Nutr. *108:* 926–935 (1978).

46 Rogers, Q. R.; Phang, J. M.: Deficiency of pyrroline-5-carboxylate synthase in the intestinal mucosa of the cat. J. Nutr. *115:* 146–150 (1985).

47 Söling, H. D.; Kleinicke, J.: Species dependent regulation of hepatic gluconeogenesis in higher animals, in Hanson, Mehlman, Gluconeogenesis: Its regulation in mammalian species, pp. 369–462 (John Wiley, New York 1976).

48 Sunde, M. L.: Utilization of D- and DL-amino acids and analogs. Poultry Sci. *51:* 44–59 (1972).

49 Van Soest, P. J.: Nutritional ecology of the ruminant (O & B Books, Corvallis 1982).

50 Waterlow, J. C.: Observations on protein turnover; in Velazquez, Bourees, Genetic factors in nutrition, pp. 279–295 (Acad. Press, New York 1984).

51 Weiner, I. M.: Urate transport in the nephron. Am. J. Physiol. *6:* F85–F92 (1979).

52 Wolin, M. J.: Fermentation in the rumen and human large intestine. Science *213:* 1463–1468 (1981).

53 Wretlind, K. A. J.; Rose, W. L.: Methionine requirement for growth and utilization of its optical isomers. J. biol. Chem. *187:* 697–703 (1950).

54 Wright, K. E.; Hall, R. C.: Association between plasma and liver vitamin A: Levels in the calf, weaning pig, rabbit and rat and adult goat fed fixed intakes of vitamin A. J. Nutr. *109:* 1063–1072 (1979).

55 Zöllner, N.: Evaluation of non-glucose carbohydrates in parenteral nutrition; in Johnston, Advances in parenteral nutrition, pp. 61–74 (MTP Press, Lancaster 1978).

D. Giesecke, Institut für Physiologie, Physiologische Chemie und Ernährungsphysiologie, Universität München, Veterinärstr. 13, D-8000 München 22 (FRG)

Dietze, Grünert, Kleinberger, Wolfram (eds.), Clinical Nutrition and Metabolic Research. Proc. 7th Congr. ESPEN, Munich 1985, pp. 329–332 (Karger, Basel 1986)

Requirements of Energy and Essential Nutrients with Regard to Body Mass

H. Hackbarth, K. Gärtner

Institute for Animal Experiments and Central Animal Laboratory, Medical School Hannover, FRG

Experiments on laboratory animals always involve the problem of extrapolating experimental results to other species and finally to man. One of the most obvious problems which has to be dealt with, in addition to many others, are differences in body size and mass. These differences raise the question of how results obtained from small sized laboratory animals can be extrapolated to man.

About 100 years ago Rubner [9] normalized the energy metabolism of different sized dogs by relating their energy metabolism to body surface area, expressed and calculated with the surface rule of Meeh [7] as the two-third power of body weight. Thus large animals need less energy per kilogram body weight than small ones. For more than 50 years thereafter body surface area was considered to be a common basis for energy metabolism and energy-related functions. In 1932, Kleiber published his famous paper 'Body Size and Metabolism,' where he compared the heat production of animals ranging in size from rats to steers, i.e. from 0.15 to 679 kg [6]. Based initially on his findings, it is now well accepted that energy metabolism is neither a linear function of body mass, nor does energy metabolism follow the surface rule as postulated by Rubner in 1883. By expressing the heat production as a function of body mass in a double logarithmic system, the best fit for Kleiber's data was described by the following allometric equation:

$$\text{Metabolic rate} = 73.3 \times \text{body mass}^{3/4}$$

This allometric equation is represented by a straight regression line with a slope of 0.74 when the data are plotted on logarithmic coordinates. If the metabolic rate were a direct function of the body surface area, the slope and the expected mass exponent would be 0.67. These findings of Kleiber were confirmed by Brody et al. [3] as well as by Benedict [2] with studies of many additional species ranging from mice to elephants. Nevertheless it is still a matter of debate whether the mass exponent of about 0.75 as determined by Kleiber is valid or not. Heusner [4] found that the mass exponent within any single species is 0.67, but that the proportionality coefficient, a, changes from small animals to large animals and that, therefore, the intraspecies regression lines seem to be shifted. Combining these intraspecific relationships with an interspecies relationship results in a mass exponent of 0.75. These results were also confirmed by our own findings; the total food consumption over 24 h by different strains of rats of both sexes were plotted in a double logarithmic system versus body weight and gave a mass exponent of 0.70, which is closer to 0.67 than to 0.75. Thus for intraspecies comparison an exponent of 0.67 should be used, while for interspecies comparison an exponent of 0.75 seems to be more suitable.

Further discussion about the validity of the body mass exponent was initiated by Bartels [1]. He found that the smallest mammals have metabolic rates which are above the general regression line. For animals between 0.26 and 3800 kg he found a slope of 0.76, while for animals between 2.4 and 260 g the slope was 0.42. Combining these data resulted in a slope of 0.66. Extrapolation from small laboratory animals of less than 260 g to larger species such as man must therefore be done very carefully.

Summarizing these general points results in the following conclusions:

(1) Comparison of different species should be done with the 0.75 power of body weight.

(2) Comparison of individuals of a single species should be done with the 0.67 power of body weight.

(3) Extrapolation from animals less than 260 g to larger species should be done very carefully.

Taking all these considerations into account, requirement of energy can be compared within as well as between species and can be extrapolated from laboratory animals to larger species such as man with reasonable precision. Protein needs as a part of energy requirement is also correlated with body weight with a body mass exponent of 0.73 as reported by Payne [8]. This mass exponent seems to be independent of whether the animal is just on maintenance, growing, pregnant, or lactating. What again differs is the proportionality coefficient, a, which is:

1.6 g protein/day per kg body weight$^{0.73}$ for maintenance;
4.7 g protein/day per kg body weight$^{0.73}$ for growing individuals;
6.0 g protein/day per kg body weight$^{0.73}$ for pregnant animals;
13 g protein/day per kg body weight$^{0.73}$ for lactation.

These differences in the proportionality coefficient shift the regression lines in a parallel way. This means that comparisons are reliable only when they are done between animals in the same condition.

Minerals and vitamin requirements have not been investitated by these allometric methods. Based on requirements for energy and protein, most diets are composed for different species on the assumption of an overall requirement based on the 0.75 power of body mass. For minerals such as sodium (Na) and chloride (Cl) which are involved in water metabolism and therefore closely correlated to energy metabolism, this assumption seems to be justified. For calcium (Ca) and phosphorus (PO_4) this assumption is almost certainly wrong, because skeletal weight increases with body mass by a mass exponent of 1.13 [5]. Thus large animals have a relative skeleton weight of more than three times that of smaller animals (elephant 37%, mouse 7% of body weight). The need for calcium and phosphorus therefore does not follow the 0.75 but the 1.13 power of body mass. Diets designed for different sized animals should therefore have a different relation between energy and calcium/phosphorus content. Similar conditions may exist for other minerals and vitamins. Unless their exact allometric relationship to body weight is known, comparison of experimental results within as well as between species have a high probability of error and extrapolation to other species and to man are often not valid.

Summarizing these points it can be concluded that energy and energy-related processes do follow the general allometric rules of the 0.75 power of body weight between species and the 0.67 power of body weight within species. Nutrients which are related to skeletal weight follow the 1.13 power of body weight. Other nutrients may follow other allometric relationships. In addition to these general conclusions, it must always be borne in mind that laboratory animals have their own species pecularities. Some of them hibernate (hamsters), some show coprophagia and burrowing (rabbit), some are adapted to high altitude (guinea pig), and in some digestion, storage of food, and energy intake is simply regulated in a different way compared to man. All these points have to be considered before experimental results obtained from laboratory animals are compared with the situation in man.

References

1 Bartels, H.: Metabolic rate of mammals equals the 0.75 power of their body weight? Expl Biol. Med. *7:* 1–11 (1982).
2 Benedict, F. G.: Vital energetics. A study in comparative basal metabolism (Carnegie Inst. of Washington, Washington, D.C. 1938).
3 Brody, S.; Procter, R. C.; Ashworth, U. S.: Basal metabolism, endogenous nitrogen, creatinine and neutral sulphur excretions as functions of body weight. Missouri Agr. Exp. Sta. Res. Bull. *220:* 1–40 (1934).
4 Heusner, A. A.: Energy metabolism and body size. I. Is the 0.75 mass exponent of Kleiber's equation a statistical artifact? Resp. Physiol. *48:* 1–12 (1982).
5 Kayser, Ch.; Heusner, A.: Etude comparative du métabolisme énergétique dans la série animale. J. Physiol., Paris *56:* 489–524 (1964).
6 Kleiber, M.: Body size and metabolism. Hilgardia *6:* 315–353 (1932).
7 Meeh, K.: Oberflächenmessungen des menschlichen Körpers. Z. Biol. *15:* 425–458 (1879).
8 Payne, P. R.: The relationship between protein and calorie requirement of laboratory animals; in Conalty, Husbandry of laboratory animals (Academic Press, London, New York 1967).
9 Rubner, M.: Über den Einfluß der Körpergröße auf Stoff- und Kraftwechsel. Z. Biol. *19:* 535–562 (1883).

PD. Dr. Hansjoachim Hackbarth, Institut für Versuchstierkunde und Zentrales Tierlaboratorium der Medizinischen Hochschule Hannover, Konstanty-Gutschow-Str. 8, D-3000 Hannover 61 (FRG)

Dietze, Grünert, Kleinberger, Wolfram (eds.), Clinical Nutrition and Metabolic Research. Proc. 7th Congr. ESPEN, Munich 1985, pp. 333–342 (Karger, Basel 1986)

Specificity of Animal Models in Liver Research

P. Soeters, J. E. G. de Boer

Dept. of Surgery, Hospital St. Annadal, University of Limburg, Maastricht, The Netherlands

Introduction

Several authors have outlined requirements for a suitable animal model for hepatic failure. Terblanche [1], for instance, writes that the hepatic lesion must be potentially reversible if the effects of treatment regimens are to be meaningfully tested. Thus the anhepatic and vascular occlusion models fail to meet this criterion. Secondly, as mortality is the most easily measured end point, the animals should consistently die within a narrowly defined period. Further, death should follow a period of coma and should be the direct consequence of fulminant hepatic failure and its complications. For practical reasons the animal must have a blood volume large enough to permit serial biochemical measurements and therapeutic interventions. Finally, it is desirable to employ agents which are not hazardous to personnel.

Schafer [2] defined during the Fifth Ammonia Symposium in Semmering the attributes of an ideal hepatotoxin. Some of them are similar to the requirements described by Terblanche. The ideal hepatotoxin should:

– be safe;

– be specific for the liver. Extra hepatic effects leave doubt concerning the relationship of the experimental findings to liver injury;

– be capable of producing graded liver injury;
– have a reliable dose response curve;
– be easy to administer;
– be active in a variety of common laboratory animals;
– produce coma and coagulopathy secondary to liver failure;
– be inexpensive and commercially available in a pure form;
– have a known mechanism of action.

In addition, we think that the model should exhibit as precisely as possible the special metabolic derangement that is to be studied. To ensure this, the animal model should be carefully defined and methods should be developed to quantitate and qualify the liver damage induced in the model.

Animal models

There are many ways of interfering with liver function. The models achieved can be roughly divided into two categories: the drug-induced models and the surgically induced models. A few of them will be mentioned and some problems attached to them will be discussed.

Drug-Induced Animal Models (Hepatotoxins)

Carbon Tetrachloride in Acute and Chronic Liver Failure

Carbon tetrachloride causes liver injury but used alone, is unreliable in its dose-response relation. If animals are pretreated with a cytochrome P450 inducer such as phenobarbital, both the reproducibility and the severity of the damage is promoted [3]. If, however, the pathogenesis of encephalopathy is studied, it is a disadvantage that phenobarbital interferes with receptor studies.

Nitrosamines

Nitrosamines are potent hepatotoxins and can be used to create both acute and chronic liver failure [4]. They have, however, other target organs; they have carcinogenic actions and are potentially harmful for laboratory personnel.

Galactosamine in Acute Liver Failure [1]

Galactosamine is a selective hepatotoxin active in a variety of laboratory animals and is considered to be one of the most suitable hepatotoxins to achieve acute hepatic failure in liver research. It is, however, expensive and only reproducible in inbred strains of animals.

Thioacetamide

Thioacetamide can be used both to produce acute and chronic liver failure [5]. It is however a carcinogen [6].

Ammonia, Methanethiol, Octanoic Acid [7]

Obviously these compounds are not hepatotoxins. Still they deserve some comment as they are commonly used to create coma and when doing so are claimed to be 'culprits' or causative agents in the genesis of hepatic encephalopathy. It is acceptable to administer these compounds to experimental animals and then to study effects on amino acid levels, hormone profiles, etc., but it goes one step too far to conclude that when coma is induced these compounds are the real causative agents in the genesis of chronic hepatic encephalopathy, especially because chronic hepatic encephalopathy is different from ammonia encephalopathy encountered in infants with inborn errors of metabolism. Koch's postulates may not apply to this situation. Artificial elevation of NH_3, methanethiol, and octanoic acid may be a completely different situation compared to the sequence of metabolic disturbances during chronic liver failure of which these compounds are just reasonably accurate parameters.

Surgically Induced Animal Models

Portacaval Shunt (PCS)

PCS is a widely employed surgical procedure to study aspects of liver disease resulting in spontaneous portasystemic shunting. This will be discussed in more detail in a later part of this contribution.

Acute Hepatic Artery Occlusion

Reports on this procedure both in experimental animals and in patients vary widely. If, however, the procedure is carried out according to high standards of asepsis and surgical technique, no hepatic failure is achieved.

Acute Vascular Occlusion

Acute vascular occlusion of both portal and arterial inflow rapidly results in liver necrosis and liver failure. The experimental setup is hardly accessible to therapeutic measures as the animals invariably die after 16–36 h. Furthermore the portal congestion that results confuses the clinical picture.

Hepatic Artery Occlusion

Therefore hepatic artery occlusion has been preceded by a first stage PCS. This solves the problem of portal congestion but permanent occlusion of the arterial inflow sooner or later also results in death despite therapeutic maneuvers. To circumvent this problem techniques for temporary hepatic artery occlusion have been developed. The amount of necrosis and the grade of hepatic failure achieved are unpredictable, however, and quantitation is difficult. This will be dealt with later in this chapter.

We will not discuss all these methods but would rather like to point out that whatever model is used, it should be carefully defined to know what we are studying. We will illustrate this by discussing three or four frequently employed animal models in liver research.

Models in Chronic Hepatic Failure

Some fifteen years ago Fischer has proposed the 'amino acid – neurotransmitter theory' concerning the pathogenesis of hepatic encephalopathy [8]. Since then interest in amino acid metabolism has greatly increased in liver research but also in other fields. We also have been interested directly or indirectly in this matter and especially in BCAA. The AA-neurotransmitter hypothesis was based upon the observation in patients with liver disease that plasma BCAA were generally decreased and plasma AAA elevated. As it turned out later these data were not very carefully controlled because plasma BCAA were only decreased in chronic hepatic failure but not in acute hepatic failure where they were normal or even elevated [9]. Record even suggested from his data in patients with acute fulminant hepatitis that elevated plasma BCAA had bad and low plasma BCAA had good prognostic significance [10]. Already at that time, however, the Fischer ratio was introduced as an indicator for the grade of encephalopathy. The lower the BCAA over AAA ratio the more severe the state of encephalopathy. Again, in less well controlled studies with PCS dogs, it appeared that encephalopathy coincided with a low ratio. Correction of the ratio by infusion of BCAA-enriched solution appeared thereafter to improve encephalopathy in dogs, supporting the prognostic value and the causal relation of the BCAA over AAA ratio [11]. Although in these dog studies infusions of BCAA-enriched AA mixtures clearly appeared to improve mental state, the significance of the ratio should be questioned because in later better controlled studies we found that the Fischer ratio decreased after PCS but increased again in the state of encephalopathy (table I). The conclusion should be that, if AA concentrations are considered as parameters for certain aspects of hepatic failure, it should be done in carefully designed and executed studies. In patients this is almost impossible because a variety of additional factors generally influence plasma AA concentrations, like the effects of nutrition, diabetes, obesity, malnutrition, sepsis, uremia, hydration, etc. [12]. Even in inbred rat strains this can be demonstrated where we found that neutral amino acids vary widely after PCS [13].

For years we have been interested in BCAA metabolism, specifically in the mechanism by which plasma BCAA levels are decreased in patients with chronic liver disease and in experimental animals with PCS. Munro

Table I. $\frac{\text{Leucine + Isoleucine + Valine}}{\text{Phenylalanine + Tyrosine}}$ molar ratios before portacaval anastomosis, 1 week and 4 weeks after portacaval anastomosis, and in hepatic encephalopathy

Dog number	Pre-shunt	1 week	4 weeks	Encephalopathy
1	4.14		1.07	1.55
2	4.09	1.96	1.17	1.32
3	3.40	1.58	1.21	1.21
4	3.62	1.29	1.06	1.36
5	3.32		0.94	1.19
6	3.32	1.61	1.18	1.28
7	4.74	1.49	0.74	0.74
8	3.84	2.32	0.98	1.28
$\bar{x}$	3.81*	1.71*	1.04*	1.24*
SEM ±	0.18	0.15	0.06	0.08
n	8	6	8	8

* All differences significant at the $p < 0.01$ level at minimum.

and several others in the past have suggested that hyperinsulinemia present in such patients and experimental animals might promote the peripheral uptake of BCAA [14]. Quantitatively by far the most important organs to take up BCAA are muscle and adipose tissues [15]. We wanted to study the in vitro handling of BCAA by muscle and adipose tissues of PCS rats and controls. From data in the literature and from our own experience, it appeared that we could safely use button-shunted rats 4–6 weeks after the shunt. To our disappointment we could not find differences in the in vitro metabolism of BCAA in adipose tissue and diaphragm of such rats, although in previous pilot studies such differences had been found. After trial and error we decided to better define our button PCS rat model. First of all it turned out that not all PCS rats showed normal growth as has also been found in the literature [16]. Indeed, in many reports in the literature and also in some of our series, rats do not grow at all so that they are virtually malnourished at the time of the experiment. Malnutrition in itself has been shown to lead to low AA levels including the BCAA [17]. It was therefore mandatory to try to create a PCS rat with a favorable growing curve. This can be achieved with the button shunt when optimal conditions are established. PCS rats can grow although not as fast as sham-operated rats [13].

Secondly, better definition of the PCS model revealed that PCS rats exhibit low plasma BCAA levels and hyperinsulinemia only until 3–4 weeks after the shunt [13]. After 4 weeks already these values tend to normalize. At 5 and 6 weeks values are completely normalized. To get an insight into the potential mechanism, we performed splenoportography at different time periods after the shunt, obviously in different rats. PCS rats that gained weight had 2½ weeks postoperatively open shunts and no clear collaterals, while the liver was not visualized. In contrast in rats that did not gain weight a clear obstruction of the shunt 2½ weeks postoperatively was visualized as well as collaterals to the stomach and esophagus but not to the liver, evidenced by abscence of contrast in the liver. All rats subjected to splenoportography 4½ weeks postoperatively gained weight including rats that did not gain weight at 2½ weeks postoperatively. All these rats had large collaterals and contrast in the liver, independent of an obstruction of the shunt. Rats, portacaval-shunted according to the 'suture' technique, lost more weight than 'button'-shunted rats.

When trying to compare in vitro handling of tissues of PCS rats with sham-operated rats, we should therefore have growing rats that exhibit at the time of the experiment the phenomena that we want to study, notably

Table II. Tissue DNA content in diaphragm and epididymal adipose tissue from control rats (non-operated and sham-operated) and PCS-operated rats; mean ± SD (n = 50)

	Tissue DNA content (μg DNA/mg wet weight)	
	adipose tissue	muscle
Sham-operated and non-operated	0.31 ± 0.04	1.69 ± 0.11
PCS-operated	0.45 ± 0.07	2.33 ± 0.31

low BCAA and high insulin levels. Furthermore, because growing PCS rats still grow at a slower rate than sham-operated controls, results should be expressed per unit weight of DNA. This has a considerable impact on the results (table II). One might even go so far as to say that if a chronic, stable, not too ill animal model is wanted, a certain growth rate should be present. If the animals do not grow at all, they are most probably more ill and malnourished and cannot be compared with animals that exhibit more favorable growth rates. Proctor has turned this notion around and has used it to advantage to create experimental cirrhosis [3]. Carbon tetrachloride is a potent selective hepatotoxin but the dose-response relationship is unpredictable. Proctor could titrate liver damage by tailoring carbon tetrachloride dosages to body weight change response. If administration of CCl_4 resulted in a steep drop in body weight, the next dosage was diminished and vice versa. In this way experimental graded cirrhosis could be achieved in rats that were not too ill, that showed some growth, and gradually developed all signs of chronic cirrhosis with most of the sequelae also encountered in humans.

Models of Acute Liver Failure

Thus far we have discussed in more detail two chronic animal models for liver research and we feel that the chronic model, although difficult to achieve, is the more suitable model to study aspects of liver disease like hepatic encephalopathy, clotting abnormalities, formation of ascites, albumin kinetics, immune response, etc. First of all, acute fulminant hepatic failure, either due to hepatitis or due to paracetamol poisoning, is much less common than chronic liver disease. In addition it appears that survival is much more related to the severity of the primary insult to the liver than to specific therapeutic interventions other than supportive treatment. Still, the acute model may serve useful purposes if the goals are neatly specified and the disturbance under study can be reliably reproduced. We have tried to establish a reproducible dog model of acute liver ischemia and were disappointed with the results. First we performed an end-to-side portacaval shunt and completely devascularized the liver with the exception of the hepatic artery inflow. At the same time, an occluder was put around this artery that could block arterial inflow as desired at a later stage, after recovery from the operation in a non-stressed situation. Several parameters commonly used to assess hepatic function were measured and we tried to quantitate liver damage by sequential measurements of alanine aminotransferase (ALT) and aspartate aminotransferase (AST). To our disappointment quantitation of ischemic damage did not correspond with survival and with other commonly used parameters for liver failure like hypoglycemia, amino acid ratios, NH_3, ketone body ratio, etc. Only lactate and catecholamines could, in an early stage, roughly predict outcome but the standard deviation is enormous so that, for the individual dog, the predicting parameter is useless. Also occlusion did not create comparable disturbances in every dog. Finally, if death occurred this did not only appear to be due to liver failure but also to multiple organ failure. Therefore if we want to study, for instance, a specific therapeutic modality in such a model, we should try to carefully quantitate the damage done and the degree of failure that we started with, otherwise the effect of treatment can never be estimated. As demonstrated, however, this is almost impossible. Therefore research in the area of acute hepatic encephalopathy should be carefully undertaken and the results interpreted with caution. Especially one should beware of extrapolation of results in acute encephalopathy to chronic encephalopathy. Indeed acute and chronic encephalopathy have been found to have differing characteristics but still the distinction is not always made. Galactosamine-induced fulminant hepatic failure in the rabbit has been used as a model from which the GABA hypothesis has resulted. In a careful study of Blitzer et al. the model was defined, and it was shown that many metabolic disturbances very closely resembled the disturbances encountered in human acute hepatic failure [18]. Also nicely described, however, was that the rabbit has a partly necrotic liver after galactosamine treatment. Being interested in metabolic aspects of severely ill patients in the intensive care situation, it became clear to us that any necrotic tissue, as long as it is still perfused to some degree, creates the same sequence of events, namely, multiple systems organ failure (MSOF). New insights in the syndrome reveal that not really organs fail but rather cells fail. Cellular and membrane integrity is lost and especially the more active energy-dependent processes are disturbed. The severely septic patient, the patient with crush injuries, a dead leg, a dead pancreas, a dead segment of bowel, they all develop MSOF rapidly and many of them are encephalopathic and sometimes severely comatose. Therefore, acute damage to the liver leading to necrosis proceeds, in our opinion, to a syndrome which is a combination of diminished liver function and MSOF as a more general sequel to the presence of necrotic tissue. The last aspect may very well be responsible for the increased permeability of the blood-brain barrier observed by Schafer, Jones, etc. [19]. Still, the galactosamine-treated rabbit may be a useful model for acute fulminant hepatic failure but again it should be realized what we are studying and that we cannot extrapolate these data to chronic hepatic failure where we are mainly dealing with diminished organ function per se, without the confusing and overwhelming effects of necrosis.

References

1 Terblanche, J.; Hickman, R.; Miller, D. et al.: Animal experience with support systems: Are there appropriate animal models of fulminant hepatic necrosis?; in Williams, Murray-Lyon, Artificial liver support, pp. 163–172 (Pitman, London 1975).
2 Schafer, D.: Toxin models of acute liver failure; in Kleinberger, Ferenci, Riederer, Thaler, Advances in hepatic encephalopathy and urea cycle diseases. 5th Int. Symp. Ammonia, Semmering 1984, pp. 57–62 (Karger, Basel 1984).
3 Proctor, E.; Chatamra, K.: High yield micronodular cirrhosis in the rat. Gastroenterology *83:* 1183–1190 (1982).
4 Aguirre, A.; Yoshimura, N.; Westman, T.; Fischer, J.: Plasma amino acids in dogs with two experimental forms of liver damage. J. surg. Res. *16:* 339–345 (1974).
5 Trennery, P.; Waring, R.: Early changes in thioacetamide-induced liver damage. Toxicol. Lett. *19:* 299–307 (1983).
6 Fitzhugh, G.; Nelson, A.: Liver tumors in rats fed thiourea or thioacetamide. Science *108:* 626–629 (1948).
7 Zieve, F.; Zieve, L.; Doizaki, W. et al.: Synergism between ammonia and fatty acids in the production of coma: Implications for hepatic coma. J. Pharmac. exp. Ther. *191:* 10–16 (1974).
8 Fischer, J.; Baldessarini, R.: False neurotransmitters and hepatic coma; in Schaffner, Popper, Progress in liver disease, vol. 5, pp. 211–223 (Grune & Stratton, New York 1976).
9 Rosen, H.; Yoshimura, N.; Hodgman, J. et al.: Plasma amino acid patterns in hepatic encephalopathy of differing aetiology. Gastroenterology *72:* 483–487 (1977).

10 Record, C.; Buxton, B.; Chase, R.; Curzon, G.; Murray-Lyon, I.; Williams, R.: Plasma and brain amino acids in fulminant hepatic failure and their relationship to hepatic encephalopathy. Eur. J. clin. Invest. *6:* 387–394 (1976).
11 Fischer, J.; Funovics, J.; Aguirre, A.; James, H.; Keane, J.; Wesdorp, R.; Yoshimura, N.; Westman, T.: The role of plasma amino acids in hepatic encephalopathy. Surgery *78:* 276–290 (1975).
12 Soeters, P.; de Boer, J.: Why are plasma branched chain amino acid levels diminished in patients with liver cirrhosis?; in Adibi, Fekl, Langenbeck, Schauder, Branched chain amino and keto acids in health and disease. Int. Symp. Branched Chain Amino and Keto Acids in Health and Disease, Göttingen 1983, pp. 483–497 (Karger, Basel 1984).
13 De Boer, J.; Oostenbroek, R.; van Dongen, J.; Janssen, M.; Soeters, P.: Sequential metabolic characteristics following portacaval shunt in rats. Eur. surg. Res. (in press).
14 Munro, H.; Fernstrom, D.; Wurtman, R.: Insulin, plasma amino acid imbalance and hepatic coma. Lancet *i:* 722–724 (1975).
15 De Boer, J.: Branched chain amino acid metabolism in portal-systemic shunting; Experimental studies in the rat; thesis Limburg (1984).
16 Rossouw, J.; Labadarios, D.; Vink, A. et al.: Liver glycogen after porta-caval shunt in rats. Metabolism *27:* 1067–1073 (1978).
17 Holt, E.; Snyderman, S.; Norton, P.; Roitman, E.; Finch, J.: The plasma aminogram in kwashiorkor. Lancet *ii:* 1343–1348 (1963).
18 Blitzer, B.; Waggoner, J.; Jones, E. et al.: A model of fulminant hepatic failure in the rabbit. Gastroenterology *74:* 664–671 (1978).
19 Horowitz, M.; Schafer, D.; Molnar, P.; Jones, E.; Blasberg, R.; Patlak, C.; Waggoner, J.; Fenstermacher, J.: Increased blood-brain transfer in a rabbit model of acute liver failure. Gastroenterology *84:* 1003–1011 (1983).

Peter B. Soeters, MD, Hospital St. Annadal, University of Limburg, Dept. of Surgery, P.O. Box 1918, 6201 BX Maastricht (The Netherlands)

Dietze, Grünert, Kleinberger, Wolfram (eds.), Clinical Nutrition and Metabolic Research. Proc. 7th Congr. ESPEN, Munich 1985, pp. 343–374 (Karger, Basel 1986)

Animal Models of Hepatic Failure. Metabolic Characteristics and Effects of TPN

E. Holm, F. Behne, H. Leweling, U. Staedt, J.-P. Striebel, A. Tschepe

Dept. of Pathophysiology, Medical Clinic I Mannheim, University of Heidelberg, FRG

'It is just as destructive to the spirit to have a system as to have no system; undoubtedly, one must accept the need to combine both.' This quotation from F. Schlegel may be considered an appropriate maxim for the reasoning behind the present contribution, which not only describes phenomena but also tries to systemically interpret the concentrations of several substances – or groups of substances – as well as central nervous effects of ammonia[1]. In 1960, Kitani published some electrophysiological results of animal experiments from which he concluded that two factors are likely to be operative in the pathogenesis of hepatic encephalopathy: the so-called hyperammonemic factor and the liver insufficiency factor [64]. In the light of current knowledge, this merely dualistic view appears to be an oversimplification. Nevertheless, Kitani's hypothesis has been helpful in classifying various pathophysiological alterations in brain electrical activity [18, 37, 39, 87, 123] and can, most probably, also be applied to some metabolic processes in peripheral tissues. When comparing animal models of hepatic failure with clinical diseases, the suggestion made by Kitani may serve as the leading principle.

The experimental data presented in the first and third section was obtained in our department. This holds true for hyperammonemia caused in healthy rats by infusion of ammonium salts [50, 69, 109; Tschepe, in prep.], for portacaval anastomosis (PCA) in three species of animals [16, 41, 42, 47, 50, 68, 71, 108, 109; Staedt, in prep.; Tschepe, in prep.], and

[1] In this paper the term 'ammonia' is used to mean either NH_3, or the sum of $NH_3 + NH_4^+$.

finally, for thioacetamide-induced liver cell damage in rats (Tschepe, in prep.) as well as in cats [17, 38, 40, 49]. Findings concerning human idiopathic portal hypertension are from Iwasaki and coworkers [57], those on fulminant hepatic failure (FHF) from Kleinberger [pers. communication 1983], and the liver cirrhosis data from our group [50, 109, 119]. With regard to intracellular amino acid concentrations in various clinical

Table I. Conventional laboratory data (means; for SD and SEM see references) in rats with exogenous hyperammonemia (HA; 6 h infusions of an ammonium acetate/bicarbonate mixture; each salt 1.4 mmol/kg × h), in animals given a portacaval anastomosis (PCA; biochemical analyses in the rats, rabbits, and cats 6 weeks, 2 weeks, and 6 weeks, respectively, after the operation), and in animals which had received thioacetamide (TAA; rats: 3 × 50 mg/kg i.p.; cats: 2 × 50 mg/kg i.p.; 24-h intervals between the injections). In each pair of figures, control values are shown above, while the values brought about by the experimental procedures are indicated below. References: [Tschepe et al., in prep.] (HA and TAA in rats), [16] (PCA in rats), [Staedt et al., in prep.] (PCA in rabbits), [47] (PCA in cats), [38, 49] (TAA in cats)

Variables	HA	Portacaval anastomosis			Thioacetamide	
	rats	rats	rabbits	cats	rats	cats
Ammonia, μg/dl	44	57	73	72	67	67
	641	295	275	348	439	352
GPT, U/l	26	15	28	21	26	21
	28	25	34	38	2375	3400
GOT, U/l	49		8	8	38	16
	40		11	22	3217	4989
Albumin, g/l	26	37	38	27		27
	27	26	35	24		30
Cholinesterase, U/l				1725		
				1055		
Quicks' test %				100		100
				100		5
Bilirubin, mg/dl	0.13	0.11	0.10	0.25	0.11	0.29
	0.11	0.13	0.12	0.34	0.61	1.12
Alkaline phosphatase, U/l	186		100	56	132	56
	161		54	65	286	218
Urea, mg/dl	43	39	38	48	34	38
	57	30	41	38	59	37
Creatinine, mg/dl	0.5	0.5	1.2	1.1	0.5	1.1
	0.4	0.6	1.4	1.1	0.7	1.1
n	11	8	18	20	10	26
	8	11	32	31	9	10

conditions, i.e. liver cirrhosis, hepatoportal encephalopathy, and FHF, Roth and his colleagues will be referred to [100].

Conventional biochemical variables which characterize the animal models under consideration are listed in table I. In each pair of figures, control values are given above, while values brought about by the experimental procedures are indicated below. Hyperammonemia was, of course, a consistent finding in all models. The activity of the transaminases was hardly affected in the ammonium-infused and PC-shunted animals but showed an excessive rise following thioacetamide administration. Overall hepatic function, as assessed by measuring the prothrombin time (Quick's test), bilirubin, and alkaline phosphatase, also proved to be largely resistant to exogenous hyperammonemia and portal-systemic shunting, whereas with thioacetamide a severe impairment of the liver became obvious. As to the decline of the albumin and cholinesterase values in the shunted animals, these changes are best explained by a worsening of the nutritional state [47], the fall in the albumin level being by far most pronounced in the rats. The parameters indicative of kidney function showed a very slight involvement of this organ in the rats which had received thioacetamide.

Plasma and Muscle Amino Acid Concentrations

Postabsorptive Values

Methionine and phenylalanine (fig. 1) are representative of those amino acids, the plasma levels of which depend primarily on the functional capacity of the liver [33, 41], allthough catabolic states contribute to raised concentrations [60, 98, 106]. During short-term exogenous hyperammonemia, normal plasma levels were maintained. Normal concentrations have also been observed in patients with idiopathic portal hypertension, a disease with minimal hepatic lesions and chronic hyperammonemia, the latter being ascribed to extensive portal-systemic collaterals [12, 85]. By contrast, FHF, both in animals and in patients, was associated with extremely high values of methionine and phenylalanine. Liver cirrhosis, not included in figure 1, ranges between idiopathic portal hypertension and FHF [57, 99]. The effects of experimental PCA – particularly on phenylalanine – are likely to be due either to mild hepatic injury brought about by the shunt operation or to protein catabolism or to

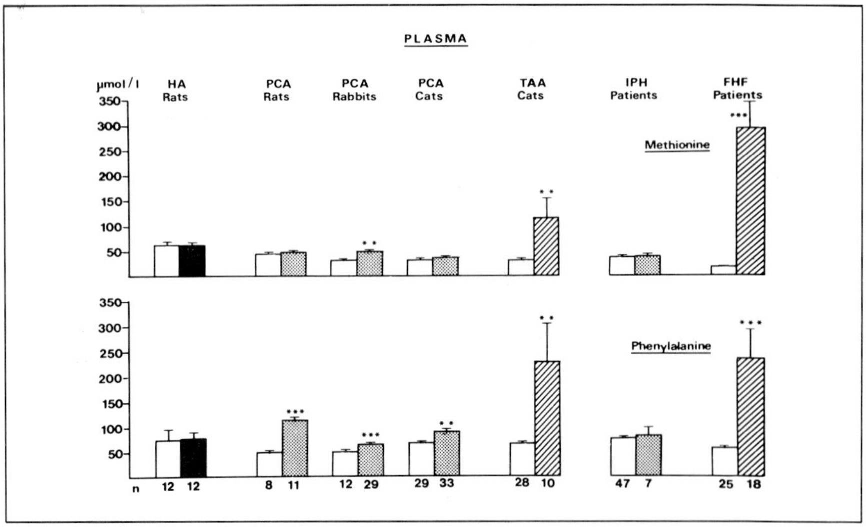

Fig. 1. Plasma levels of methionine and phenylalanine (mean ± SEM) in rats with exogenous hyperammonemia (HA), in animals given a portacaval anastomosis (PCA), in cats which had received thioacetamide (TAA) as well as in patients with idiopathic portal hypertension (IPH) or fulminant hepatic failure (FHF). For experimental details see legend to table I. Calculation of error probabilities by means of the U-Test. ** $p \leq 0.01$, *** $p \leq 0.001$, as compared to controls. References: [69] (HA in rats), [16, 68, 71] (PCA in rats), [Staedt et al., in prep.] (PCA in rabbits), [41, 47, 108] (PCA in cats), [38, 40, 49] (TAA in cats), [57] (IPH in patients), [Kleinberger, pers. communication 1983] (FHF in patients).

both [41, 47, 62]. Portal-systemic shunting per se does not increase phenylalanine in plasma [41, 57].

Valine and leucine (fig. 2) had decreased concentrations in the ammonium-infused rats, in all groups of PC-shunted animals as well as in patients with idiopathic portal hypertension. As reported in countless papers, the same alterations are typical of cirrhotic patients. However, thioacetamide administration and clinical FHF increased branched chain amino acid (BCAA) levels. From the data in figure 2, one can infer that hyperammonemia as well as portal-systemic shunting per se cause a deficit of BCAA in plasma, even when the liver is impaired to a slight degree, whereas very severe damage to the organ exerts the opposite effect.

Our view as to the basic conditions determining the plasma levels of methionine, phenylalanine, and BCAA is strongly backed by the results of the very differentiated investigations done by Karavias in rats [62].

Regarding alanine, a pattern very similar to that of the BCAA was observed (fig. 3). The increase of alanine found – as an exception – in the PCA rats may be attributed to the catabolic state of these animals (table I), which has already been mentioned and which will once again be referred to in connection with the intracellular amounts of alanine. Patients with liver cirrhosis exhibit low, normal, or high plasma alanine concentrations [46].

In answer to the main question of this paper, it can at first be stated that, so far as the amino acids represented in figures 1–3 are concerned, exogenous hyperammonemia gives rise to plasma levels similar to those seen in patients with idiopathic portal hypertension. Secondly, PC-shunted animals appear to be a suitable model of human liver cirrhosis with respect to the amino acids under debate. Finally, the changes of the amino acid pattern in thioacetamide-injected animals parallel those found in clinical FHF.

Before turning to intracellular amino acid levels, some pathophysiological and biochemical suggestions should be outlined which, in our

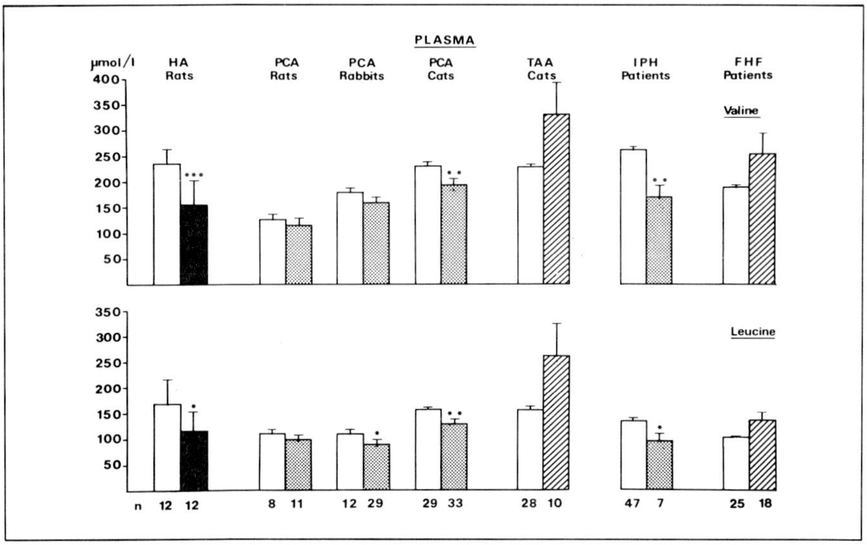

Fig. 2. Plasma levels of valine and leucine (mean ± SEM) in rats with exogenous hyperammonemia (HA), in animals given a portacaval anastomosis (PCA), in cats which had received thioacetamide (TAA) as well as in patients with idiopathic portal hypertension (IPH) or fulminant hepatic failure (FHF). For experimental details see legend to table I; for statistics and references see legend to figure 1. * $p \leq 0.05$, ** $p \leq 0.01$, *** $p \leq 0.001$, as compared to controls.

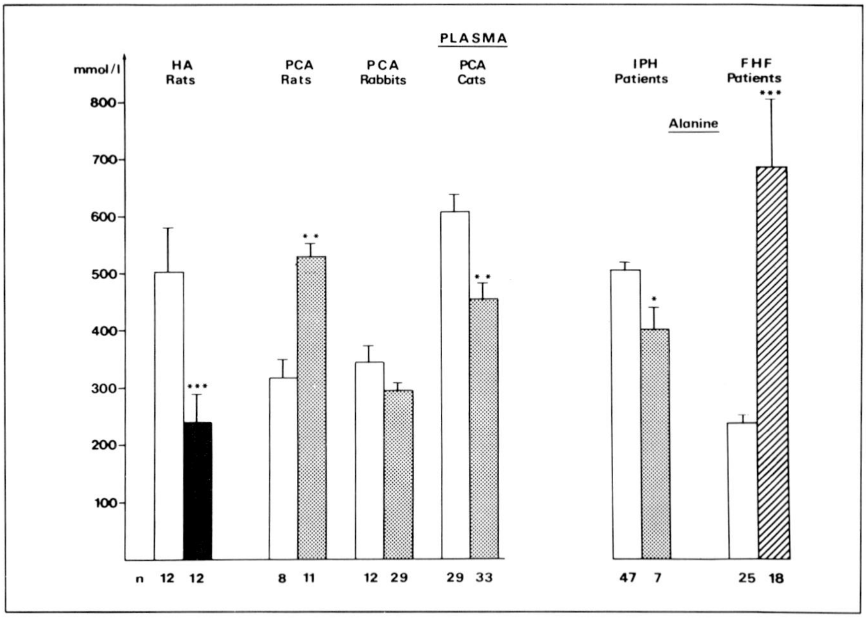

Fig. 3. Plasma levels of alanine (mean ± SEM) in rats with exogenous hyperammonemia (HA), in animals given a portacaval anastomosis (PCA) as well as in patients with idiopathic portal hypertension (IPH) or fulminant hepatic failure (FHF). For experimental details see legend to table I; for statistics and references see legend to figure 1. * $p \leq 0.05$, ** $p \leq 0.01$, *** $p \leq 0.001$, as compared to controls.

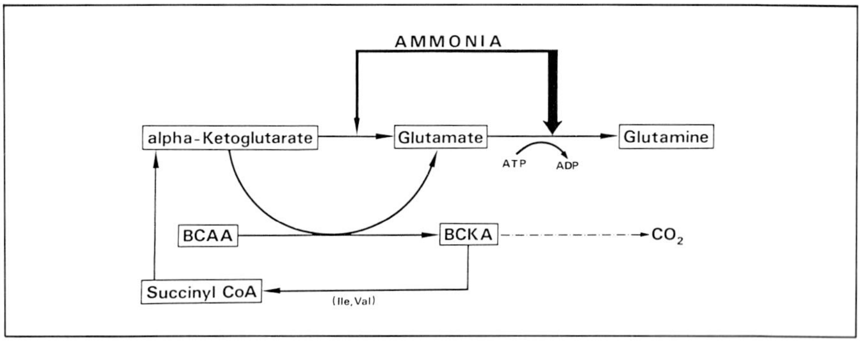

Fig. 4. Suggested influence of ammonia on the metabolism and, thereby, on the plasma levels of BCAA. Further comments are given in the text.

opinion, at least partly explain the deficit of BCAA and of alanine in hyperammonemic animals with largely preserved liver function as well as in patients with idiopathic portal hypertension or liver cirrhosis.

A factor pattern based on data which had been obtained in 208 cirrhotics (table II) failed to demonstrate a relationship between hyperammonemia and parameters of overall hepatic function (albumin, Quick's test, cholinesterase, bilirubin). Instead, co-variations of plasma ammonia, serum glucose, and the number of thrombocytes were revealed (table II). Portal hypertension most likely brought about these CO-Variations, since it causes hypersplenism and a collateral circulation which, for its part, is associated with increased gluconeogenesis [13, 103, 107] and hyperammonemia (table I) [5, 7, 12, 37, 55, 63, 110]. Thus, the plasma ammonia level in liver cirrhosis can be considered as predominantly determined by the degree of portal-systemic shunting. The same holds true for BCAA levels [41, 42].

We put forward the hypothesis that hyperammonemia lowers the concentrations of BCAA by stimulating glutamine synthesis (fig. 4). The excessive formation of glutamine may reduce the glutamate pool size

Table II. Factor pattern of biochemical variables and the number of thrombocytes in 208 patients with liver cirrhosis. Principal component method. Varimax rotation. Only loadings of ± 0.40 and above are indicated. The first 5 eigenvalues of the correlation matrix were 2.8, 2.3, 1.5, 1.4, and 1.2. The 5 factors developed account for 70.4% of the total variance [48]

Variables	Factors				
	1	2	3	4	5
GPT	+ 0.95				
GOT	+ 0.92				
Albumin		+ 0.68			
Quick's test		+ 0.76			
Cholinesterase		+ 0.80			
Bilirubin	+ 0.57	− 0.43			
Alk. phosphatase			+ 0.73		
Gamma-GT			+ 0.85		
Ammonia			+ 0.68		− 0.40
Glucose					− 0.48
Thrombocytes					+ 0.81
Urea				+ 0.90	
Creatinine				+ 0.90	

which is likely to be restored, to a large extent, by an intensified BCAA transamination [42, 43, 70]. Besides this transamination process, a supply – via succinate – of the alpha-ketoglutarate carbon skeleton by degradation of valine and isoleucine could, theoretically, in addition contribute to replenishing the glutamate pool (fig. 4). However, there is hardly enough evidence in support of this metabolic pathway playing a quantitatively decisive role, the problem becoming even more complicated, since normal plasma levels of the branched chain ketoacids were recently established in patients with liver cirrhosis [117].

As reported by Chang and Goldberg, an in vitro increase of glutamine production is coupled with a decline in alanine production [6]. In vivo, this is reflected by a shift in the arteriovenous differences for glutamine and alanine, as the peripheral release of these two substances is mainly accounted for by de novo synthesis [25, 101]. The figure 5 data refer to two groups of human subjects (healthy controls and cirrhotic patients) as well as to cats before and after a portacaval shunt operation. The values depicted represent the arteriovenous difference for alanine minus that for glutamine, thus showing to what extent one of the two arteriovenous differences was greater. While the healthy subjects had predominantly negative values, positive values were obtained in almost all cirrhotics. Even more marked was the shift from negative to positive values caused by the shunt operation in the cats. Considering the human subjects, it is necessary to state that ignoring the cirrhosis-induced increase in blood flow [65, 67] results in an underestimation of the difference between the healthy controls and the patients. Observations made by several groups of authors in cirrhotics confirm our findings [24, 31, 56]. Thus, more glutamine than alanine is released by peripheral tissues in hyperammonemic states [43].

In intracellular water of muscle (fig. 6), glutamine levels above normal and glutamate as well as alanine levels below normal could not necessarily be predicted by, but would be in excellent agreement with, the hypothesis illustrated in figure 4. In fact, such concentrations occurred in rats with acute exogenous hyperammonemia as well as in PC-shunted rabbits with chronic hyperammonemia. The shunted cats displayed a similar pattern, although less clearly. In the rats with PCA, only an insignificant fall in the glutamate level was noted (fig. 6). Most probably, as a consequence of malnutrition, ammonia-induced stimulation of glutamine synthesis had been overcome by a shortage of energy in these animals [22].

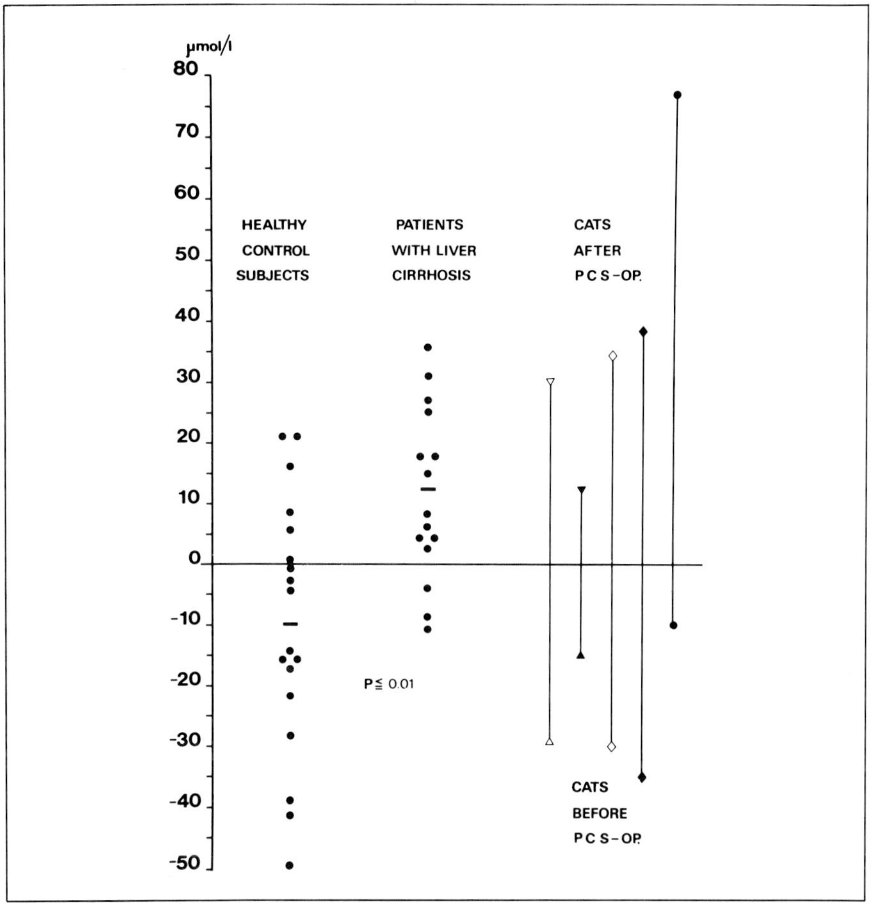

Fig. 5. Arteriovenous concentration differences for alanine minus those for glutamine in 18 healthy subjects and 15 cirrhotic patients as well as in 5 cats before and 2 weeks after portacaval shunt (PCS) operation. Measurements were done in plasma. On average, the patients displayed twice the normal plasma ammonia level, while the ammonia values of the shunted cats exceeded the reference range by nearly 500%.

Nevertheless, glutamine as a percentage of total glutamate and glutamine in the cells was found to be raised in each of the four models (table III). It has been ascertained by Roth and coworkers that this percentage value is also increased in human liver cirrhosis, hepatoportal encephalopathy, and even in FHF [100]. In this respect, there are thus strikingly similar changes in animals and patients.

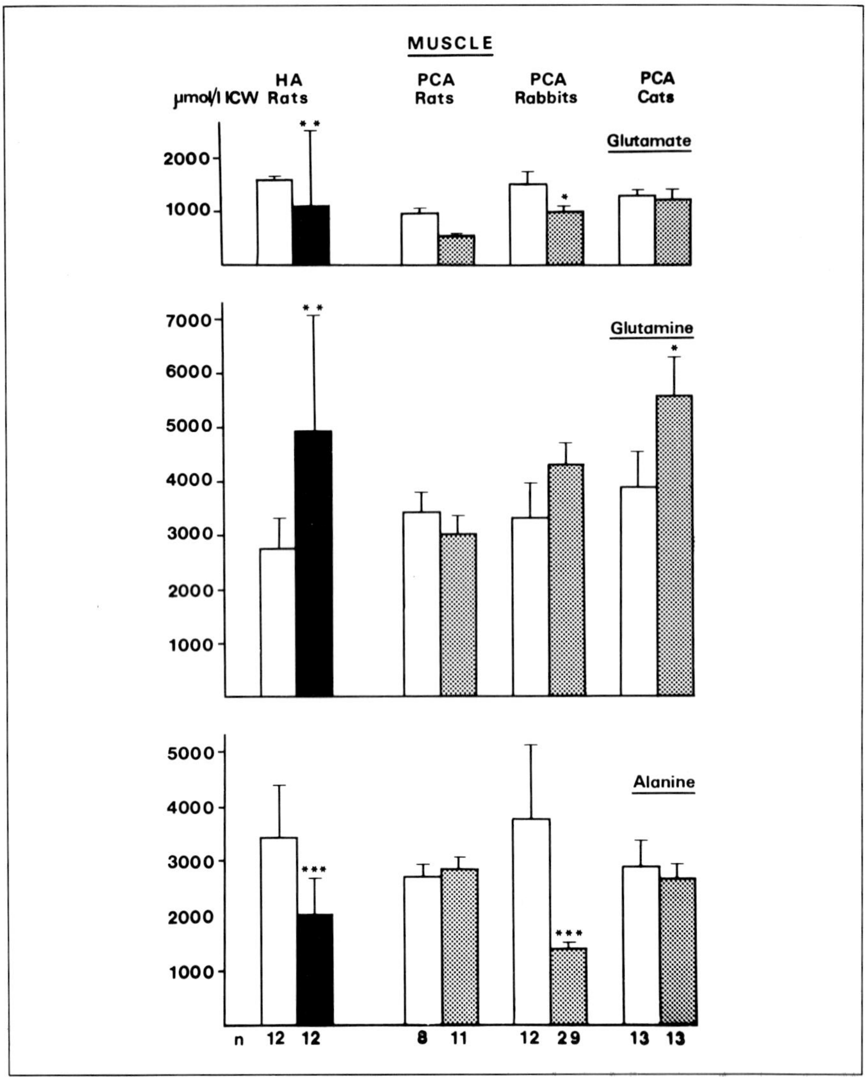

Fig. 6. Concentrations of glutamate, glutamine, and alanine (mean ± SEM) in intracellular water (ICW) of muscle in rats with exogenous hyperammonemia (HA) and in animals given a portacaval anastomosis (PCA). For experimental details see legend to table I. Calculation of error probabilities by means of the U-Test. ** $p \leq 0.01$, *** $p \leq 0.001$, as compared to controls. References: [69] (HA in rats), [16, 68, 71] (PCA in rats), [Staedt et al., in prep.] (PCA in rabbits), [42, 108] (PCA in cats).

Table III. Glutamine concentration in intracellular water of muscle as % of total glutamate and glutamine in rats with exogenous hyperammonemia (HA), in animals given a portacaval anastomosis (PCA) as well as in patients with liver cirrhosis (LC), hepato-portal encephalopathy (HPE), or fulminant hepatic failure (FHF). References for the experimental data as in figure 6. (Results obtained in the patients are from Roth et al. [100])

Species	Control values	n	Pathological state		n
Rats	63.4	12	HA	81.8	12
Rats	77.6	8	PCA	84.5	11
Rabbits	68.9	12	PCA	81.2	29
Cats	77.0	13	PCA	84.3	13
Humans	83.7	16	LC	88.8	7
	83.7	16	HPE	89.8	3
	83.7	16	FHF	95.3	3

Although it is suggested in this paper – and supported by the findings described – that acute as well as chronic hyperammonemia is likely to initiate a sequence of metabolic events which ultimately result in lowered plasma BCAA levels, one should not overlook the potential role of raised insulin concentrations. Insulin has been thought to remove BCAA from plasma into muscle, thereby reducing their plasma levels [60, 82]. In addition, insulin is known to stimulate branched chain ketoacid dehydrogenase, i.e. the rate-limiting enzyme complex in the degradation of BCAA [27]. Arguments for an at least long-term effect of insulin on plasma BCAA have been delineated by Soeters et al. [104, 105].

Effects of TPN

With regard to the proportional amounts of amino acids in total parenteral nutrition (TPN) regimens, there is ongoing debate on the question of whether a conventional or a so-called Hepa solution should be administered in cirrhosis and other forms of hepatic failure [19, 26, 45]. In rats given a PCA and receiving TPN (fig. 7), a conventional amino acid mixture brought about an excess of methionine in both plasma and muscle; high values of phenylalanine were maintained. By contrast, a transfer-adapted Hepa solution induced largely balanced extra- and intracellular amino acid patterns. This issue has been thoroughly discussed at former congresses [3, 19, 20, 41, 43].

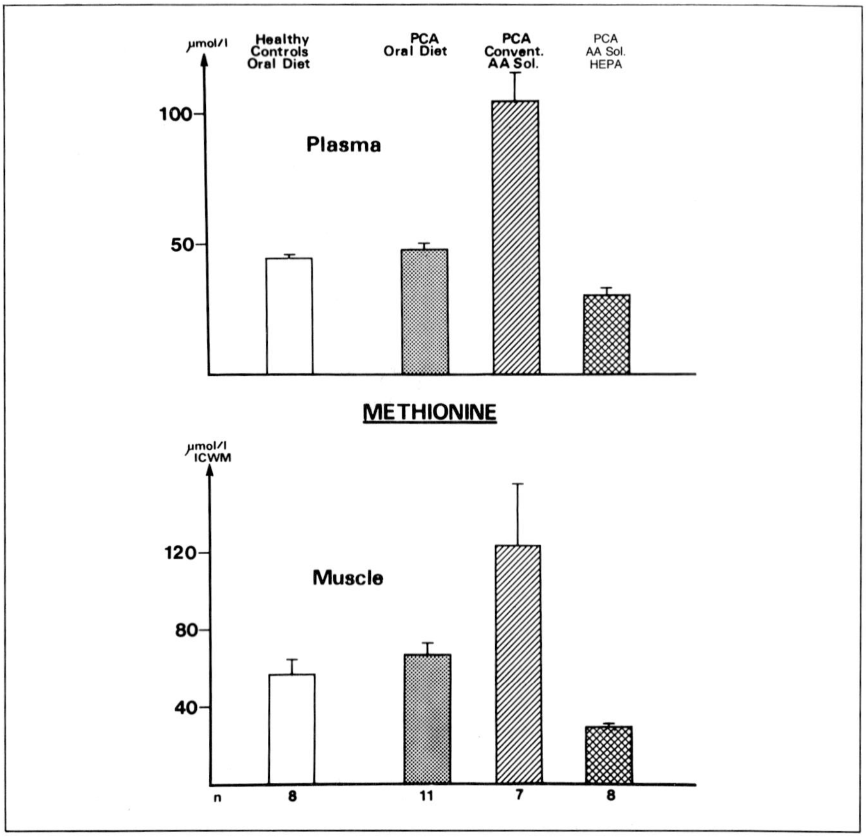

a

Fig. 7a and b. Concentrations of *a* methionine and *b* phenylalanine (mean ± SEM) in plasma and intracellular water (ICW) of muscle in 4 groups of rats. Two groups received total parenteral nutrition which included either a conventional amino acid solution or a transfer-adapted Hepa solution. PCA = portacaval anastomosis. Results obtained by Leweling et al. [68, 71].

Brain and Cerebrospinal Fluid Amino Acid Concentrations, Energy State of the Central Nervous System

Table IV indicates alterations of amino acid levels in brain and cerebrospinal fluid as observed by 35 groups of authors in various animal models of hepatic failure as well as in patients. First of all, it is well known and obvious from the upper four rows of symbols that experimental PCA,

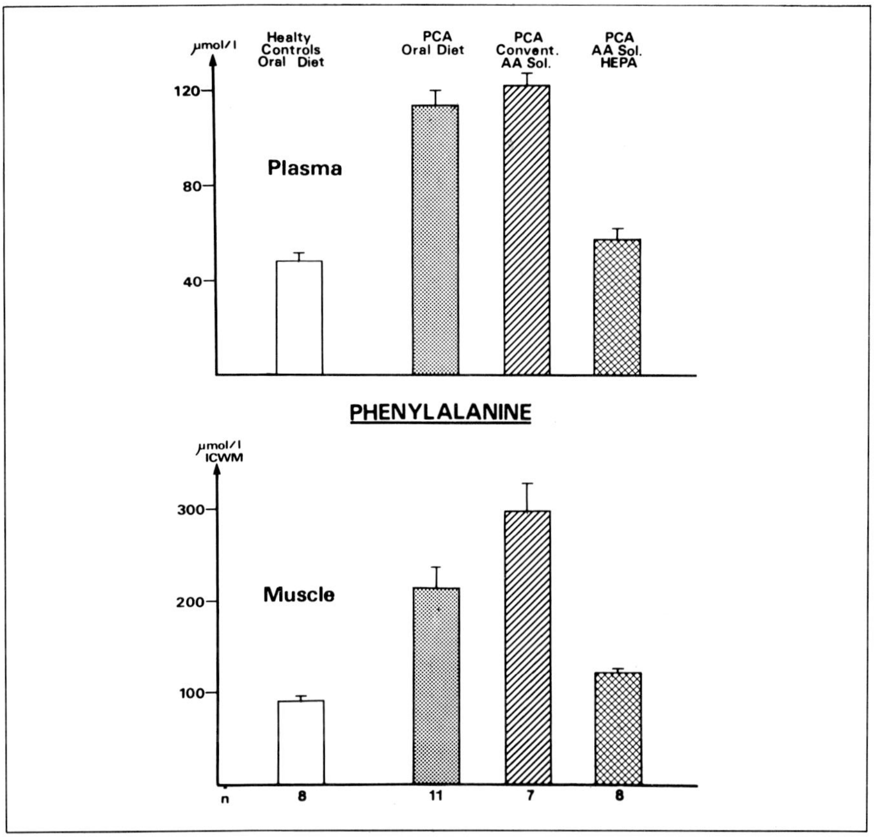

b

hepatectomy, liver devascularization, and toxic liver cell damage result in elevated concentrations of methionine, phenylalanine, tyrosine, and tryptophan in brain and cerebrospinal fluid. Whatever that may mean, there is good agreement with findings obtained in patients who suffered from liver cirrhosis or FHF. Leaving aside exogenous hyperammonemia, the BCAA mostly showed either a clear-cut increase or a tendency towards an increase; however, normal levels also occurred. The latter finding has been explained by an intensified metabolism following enhanced uptake into the brain [58]. An excess of glutamine was seen in each animal model and in each group of patients with hepatic failure. The neurotransmitter amino acids glutamate and aspartate tended to be reduced in brain tissue and cerebrospinal fluid of animals and patients, the decrease of aspartate

Table IV. Changes in the concentrations of brain and cerebrospinal fluid (CSF) amino acids induced in animals by exogenous hyperammonemia (HA), portacaval anastomosis (PCA), and other experimental procedures as well as in patients by liver cirrhosis (LC) and fulminant hepatic failure (FHF)

Amino acids	HA		PCA		Hepa-tectomy	Liver devasc.	Galactos-amine, CCl_4	LC patients		FHF patients	
	brain	CSF	brain	CSF	brain	brain	brain	brain	CSF	brain	CSF
Met		–	↑ •	↑	↑	↑	↑	(↑)	(↑)	↑	↑
Phe		–	↑ •	↑	↑	↑	↑	(↓)	↑	↑	↑
Tyr		–	↑	↑	↑	↑	↑	(↑)	↑	↑	↑
Try			↑		↑	↑	↑	↑	(↑)	↑	
Val		↓	(↑)	↑	(↑)	(↑)	↑	–	?	↑	↑
Leu		↓	(↑)	↑	(↑)	(↑)	↑	–	?	↑	↑
Ile		↓	(↑)	(↑)	(↑)	(↑)	↑	↑	?	↑	↑
Gln	↑	↑	↑ •	↑	↓	↓		↑	↑	↑	↑
Glu	–	–	(↓) •	↓	↓	(↓)	–	(↓)	?	?	↑
Asp	↓		? •		↓	↓		(↓)	?	(↓)	(↓)
Ala	↑	(↓)	(↓)	(↓)	↑	↑		–	↑	↑	↑
References	[30, 34, 72]	[102]	[1, 8, 10, 14, 32, 36, 53, 58, 59, 61, 75, 98, 121]	[102]	[21, 32, 52, 115, 116]	[9, 11, 23, 75, 76, 122]	[66, 122]	[93, 120]	[4, 54, 86, 95, 111, 113, 118]	[92]	[92, 118]

* ↑, ↓ largely consistent results;
(↑), (↓) only minor changes or deviations not consistently observed;
– normal concentrations or concentrations classified as normal in the majority of the pertinent studies;
? inconsistent results;
• concentrations measured by most authors in brain tissue and by Eriksson et al. [14] in the extracellular space of the brain

probably resulting from 'concerted transamination' between pyruvate and aspartate [36].

Focussing on ammonia, ammonia-related amino acids, and the central nervous energy state, we would like to address two topics which have best been elucidated by animal experiments. Mechanisms of ammonium/ammonia actions on brain activity are the first of these topics. Ammonia appears to alter brain function on three levels. In the first and lowest level, the ammonium ion by itself reduces postsynaptic inhibition by inactivating the extrusion of chloride from neurons [74, 79, 89, 90]. Such an effect is not exerted by aspartate – an excitatory, sodium channels activating transmitter – the concentration of which was seen to be decreased in tissue but increased in the extracellular space of the brain during hyperammonemia (tables IV and V). Neither is such an effect brought about by a change in the energy state (table V). Raabe has most elegantly demonstrated that the earliest action of ammonium, i.e. a reversible impairment of the efficacy of postsynaptic inhibition, occurs with concomitant alterations of the EEG, the latter finding proving a disturbance in brain function [88, 90]. Holm et al. infused cats with ammonium salts at amounts similar to those used by Raabe; the infusions influenced only the cerebral cortex and other structures above the brainstem, while the reticular activating system remained resistant to the ammonia levels reached. This was clearly documented by the spontaneous and activated EEG, by evoked potentials following sensory and central stimulation, and by single unit discharge frequencies [37, 39]. On the second level of ammonia intoxication, represented in table V by chronic hyperammonemia, the ammonia-induced fall in tissue concentrations of glutamate and/or aspartate may further affect brain activity without interfering with energy metabolism. When acute-on-chronic hyperammonemia causes not only precoma but coma, the third level is reached; it is characterized by an energy deficit in the central nervous system (table V).

Neuronal tolerance to ammonia, as investigated by Raabe and Onstad [91], is our second topic in this connection. It is of utmost clinical importance. In cats which had not yet undergone surgical portal-systemic shunting, disinhibition of antidromic action potentials – the earliest event in ammonia intoxication – occurred when 2.7 mmol of ammonium acetate/kg were administered (table VI). This ammonium load increased the tissue levels of ammonia and glutamine. After the shunt operation, only 0.6 mmol of ammonium acetate/kg were required to produce disinhibition and the tissue glutamine content did not change (table VI). Raabe and

Table V. Mean concentrations of ammonia, glutamine, and ammonia-related amino acids as well as variables indicative of the energy state in the central nervous system (CNS) of animals with various degrees and courses of hyperammonemia (HA) caused by ammonium injection or infusion (acute HA), portacaval anastomosis (PCA) or hepatectomy (chronic HA), or by an acute ammonium load following a shunt operation.

States of experimental hyperammonemia (HA)	CNS tissue concentrations							
	ammonia	glutamine	glutamate	aspartate	alanine	ATP	ATP/ADP	energy charge
Acute HA, 5 min	0.2	6.7	11.6	2.8	0.4	2.5		
Hawkins et al. [30]	1.5**	8.4**	11.3	2.3**	0.6**	2.5		
Acute HA, 30 min	0.1	5.0	11.4	3.3		2.4		0.928
Lin and Raabe [72]	5.1***	9.7***	9.9	2.3*		2.3		0.911
Chronic HA, PCA	0.3	5.4	10.7	2.7	0.5			
Hindfelt et al. [36]	0.6	14.0***	9.1*	2.8	0.5			
Chronic HA, Hepatectomy		11.7	10.7	2.6	0.6	2.8		0.945
Holmin et al. [52]		19.2**	9.5*	1.7*	0.8*	2.9*		0.952**
Acute-on-chronic HA,	0.5	12.0	9.5	2.8	0.5	2.7	11.9	
PCA + Injection of NH_4^+	2.5***	12.3	9.2	1.8***	0.6	2.6	11.6	
Hindfelt et al. [36]	3.4***	15.5***	8.1***	1.8***	2.0***	2.4*	8.5*	

* $p \leq 0.05$, ** $p \leq 0.01$, *** $p \leq 0.001$, as compared to control values

Table VI. Mean ammonium loads required for disinhibition of antidromic action potentials before and after surgical portal-systemic shunting (SPSS) in cats. Furthermore, the mean cerebral concentrations of ammonia and glutamine during these experiments are indicated.

State of the animals	Load of ammonium acetate required for disinhibition (mmol/kg)	Cerebral concentrations (μmol/g) before and during disinhibition of antidromic action potentials			
		ammonia		glutamine	
		control	disinhibition	control	disinhibition
Before SPSS	2.7	0.20	0.73**	3.1	5.6*
After SPSS	0.6	1.13	1.61	13.8	13.7

* $p \leq 0.01$, ** $p \leq 0.001$, as compared to control values. (Results obtained by Raabe and Onstad [91])

Onstad concluded that, in chronic hyperammonemia, the central nervous system is utilizing ammonia removal mechanisms at maximum capacity, so that a small additional ammonia load has a very sharp effect [91]. The clinical parallels of these findings need not be outlined.

Levels of Energy-Yielding Substrates in Whole Blood/Plasma/Serum

Postabsorptive Values

In the experimental and clinical states investigated, glucose concentrations were, in general, much less characteristic than the lactate values (fig. 8). Glucose tended to be increased in ammonium-infused rats, in PC-shunted cats, and in cirrhotic patients but was decreased in animals and patients with FHF. Following surgical portal-systemic shunting, rats and rabbits – in contrast to the cats – had significant hypoglycemia. Thus, among the experimental procedures used, only toxic liver damage represented a suitable model of the corresponding clinical disease (fig. 8).

Lactate is of special interest. Its level significantly declined in acute exogenous hyperammonemia (fig. 8). Based on in vitro findings, McKhann and Tower have postulated that oxidative decarboxylation of pyruvate is reduced by ammonia [77]. This hypothesis has, to our knowledge, never been confirmed. Instead, Häussinger and coworkers have

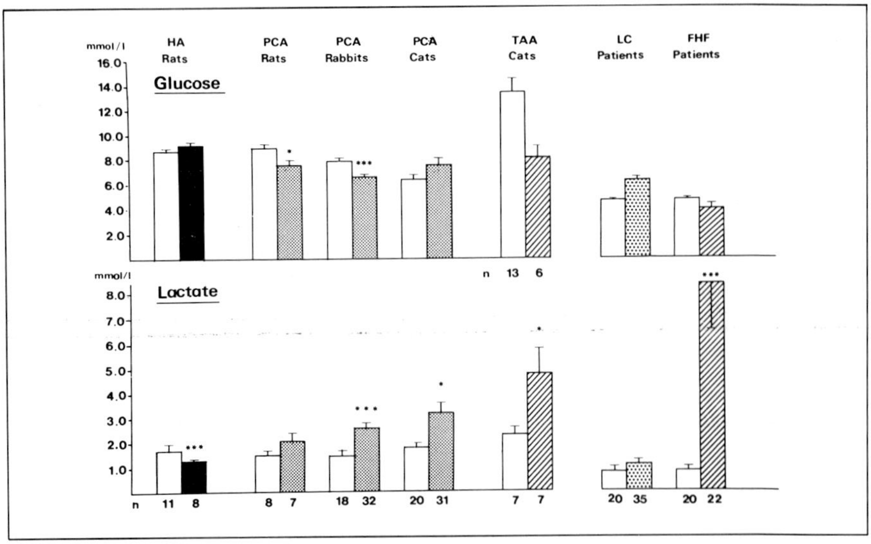

Fig. 8. Concentrations of glucose and lactate (mean ± SEM) in rats with exogenous hyperammonemia (HA), in animals given a portacaval anastomosis (PCA), in cats which had received thioacetamide (TAA) as well as in patients with liver cirrhosis (LC) or fulminant hepatic failure (FHF). The substrates were measured in whole blood (HA, rats; PCA, rats and rabbits) or serum (PCA and TAA, cats; LC and FHF, patients). For experimental details see legend to table I. Calculation of error probabilities by means of the U-Test. * $p \leq 0.01$, *** $p \leq 0.001$, as compared to controls. References: [Tschepe et al., in prep.] (HA and PCA in rats), [Staedt et al., in prep.] (PCA in rabbits), [47] (PCA in cats), [17] (TAA in cats), [119] (LC in patients), [Kleinberger, pers. communication, 1983] (FHF in patients).

observed an enhanced activity of pyruvate dehydrogenase after ammonium addition to perfused rat liver [28], a result which could explain the fall in lactate concentration seen in the ammonium-infused animals. Since changes of the lactate levels in the opposite direction were found not only in experimental and clinical FHF but also in animals with PCA and in cirrhotic patients (fig. 8), it can be concluded that even slight or moderate hepatic lesions are sufficient to overcome the action of ammonia. Obviously, lactate is a very sensitive indicator of an impairment of hepatic function.

The concentration of triglycerides (fig. 9) was not influenced by exogenous hyperammonemia but was consistently lowered by experimental portal-systemic shunting as well as by toxic liver injury. Cirrhotic

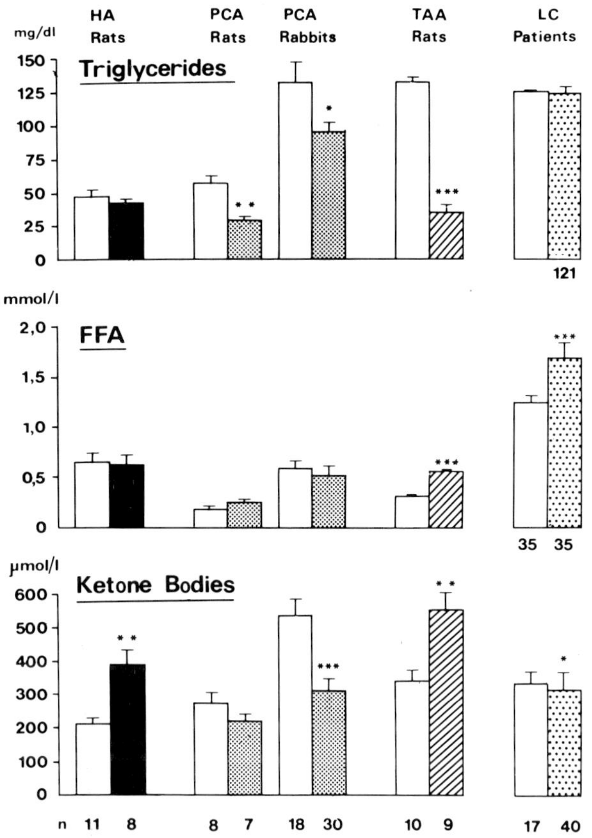

Fig. 9. Concentrations of serum triglycerides, serum free fatty acids (FFA), and whole blood ketone bodies (mean ± SEM) in rats with exogenous hyperammonemia (HA), in animals given a portacaval anastomosis (PCA), in rats which had received thioacetamide (TAA) as well as in patients with liver cirrhosis (LC). For experimental details see legend to table I. Calculation of error probabilities by means of the U-Test. * $p \leq 0.05$, ** $p \leq 0.01$, *** $p \leq 0.001$, as compared to controls. References: [50, 109] (HA in rats, PCA in rats and rabbits, LC in patients), [Tschepe et al., in prep.] (TAA in rats).

patients had, on average, normal triglyceride levels, most probably because the effect of portal-systemic shunting is counteracted by alcohol.

Free fatty acid (FFA) levels (fig. 9) also remained unchanged during the ammonium infusions. Experimental portal-systemic shunting had varying effects, whereas thioacetamide-induced liver insufficiency increased the sum of FFA. Although liver cirrhosis was likewise associated with a rise in FFA concentrations, this – according to findings of Riggio et al. [94] and of our group [50, 109] – cannot be attributed to hepatic failure; in fact, it is more likely that the nutritional state plays a primary role in cirrhosis [94].

The amount of ketone bodies in whole blood (fig. 9) was markedly raised by ammonia. The intensified ketogenesis was most probably mediated, at least in part, by a deficit of oxaloacetate [73, 83]. We can assume that such a deficit is caused by the interference of ammonia with the tricarboxylic acid cycle [35, 36] and by increased gluconeogenesis [112]. In addition, ammonia reduces the muscular de novo-synthesis, the peripheral release, and the plasma level of alanine (fig. 3) [6, 69]; since alanine suppresses ketone body production in the liver [84], the latter process may be disinhibited by hyperammonemia. Portal-systemic shunting caused a decline in the ketone body concentration. It has been suggested that the reduction in hepatic blood flow and, thus, the availability of FFA to the hepatocytes is the mechanism of this phenomenon [15]. Since the ketone body level is increased by hyperammonemia and decreased by portal-systemic shunting, varying concentrations are the result in human cirrhosis.

Effects of TPN

The last part of this contribution concerns TPN in PC-shunted rabbits. As evidenced by the values of glucose, pyruvate, and lactate in figure 10, glucose intolerance failed to occur in the PCA animals. However, most cirrhotic patients display glucose intolerance [2, 78, 80].

The clearance of triglycerides was excellent in the shunted rabbits (fig. 11), as it is in patients with liver cirrhosis [29, 44, 50, 81, 96, 97]. The reduction in the ketone body level (fig. 11) also parallels observations made in cirrhotic patients [50, 114]. With regard to the FFA, there is no agreement between the results obtained in the animals (fig. 11) and those

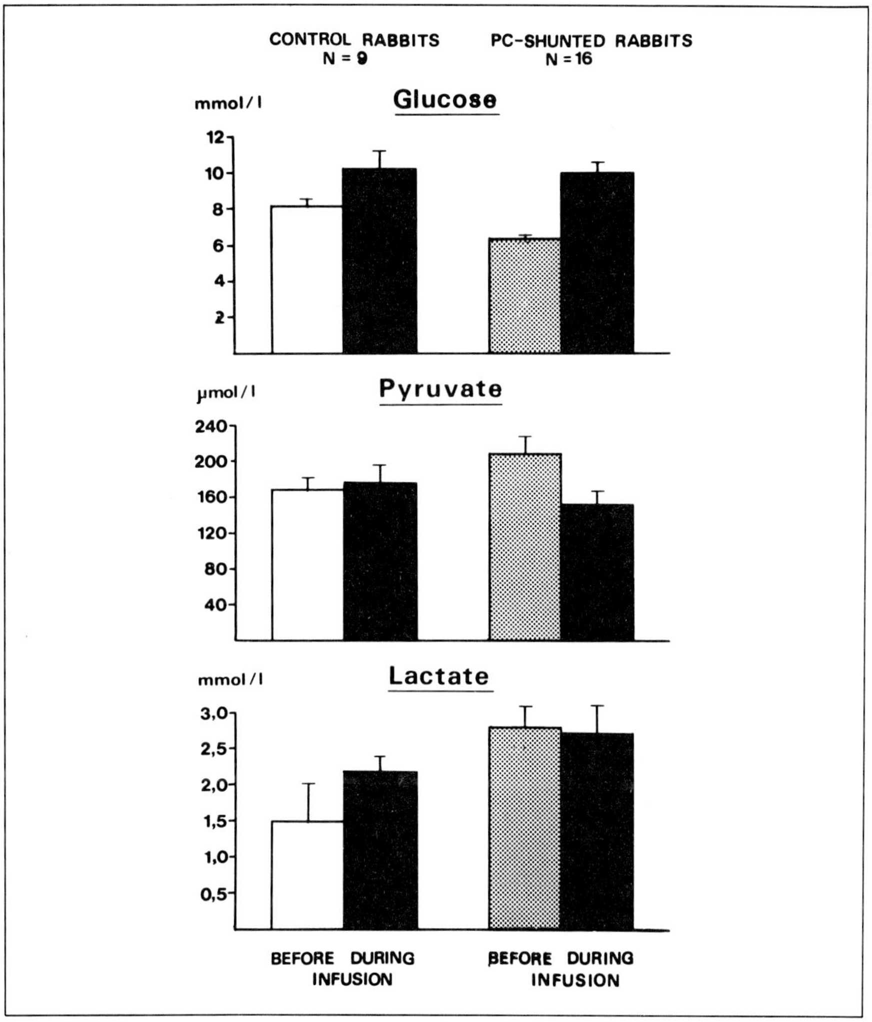

Fig. 10. Concentrations of whole blood glucose, pyruvate, and lactate (mean ± SEM) in rabbits without and with a portacaval shunt, in each instance both before and during total parenteral nutrition. Results obtained by Staedt et al. (in prep.)

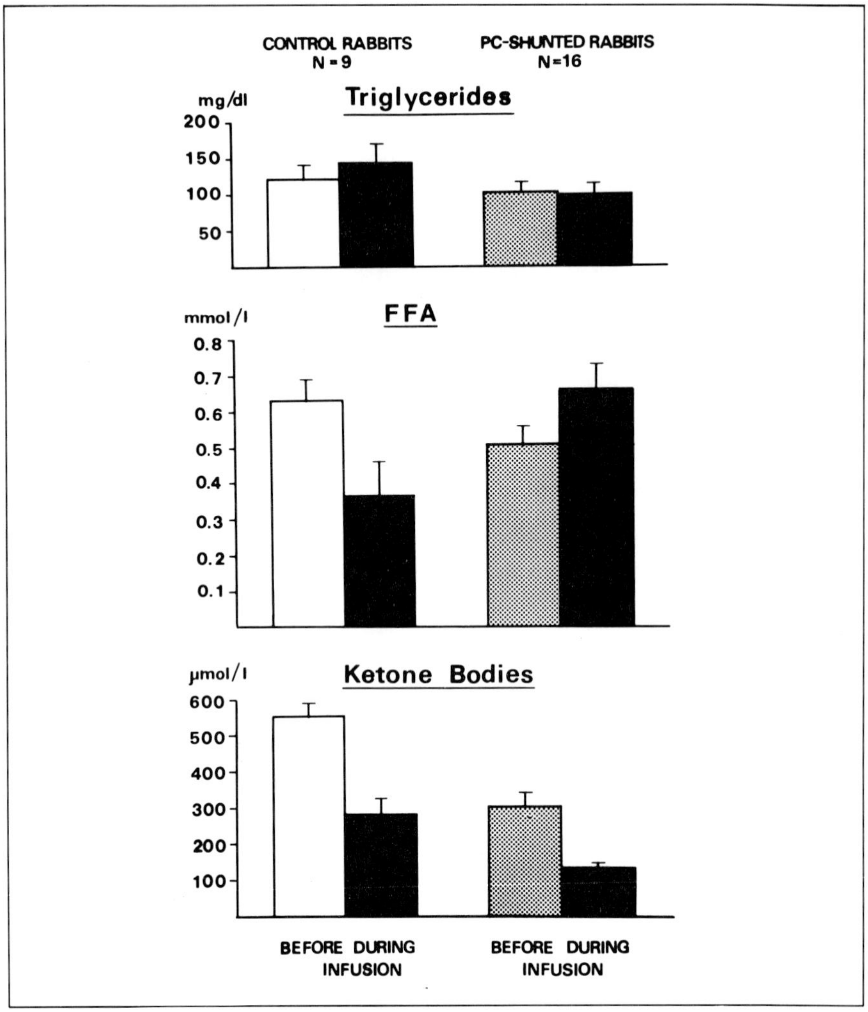

Fig. 11. Concentrations of serum triglycerides, serum free fatty acids (FFA), and whole blood ketone bodies (mean ± SEM) in rabbits without and with a portacaval shunt, in each instance both before and during total parenteral nutrition. Results obtained by Staedt et al. (in prep.).

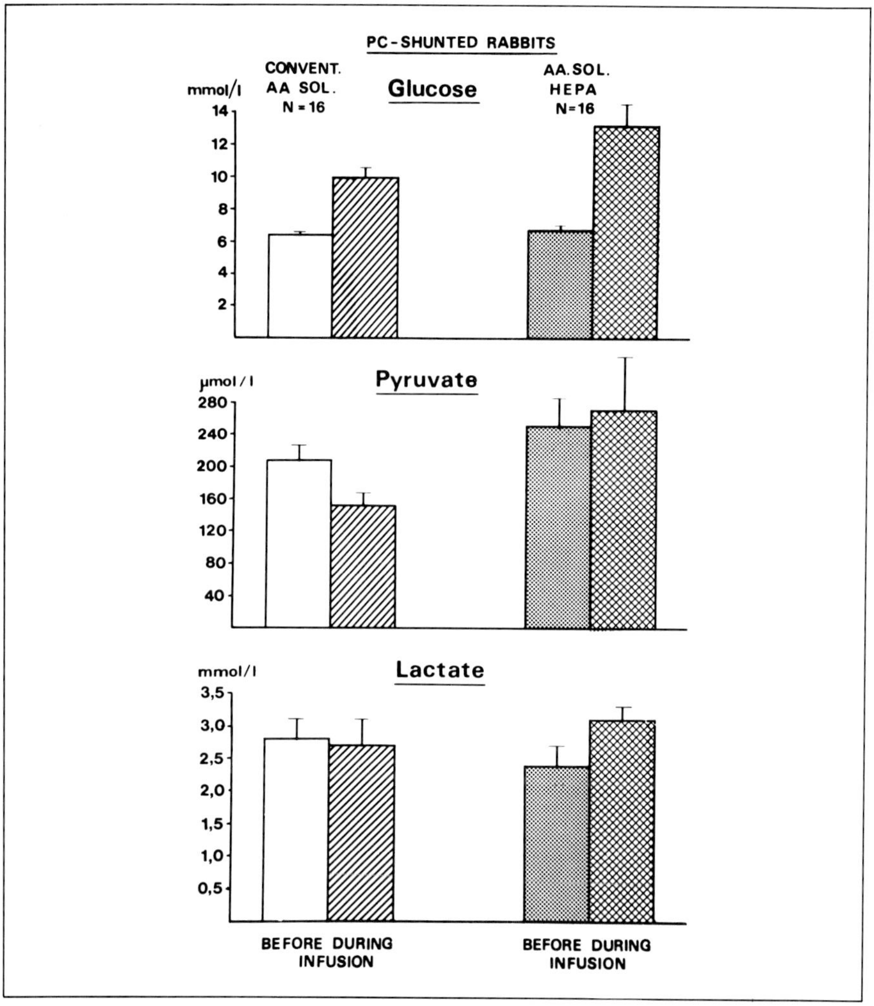

Fig. 12. Concentrations of whole blood glucose, pyruvate, and lactate (mean ± SEM) in rabbits with a portacaval shunt before and during total parenteral nutrition which included either a conventional amino acid solution or a so-called Hepa solution. Results obtained by Staedt et al. (in prep.).

reported for patients [50, 114]. Pronounced shunting of FFA around the liver in the rabbits may be the reason for this discrepancy.

In PCA rabbits, the effects of different amino acid solutions, namely of a conventional and of a so-called Hepa solution, on glucose tolerance were compared (fig. 12). As indicated by the glucose, pyruvate, and lactate levels, the Hepa solution clearly impaired glucose tolerance. Goldberg and Chang have reported that leucine inhibits pyruvate decarboxylation [27]. In the clinical setting, impaired glucose tolerance due to the use of a Hepa solution has not yet been described; however, from the experimental results, this phenomenon may be predicted. A lipid system of TPN appears to be the best therapeutic answer to this problem [114].

Acknowledgments

The authors wish to thank Prof. Dr. K. H. Bässler and Mrs. Cornelia Kunz for the analysis of free fatty acids by gas chromatography. Furthermore, we are grateful to Mrs. Ingeborg Mennicke and Mrs. Sybille Rienmüller for technical assistance.

References

1 Baldessarini, R. J.; Fischer, J. E.: Serotonin metabolism in rat brain after surgical diversion of the portal venous circulation. Nature new Biol. *245:* 25–27 (1973).

2 Berkowitz, D.: Glucose tolerance, free fatty acid, and serum insulin responses in patients with cirrhosis. Am. J. dig. Dis. *14:* 691–699 (1969).

3 Capocaccia, L.; Fischer, J. E.; Rossi-Fanelli, F. (eds.): Hepatic encephalopathy in chronic liver failure (Plenum Press, New York, London 1984).

4 Cascino, A.; Cangiano, C.; Fiaccadori, F.; Ghinelli, F.; Merli, M.; Pelosi, G.; Riggio, O.; Rossi-Fanelli, F.; Sacchini, D.; Stortoni, M.; Capocaccia, L.: Plasma and cerebrospinal fluid amino acid patterns in hepatic encephalopathy. Dig. Dis. Sci. *27:* 828–832 (1982).

5 Van Caulaert, C.; Deviller, C.: Ammoniémie expérimentale après ingestion de chlorure d'ammonium chez l'homme à l'état normal et pathologique. C. r. Séanc. Soc. Biol. *111:* 50–52 (1932).

6 Chang, T. W.; Goldberg, A. L.: The origin of alanine produced in skeletal muscle. J. biol. Chem. *253:* 3677–3684 (1978).

7 Conn, H. O.: Ammonia tolerance in liver disease. J. Lab. clin. Med. *55:* 855–871 (1960).

8 Cremer, J. E.; Heath, D. F.; Teal, H. M.; Woods, M. S.; Cavanagh, J. B.: Some dynamic aspects of brain metabolism in rats given a portocaval anastomosis. Neuropathol. appl. Neurobiol. *3:* 293–311 (1975).

9 Cummings, M. G.; James, J. H.; Soeters, P. E.; Keane, J. M.; Foster, J.; Fischer, J. E.:

Regional brain study of indoleamine metabolism in the rat in acute hepatic failure. J. Neurochem. *27:* 741–746 (1976).

10 Cummings, M. G.; Soeters, P. B.; James, J. H.; Keane, J. M.; Fischer, J. E.: Regional brain indoleamine metabolism following chronic portacaval anastomosis in the rat. J. Neurochem. *27:* 501–509 (1976).

11 Curzon, G.; Kantamaneni, B. D.; Winch, J.; Rojas-Bueno, A.; Murray-Lyon, I. M.; Williams, R.: Plasma and brain tryptophan changes in experimental acute hepatic failure. J. Neurochem. *21:* 137–145 (1973).

12 Datta, D. V.; Agarwalla, M. L.; Narang, A. P. S.; Samanta, A. K. S.; Chuttani, P. N.: Ammonia tolerance test in liver disease with special reference to non-cirrhotic portal fibrosis. Indian J. med. Res. *70:* 825–832 (1979).

13 Dudley, F. J.; Alford, F. P.; Chisholm, D. J.; Findlay, D. M.: Effect of portasystemic venous shunt surgery on hyperglucagonaemia in cirrhosis: Paired studies of pre- and post-shunted subjects. Gut *20:* 817–824 (1979).

14 Eriksson, L. S.; Delin, A.; Tossman, U.; Ungerstedt, U.: Alterations in extracellular brain amino acid concentrations in PC-shunted rats. Clin. Nutr. 2, special suppl., O. 67 (1983).

15 Federspil, G.; Boninsegna, A.; Picchi, G.; Zanon, G.; de Palo, C.: Effect of portacaval shunt on circulating free fatty acids and ketone bodies in rats. Metabolism *29:* 495–497 (1980).

16 Ferreira dos Santos, Ch.; Fezer, M.: Auswirkungen der portokavalen Anastomose und parenteraler Ernährungen mit verschiedenen Aminosäurengemischen auf biochemische Parameter des Plasmas, der Muskulatur und der Leber bei Ratten. Med. diss. Heidelberg/Mannheim (1984).

17 Fischer, B.; Bindert, R.; Burkhardt, H.; Stegaru, B.; Regula, H.: Akute Leberschädigung durch Thioacetamid. Biochemische Veränderungen bei Katzen; in Holm, Ammoniak und hepatische Enzephalopathie, pp. 217–243 (Fischer, Stuttgart 1975).

18 Fischer, B.; Münzenmaier, R.; Bindert, R.; Holm, E.; Wyrwoll, M.: Neurophysiologische Untersuchungen an lebergeschädigten Katzen mit Hyperammoniämie; in Imler, Szám, Neue Erkenntnisse zum Ammoniakstoffwechsel, pp. 111–122 (Witzstrock, Baden-Baden, Brüssel 1974).

19 Fischer, J. E.: Efficacy of branched-chain amino acids in the treatment of hepatic encephalopathy; in Bianchi, Gerok, Landmann, Sickinger, Stalder, Liver in metabolic diseases, pp. 184–192 (MTP Press, Lancaster 1983).

20 Fischer, J. E.: Branched chain amino acids in hepatic encephalopathy: Results of parenteral trials; in Holm, Kasper, Metabolism and nutrition in liver disease, pp. 259–273 (MTP Press, Lancaster 1985).

21 Flock, E. V.; Block, M. A.; Grindlay, J. H.; Mann, F. C.; Bollman, J. L.: Changes in free amino acids of brain and muscle after total hepatectomy. J. biol. Chem. *200:* 529–536 (1953).

22 Fürst, P.: Intracellular amino acids in muscle tissue in postoperative trauma and severe injury: The effect of parenteral nutrition; in Bottermann, Rakette, Intensivmedizinische Aspekte bei parenteraler Ernährung. Klin. Ern., vol. 8, pp. 32–45 (Zuckschwerdt, München, Bern, Wien 1982).

23 Funovics, J.: Die zerebrale Manifestation im Syndrom des Koma hepaticum. Wien. klin. Wschr. *87:* suppl. 35, pp. 3–16 (1975).

24 Ganda, O. P.; Ruderman, N. B.: Muscle nitrogen metabolism in chronic hepatic insufficiency. Metabolism *25:* 427–435 (1976).
25 Garber, A. J.; Karl, I. E.; Kipnis, D. M.: Alanine and glutamine synthesis and release from skeletal muscle. J. biol. Chem. *251:* 826–835 (1976).
26 Gerok, W.: Hepatische Enzephalopathie. Therapie mit adaptierten Aminosäuren- und Ketosäurengemischen. Therapiewoche *34:* 49–62 (1984).
27 Goldberg, A. L.; Chang, T. W.: Regulation and significance of amino acid metabolism in skeletal muscle. Fed. Proc. *37:* 2301–2307 (1978).
28 Häussinger, D.; Weiss, L.; Sies, H.: Activation of pyruvate dehydrogenase during metabolism of ammonium ions in hemoglobin-free perfused rat liver. Eur. J. Biochem. *52:* 421–431 (1975).
29 Hansen, W.: Fettoleranz und Postheparinlipasen bei Leberkrankheiten. Verh. dt. Ges. inn. Med. *81:* 1335–1336 (1975).
30 Hawkins, R. A.; Miller, A. L.; Nielsen, R. C.; Veech, R. L.: The acute action of ammonia on rat brain metabolism in vivo. Biochem. J. *134:* 1001–1008 (1973).
31 Hayashi, M.; Ohnishi, H.; Kawade, Y.; Muto, Y.; Takahashi, Y.: Augmented utilization of branched-chain amino acids by skeletal muscle in decompensated liver cirrhosis in special relation to ammonia detoxication. Gastroenterol. jap. *16:* 64–70 (1981).
32 Herlin, P. M.; James, J. H.; Craig, B. S.; Nachbauer, A.; Fischer, J. E.: Effect of total hepatectomy and administration of branched-chain amino acids on regional norepinephrine, dopamine, and amino acids in rat brain. Ann. Surg. *198:* 172–177 (1983).
33 Herz, R.; Rössle, M.; Schulte, U.; Gerok, W.: Periphere Aminosäuren-Konzentrationen bei eingeschränkter quantitativer Leberfunktion infolge Leberzirrhose. Z. Gastroenterol. *17:* 572–573 (1979).
34 Hindfelt, B.: The effect of sustained hyperammonemia upon the metabolic state of the brain. Scand. J. clin. Lab. Invest. *30:* 245–255 (1972).
35 Hindfelt, B.: Ammonia and brain energy metabolism; in Holm, Aminosäuren- und Ammoniakstoffwechsel bei Leberinsuffizienz, pp. 103–107 (Witzstrock, Baden-Baden, Köln, New York 1982).
36 Hindfelt, B.; Plum, F.; Duffy, T. E.: Effect of acute ammonia intoxication on cerebral metabolism in rats with portacaval shunts. J. clin. Invest. *59:* 386–396 (1977).
37 Holm, E. (ed.): Ammoniak und hepatische Enzephalopathie. Biochemie, Elektrophysiologie, Toxikologie (Fischer, Stuttgart 1975).
38 Holm, E.; Fiene, R.; Striebel, J.-P.; Haux, P.; Kirchmeier, J.: Spontane und infusionsabhängige Konzentrationen der Plasmaaminosäuren bei Leberinsuffizienz. Biochemische Daten und EEG; in Wewalka, Dragosics, Aminosäuren, Ammoniak und hepatische Enzephalopathie, pp. 176–191 (Fischer, Stuttgart, New York 1978).
39 Holm, E.; Hamann, K.-F.; Reith, H.-J.; Fischer, B.: Neurophysiological studies in cats with exogenous hyperammonemia; in Imler, Szàm, Neue Erkenntnisse zum Ammoniakstoffwechsel, pp. 92–110 (Witzstrock, Baden-Baden, Brüssel 1974).
40 Holm, E.; Krämer, W.; Reith, H.-J.; Magin, T.; Mezitis, N. H. E.: Electrophysiological and psychometric studies in hepatic encephalopathy; in Varró, Bálint, Creutzfeldt, Current views in gastroenterology, vol. I, pp. 597–613 (Budapest 1977).
41 Holm, E.; Leweling, H.; Staedt, U.: Metabolism and nutritional supply of amino acids in hepatic failure; in Kleinberger, Deutsch, New aspects of clinical nutrition, pp. 377–399 (Karger, Basel 1983).

42 Holm, E.; Leweling, H.; Staedt, U.; Striebel, J.-P.; Jacob, St.: The metabolic fate of branched-chain amino acids; in Capocaccia, Fischer, Rossi-Fanelli, Hepatic encephalopathy in chronic liver failure, pp. 161–181 (Plenum Press, New York, London 1984).

43 Holm, E.; Leweling, H.; Staedt, U.; Striebel, J.-P.; Tschepe, A.: Amino acids and nutrition in liver cirrhosis. BCAA-enriched intravenous and oral diets. Scand. J. Gastroent. (in press).

44 Holm, E.; Staedt, U.; Leweling, H.; Bässler, K. H.; Specker, M.; Tschepe, A.: Fettstoffwechsel und parenterale Fettzufuhr bei Leberinsuffizienz. Infusionstherapie *10:* 184–204 (1983).

45 Holm, E.; Staedt, U.; Striebel, J.-P.; Hammer, R.; Klinker, J.: Grundlagen und Effizienz der Infusionstherapie mit hepatologisch konzipierten Aminosäurenlösungen; in Holm, Kleinberger, Konzepte für Aminosäurenlösungen. Klin. Ern., vol. 18, pp. 43–69 (Zuckschwerdt, München, Bern, Wien, in press).

46 Holm, E.; Striebel, J.-P.; Bardehle, W.; Kihm, U.; Schneider, E. J.; Klimm, J.: Aminosäureninfusionen bei 73 internistischen und 25 frisch operierten Patienten mit Leberzirrhose. Parenterale Ernährung und adjuvante Komabehandlung; in Ibe, Krankheitsadaptierte Ernährungstherapie. Klin. Ern., vol. 2, pp. 51–101 (Zuckschwerdt, München 1985).

47 Holm, E.; Striebel, J.-P.; Kattermann, R.; Schick, E.; Staedt, U.: Encephalopathy resulting from portacaval anastomosis in cats. Ammonia, amino acids, and cerebral electrical activity; in Holm, Aminosäuren- und Ammoniakstoffwechsel bei Leberinsuffizienz, pp. 58–94 (Witzstrock, Baden-Baden, Köln, New York 1982).

48 Holm, E.; Striebel, J.-P.; Langhans, W.; Kattermann, R.; Werner, B.: Beziehungen zwischen Plasmaammoniak, Plasmaaminosäuren und weiteren Parametern bei Leberzirrhose. Zwei Hauptkomponentenanalysen. Verh. dt. Ges. inn. Med. *86:* 775–780 (1980).

49 Holm, E.; Striebel, J.-P.; Münzenmaier, R.; Kattermann, R.: Pathogenese der hepatischen Enzephalopathie. Leber Magen Darm *7:* 241–254 (1977).

50 Holm, E.; Tschepe, A.; Staedt, U.; Leweling, H.; Gladisch, R.; Bässler, K. H.: Fatty acid and ketone body metabolism in hepatic failure; in Kleinberger, Ferenci, Riederer, Thaler, Advances in hepatic encephalopathy and urea cycle diseases, pp. 645–666 (Karger, Basel 1984).

51 Holmin, T.; Agardh, C.-D.; Alinder, G.; Herlin, P.: Some effects of total hepatectomy upon the metabolic state of the rat brain; in Holm, Amino acid and ammonia metabolism in hepatic failure, pp. 108–111 (Witzstrock, Baden-Baden, Köln, New York 1982).

52 Holmin, T.; Agardh, C.-D.; Alinder, G.; Herlin, P.; Hultberg, B.: The influence of total hepatectomy on cerebral energy state, ammonia-related amino acids of the brain and plasma amino acids in the rat. Eur. J. clin. Invest. *13:* 215–220 (1983).

53 Holmin, T.; Siesjö, B. K.: The effect of portacaval anastomosis upon the energy state and upon acid-base parameters of the rat brain. J. Neurochem. *22:* 403–412 (1974).

54 Hutson, D. G.; Ono, J.; Dombro, R. S.; Levi, J. U.; Livingstone, A.; Zeppa, R.: A longitudinal study of tryptophan involvement in hepatic coma. Am. J. Surg. *137:* 235–239 (1979).

55 Imler, M.; Schlienger, J. L.; Brandt, C.: Modifications of blood ammonia and behaviour in rats after occlusion of the portal vein. Digestion *2:* 448–449 (1974).

56 Imler, M.; Schlienger, J. L.; Frick, A.; Stahl, A.; Chabrier, G.: Study of muscular glutamine and alanine release in cirrhotics with hyperammonemia and in ammonium infused rats; in Holm, Amino acid and ammonia metabolism in hepatic failure, pp. 33–39 (Witz-strock, Baden-Baden, Köln, New York 1982).

57 Iwasaki, Y.; Sato, H.; Ohkubo, A.; Sanjo, T.; Futagawa, S.; Sugiura, M.; Tsuji, S.: Effect of spontaneous portal-systemic shunting on plasma insulin and amino acid concentrations. Gastroenterology *78:* 677–683 (1980).

58 James, J. H.; Escourrou, J.; Fischer, J. E.: Blood-brain neutral amino acid transport activity is increased after portacaval anastomosis. Science *200:* 1395–1397 (1978).

59 James, J. H.; Hodgman, J. M.; Funovics, J. M.; Yoshimura, N.; Fischer, J. E.: Brain tryptophan, plasma free tryptophan and distribution of plasma neutral amino acids. Metabolism *25:* 471–476 (1976).

60 James, J. H.; Ziparo, V.; Jeppson, B.; Fischer, J. E.: Hyperammonaemia, plasma amino acid imbalance, and blood-brain aminoacid transport: A unified theory of portal-systemic encephalopathy. Lancet *ii:* 772–775 (1979).

61 Jeppsson, B.; James, J. H.; Hummel, R. P.; Brenner, W.; West, R.; Fischer, J. E.: Increased blood-brain transport of tryptophan after portacaval anastomoses in germ-free rats. Metabolism *32:* 4–8 (1983).

62 Karavias, Th.: Der Einfluß zweier hämodynamisch unterschiedlicher portosystemischer Anastomosen auf die hepatischen und zerebralen Funktionen der gesunden und zirrhotischen Ratte; Habschr. Berlin (1983).

63 Kirk, E.: Amino acid and ammonia metabolism in liver diseases. Acta med. scand., suppl. 77 (1936).

64 Kitani, T.: Diskussionsbeiträge zu 'Coma hepaticum'. Proc. Int. Congr. Gastro-Enterol. *30:* 465–482 (1960).

65 Klassen, G. A.; Aronoff, A.; Karpati, G.: Forearm metabolism in patients with chronic liver disease. Clin. Sci. *37:* 455–470 (1969).

66 Knott, P. J.; Curzon, G.: Tryptophan and tyrosine disposition and brain tryptophan metabolism in acute carbon tetrachloride poisoning. Biochem. Pharmac. *24:* 963–966 (1975).

67 Kontos, H. A.; Shapiro, W.; Mauck, H. P.; Patterson, J. L.: General and regional circulatory alterations in cirrhosis of the liver. Am. J. Med. *37:* 526–535 (1964).

68 Leweling, H.; Holm, E.; Staedt, U.; Feussner, H.; Zelder, O.; Striebel, J.-P.: Totale parenterale Ernährung bei Ratten mit portokavaler Anastomose. Infusionstherapie *9:* 234 (1982).

69 Leweling, H.; Holm, E.; Staedt, U.; Striebel, J.-P.; Tschepe, A.: Intra- and extracellular amino acid concentrations in ammonium-infused rats. Evidence that hyperammonemia reduces BCAA levels; in Kleinberger, Ferenci, Riederer, Thaler, Advances in hepatic encephalopathy and urea cycle diseases, pp. 552–554 (Karger, Basel 1984).

70 Leweling, H.; Holm, E.; Staedt, U.; Tschepe, A.; Striebel, J.-P.: Rational and nutritional effects of BCAA-enriched TPN regimens in patients with liver cirrhosis; in Holm, Kasper, Metabolism and nutrition in liver disease; pp. 235–257 (MTP Press, Lancaster 1985).

71 Leweling, H.; Staedt, U.; Holm, E.; Zelder, O.; Feussner, H.; Striebel, J.-P.: Plasmaammoniak und extra- sowie intrazelluläre Aminosäurenmuster portocaval-shunt-operierter Ratten bei totaler parenteraler Ernährung unter Verwendung einer 'konventionellen' und einer transfer-adaptierten Aminosäurenlösung; in Zelder, Röher, Fischer, Bode, Experimentelle und klinische Hepatologie, pp. 155–165 (Schattauer, Stuttgart, New York 1984).

72 Lin, S.; Raabe, U.: Ammonia intoxication: Effects on cerebral cortex and spinal cord. J. Neurochem. *44:* 1252–1258 (1985).

73 Lopes-Cardozo, M.: Regulation of ketogenesis in isolated rat liver mitochondria; in Söling, Seufert, Biochemical and clinical aspects of ketone body metabolism, pp. 41–49 (Thieme, Stuttgart 1978).

74 Lux, H. D.: Ammonium and chloride extrusion: Hyperpolarizing synaptic inhibition in spinal motoneurons. Science *173:* 555–557 (1971).

75 Mans, A. M.; Saunders, S. J.; Kirsch, R. E.; Biebuyck, J. F.: Correlation of plasma and brain amino acid and putative neurotransmitter alterations during acute hepatic coma in the rat. J. Neurochem. *32:* 285–292 (1979).

76 Mattson, W. J.; Iob, V.; Sloan, M.; Coon, W. W.; Turcotte, J. G.; Child, C. G.: Alterations of individual free amino acids in brain during acute hepatic coma. Surgery Gynec. Obstet *130:* 263–266 (1970).

77 McKhann, G. M.; Tower, D. B.: Ammonia toxicity and cerebral oxidative metabolism. Am. J. Physiol. *200:* 420–424 (1961).

78 Megyesi, C.; Samols, E.; Marks, V.: Glucose intolerance and diabetes in chronic liver disease. Lancet *ii:* 1051–1055 (1967).

79 Meyer, H.; Lux, H. D.: Action of ammonium on a chloride pump. Pflügers Arch. *350:* 185–195 (1974).

80 Mezey, E.: Liver disease and nutrition. Gastroenterology *74:* 770–783 (1978).

81 Milewski, B.; Szostak, W. B.; Medrzejewski, W.; Cybulska, B.; Krygier, T.: Studies on the intravenous fat tolerance test in patients with compensated liver cirrhosis and chronic aggressive hepatitis. Pol. Arch. Med. Wewn *50:* 259–261 (1973).

82 Munro, H. N.; Fernstrom, J. D.; Wurtman, R. J.: Plasma amino acid imbalance and hepatic coma. Klin. Anästh. Intensivther. *13:* 103–112 (1977).

83 Newsholme, E. A.; Start, C.: Regulation des Stoffwechsels – Homöostase im menschlichen und tierischen Organismus (Chemie, Weinheim, New York 1977).

84 Nosadini, R.; Alberti, K. G. M. M.; Johnston, D. G.; Del Prato, S.; Marescotti, C.; Duner, E.: The antiketogenic effect of alanine in normal man: Evidence for an alanine-ketone body cycle. Metabolism *30:* 563–567 (1981).

85 Okuda, K.; Kono, K.; Ohnishi, K.; Kimura, K.; Omata, M.; Koen, H.; Nakajima, Y.; Musha, H.; Hirashima, T.; Takashi, M.; Takayasu, K.: Clinical study of eighty-six cases of idiopathic portal hypertension and comparison with cirrhosis with splenomegaly. Gastroenterology *86:* 600–610 (1984).

86 Ono, J.; Hutson, D. G.; Dombro, R. S.; Levi, J. U.; Livingstone, A.; Zeppa, R.: Tryptophan and hepatic coma. Gastroenterology *74:* 196–200 (1978).

87 Pappas, S. C.; Ferenci, P.; Schafer, D. F.; Jones, E. A.: Visual evoked potentials in a rabbit model of hepatic encephalopathy. II. Comparison of hyperammonemic encephalopathy, postictal coma, and coma induced by synergistic neurotoxins. Gastroenterology *86:* 546–551 (1984).

88 Raabe, W.: Postsynaptic inhibition and the EEG in ammonia intoxication. Electroenceph. clin. Neurophysiol. *51:* 30 P (1981).
89 Raabe, W.; Gumnit, R. J.: Disinhibition in cat motor cortex by ammonia. J. Neurophysiol. *38:* 347–355 (1975).
90 Raabe, W.; Lin, S.: Pathophysiology of ammonia intoxication. Exp. Neurol. *87:* 519–532 (1985).
91 Raabe, W.; Onstad, G.: Porta-caval shunting changes neuronal tolerance to ammonia. Ann. Neurol. *8:* 106 (1980).
92 Record, C.; Buxton, B.; Chase, R. A.; Curzon, G.; Murray-Lyon, I. M.; Williams, R.: Plasma and brain amino acids in fulminant hepatic failure and their relationship to hepatic encephalopathy. Eur. J. clin. Invest. *6:* 387–394 (1976).
93 Riederer, P.; Jellinger, K.; Rausch, W. D.; Kleinberger, G.; Kothbauer, P.: Zur Biochemie der hepatischen Enzephalopathien. Z. Gastroenterol. *16:* 768–777 (1978).
94 Riggio, O.; Merli, M.; Cantafora, A.; DiBiase, A.; Lalloni, L.; Leonetti, F.; Miazzo, P.; Rinaldi, V.; Rossi-Fanelli, F.; Tamburrano, G.; Capocaccia, L.: Total and individual free fatty acid concentrations in liver cirrhosis. Metabolism *33:* 646–651 (1984).
95 Rössle, M.; Luft, M.; Herz, R.; Klein, B.; Lehmann, M.; Gerok, W.: Amino acid, ammonia and neurotransmitter concentrations in hepatic encephalopathy: Serial analysis in plasma and cerebrospinal fluid during treatment with an adapted amino acid solution. Klin. Wschr. *62:* 867–875 (1984).
96 Rössner, S.: The relation of intravenous fat solutions to lipoprotein metabolism. Acta chirurg. scand., suppl. 507, pp. 220–225 (1980).
97 Rössner, S.; Johansson, C.; Walldius, G.; Aly, A.: Intralipid clearance and lipoprotein pattern in men with advanced alcoholic liver cirrhosis. Am. J. clin. Nutr. *32:* 2022–2026 (1979).
98 Rosen, H.; Soeters, P. B.; James, J. H.; Hodgman, J.; Fischer, J. E.: Influences of exogenous intake and nitrogen balance on plasma and brain aromatic amino acid concentrations. Metabolism *27:* 393–404 (1978).
99 Rosen, H. M.; Yoshimura, N.; Hodgman, J. M.; Fischer, J. E.: Plasma amino acid patterns in hepatic encephalopathy of differing etiology. Gastroenterology *72:* 483–487 (1977).
100 Roth, E.; Funovics, J.; Karner, J.; Mühlbacher, F.; Rauhs, R.; Steininger, R.; Huk, I.; Sporn, P.; Kleinberger, G.: Muscle amino acid levels in patients with liver diseases; in Kleinberger, Ferenci, Riederer, Thaler, Advances in hepatic encephalopathy and urea cycle diseases, pp. 527–537 (Karger, Basel 1984).
101 Ruderman, N. B.; Berger, M.: The formation of glutamine and alanine in skeletal muscle. J. biol. Chem. *249:* 5500–5506 (1974).
102 Schäfer, K.; Ukida, M.; Steffen, C.; Bode, C.; Zelder, O.; Bode, J. C.: Effect of ammonia on plasma and cerebrospinal fluid amino acids in dogs with and without portacaval anastomoses. Res. exp. Med. *185:* 35–44 (1985).
103 Sherwin, R.; Joshi, P.; Hendler, R.; Felig, P.; Conn, H. O.: Hyperglucagonemia in Laennec's cirrhosis. The role of portal-systemic shunting. New Engl. J. Med. *290:* 239–242 (1974).
104 Soeters, P. B.; de Boer, J.: Why are plasma branched chain amino acid levels diminished in patients with liver cirrhosis?; in Adibi, Fekl, Langenbeck, Schauder, Branched chain amino and keto acids in health and disease, pp. 483–496 (Karger, Basel 1984).

105 Soeters, P. B.; de Boer, J. E. G.; Oostenbroek, R. J.; Janssen, M. A.: Fate of branched chain amino acids; in Kleinberger, Deutsch, New aspects of clinical nutrition, pp. 337–345 (Karger, Basel 1983).

106 Soeters, P. B.; Fischer, J. E.: Insulin, glucagon, amino acid imbalance, and hepatic encephalopathy. Lancet *ii:* 880–882 (1976).

107 Soeters, P. B.; Weir, G.; Ebeid, A. M.; Fischer, J. E.: Insulin, glucagon, portal systemic shunting, and hepatic failure in the dog. J. surg. Res. *23:* 183–188 (1977).

108 Staedt, U.; Holm, E.; Striebel, J.-P.; Gasteiger, P.: Amino acid concentrations in plasma and intracellular water of muscle in cats given a portacaval anastomosis. Effects of brief intravenous nutrition including a BCAA-enriched solution. Clin. Nutr. *1:* F 52 (1982).

109 Staedt, U.; Jacob, St.; Lenhard, B.; Klinker, J.; Holm, E.: Basic conditions determining the postabsorptive concentrations of triglycerides, free fatty acids, and ketone bodies in hepatic failure; in Holm, Kasper, Metabolism and nutrition in liver disease; pp. 129–138 (MTP Press, Lancaster 1985).

110 Stahl, J.: Studies of the blood ammonia in liver disease. Its diagnostic, prognostic, and therapeutic significance. Ann. intern. Med. *58:* 1–24 (1963).

111 Steigmann, F.; Condon, R. E.; Silverman, D. A.; Bombeck, C. T.; Alavi, I.; Dubin, A.; Hepatic coma: Newer pathogenetic and therapeutic factors. Am. J. Gastroent., N.Y. *54:* 355–362 (1970).

112 Strombeck, D. R.; Rogers, Q.; Stern, J. S.: Effects of intravenous ammonia infusion on plasma levels of amino acids, glucagon and insulin in dogs. Gastroenterology *74:* 1165 (1978).

113 Teijema, H. L.; Janssens, A. R.; Lanser, J. B. K.; Vrijland, E.; Wielaard, R.: Human hepatic encephalopathy: Plasma and CSF amino acids and ammonia; in Holm, Amino acid and ammonia metabolism in hepatic failure, pp. 17–22 (Witzstrock, Baden-Baden, Köln, New York 1982).

114 Tschepe, A.; Saeger, H.-D.; Belz, J.; Gladisch, R.; Holm, E.: Metabolic effects of various parenteral nutrition regimens (lipid systems) in patients with liver cirrhosis; in Holm, Kasper, Metabolism and nutrition in liver disease (MTP Press, Lancaster, in press).

115 Tyce, G. M.; Flock, E. V.; Owen, C. A.: Metabolism of glucose in brain after hepatectomy; in Polli, Neurochemistry of hepatic coma. Exp. Biol. Med., vol. 4, pp. 92–103 (Karger, Basel 1971).

116 Tyce, G. M.; Flock, E. V.; Owen, C. A.; Stobie, G. H. C.; David, C.: 5-hydroxyindole metabolism in the brain after hepatectomy. Biochem. Pharmac. *16:* 979–992 (1967).

117 Volz, M.; Junge, U.: Branched chain amino acids and their keto analogues in liver disease. Falk Symp. No. 41, Nutrition in Liver Disease, Freiburg i. Br. 1984 (Abstract Book).

118 Watanabe, A.; Takei, N.; Higashi, T.; Shiota, T.; Nakatsukasa, H.; Fujiwara, M.; Sakata, T.; Nagashima, H.: Glutamic acid and glutamine levels in serum and cerebrospinal fluid in hepatic encephalopathy. Biochem. Med. *32:* 225–231 (1984).

119 Weber, Th.: Fett in der parenteralen Ernährung von Patienten mit Leberzirrhose. Postabsorptive und infusionsabhängige Konzentrationen energieliefernder Substrate und ihrer Metaboliten; Med. Diss. Heidelberg/Mannheim (1983).

120 Weiser, M.; Riederer, P.; Kleinberger, G.: Human cerebral free amino acids in hepatic coma. J. neural Transm., suppl. 14, pp. 95–102 (1978).

121 Williams, A. H.; Kyu, M. H.; Fenton, J. C. B.; Cavanagh, J. B.: The glutamate and glutamine content of rat brain after portocaval anastomosis. J. Neurochem. *19:* 1073–1077 (1972).

122 Zaki, A. E. O.; Ede, R. J.; Davis, M.; Williams, R.: Experimental studies of blood brain barrier permeability in acute hepatic failure. Hepatology *4:* 359–363 (1984).

123 Zeneroli, M. L.; Ventura, E.; Baraldi, M.; Penne, A.; Messori, E.; Zieve, L.: Visual evoked potentials in encephalopathy induced by galactosamine, ammonia, dimethyldisulfide, and octanoid acid. Hepatology *2:* 532–538 (1982).

Prof. Dr. E. Holm, I. Med. Klinik, Abt. für Pathophysiologie, Theodor-Kutzer-Ufer, D-6800 Mannheim 1 (FRG)

Dietze, Grünert, Kleinberger, Wolfram (eds.), Clinical Nutrition and Metabolic Research. Proc. 7th Congr. ESPEN, Munich 1985, pp. 375–384 (Karger, Basel 1986)

Animal Models of Sepsis in Relation to Metabolism and Nutrition

B. Jeppsson, L. Hansson

Department of Surgery, University of Lund, Lund, Sweden

The study of sepsis in man in relation to metabolism and nutrition is difficult. The diversity of microorganisms involved and the individualized treatment septic patients often receive make it difficult to perform controlled clinical studies. Therefore, there is a need for animal models that simulate the clinical course of sepsis in order to decrease the number of uncontrolled variables.

The term 'sepsis' often refers to different conditions in different studies, from a low-grade infection lasting for days or weeks to a raging process leading to death within a few hours. In this paper 'sepsis' refers to an acute infection in which an animal is toxic with fever, weakness, anorexia, and lethargy because of invasive infection, and 'septic shock' is used when the effects of sepsis lead to circulatory collapse.

The requirement for a good animal model of sepsis is to have a controlled setting with a predictable time course of reasonable length and a high level of reproducibility. The animals should exhibit: overt signs of illness in a state of hyperdynamic circulation; the metabolic changes seen in humans with increased energy substrate turnover and protein metabolism; and an altered hormonal milieu [1–3] (table I). The choice of animal species must be made to fit the purpose of the intended study. There are many advantages in using small rodents since they are relatively inexpensive, available in large numbers, genetically identical, the same age and sex, on the same diet, and free of specific pathogen. This improves statistical evaluation and minimizes biological variables. A larger animal facilitates the collection of adequate samples of blood and tissues, and makes regional metabolic studies easier. The biological variation increases however. Dogs and pigs have been used the most. Pigs are in many ways

Table I. Response to sepsis

Parameter	Human [2, 3]	Parent. adm. of bacteria	Parent. adm. of bacteria [20]	Implantation models	Ischemic models
Toxic symptoms (fever, malaise, anorexia, etc.)	present	present	present	present	present
Blood cultures	frequently positive	positive	80% positive	positive	positive
White blood cells	leukocytosis during hyperphase	leukopenia [14]	leukocytosis	leukopenia [21]	leukopenia [34]
Hemodynamic response	hyperdynamic	shock	hyperdynamic	hyperdynamic [21]	hyperdynamic [29]
Metabolic rate	increase	decrease [12]	increase	increase [21]	unknown
Hormonal response					
Insulin	increase	no change [13] decrease [14, 15]	increase	unknown	increase [29]
Glucagon	increase	increase [13]	increase	unknown	unknown
Substrate changes					
Glucose prod.	no change, increase*	increase [12]	no change	unknown	decrease [31] increase [32]
Glucose oxid.	no change, increase*	unknown	no change	unknown	unknown
Ketogenesis	impaired	unknown	unknown	decrease [26]	unknown
FFA release	unknown	unknown	increase	unknown	decrease [30]
Triglyceride conc.	increase	unknown	increase	unknown	normal [10]
Protein catab.	present	present [13]	unknown	present	present [33]
Amino acid changes	present	present [13]	unknown	unknown	present [33, 34]

* decrease in agonal phase

Table II. Experimental models

(A) Endotoxin models
(B) Sepsis models
(1) Parenteral administration of bacteria (intravenous, intraarterial or intraperitoneal)
(2) Implantation of fecal material, bacteria, or infected foreign material (in peritoneum, soft tissues, fractures)
(3) Ischemic organ and perforation

more similar to man than dogs [4]. The number of pigs and dogs which can be used for experimental studies, however, is limited by the cost involved. One may be forced to study a smaller number of animals, thus reducing the significance of the results.

The three main approaches used to produce sepsis in laboratory animals have been: (1) parenteral administration of bacteria; (2) implantation of fecal material, bacteria, or infected foreign material; (3) surgical operations that create ischemic organs and perforated viscera (table II).

Endotoxin Models

Before discussing 'true' septic models, the endotoxin models must be dealt with. Although the administration of endotoxin in laboratory animals will induce some physiologic and biochemical alterations associated with gram-negative sepsis, the clinical pictures that result from gram-negative sepsis and endotoxin are quite different. Endotoxin causes shock and death when injected into various laboratory animals, quite different from the hyperdynamic circulation seen in patients [5]. Even though endotoxins may be released by gram-negative organisms, there is little support for the contention that endotoxins play a major role in clinical sepsis [6].

Endotoxin levels in septic patients are quite low, whereas doses used experimentally to produce symptoms are considerably larger [7]. Besides, since live bacteria are not injected, a sustained septicemia is not induced. Some metabolic alterations induced by endotoxin administration have been described. As far as carbohydrate metabolism is concerned, the response to endotoxin is marked by a profound hypoglycemia due to impaired gluconeogenesis and reduced peripheral glucose uptake [8]. This is in contrast to septic patients who frequently show persistent hyperglycemia and gluconeogenesis. Insulin and glucagon levels are elevated in both conditions. Fasting dogs receiving E.coli endotoxin show muscle proteolysis with elevated glycine and alanine levels in plasma and with increased oxidative decarboxylation in muscle of the branched-chain amino acids valine, isoleucine, and leucine (BCAA) also observed in septic patients [9]. Other similarities are: increased plasma lactate and pyruvate levels, and hypertriglyceridemia [10]. Although endotoxinemia share some common metabolic alterations with clinical sepsis, caution must be exercised in using endotoxin models for metabolic and nutritional studies because of the differences in carbohydrate metabolism and cardiovascular response.

Sepsis Models

Parenteral Administration of Bacteria

A number of investigators have produced sepsis by parenteral administration of concentrated live bacteria, mostly E.coli or Pseudomonas. The administration of E.coli or Pseudomonas aeruginosa in fasted animals will lead to a bacteremic shock with hypotension, low cardiac output and increased peripheral resistance, and a high mortality within 12–42 h [11–16].

Some knowledge about metabolic reactions after parenteral administration of bacteria is available (table I). Intraarterial injection of 10^{10} live E. coli in guinea pigs led to a 60% mortality before 24 h. The animals had an increased glucose production over the first 6 h and hyperglycemia was evident. At 14 h hypoglycemia ensued [12]. Dogs injected with 10^9 E.coli/kg BW exhibited hypoglycemia, increased plasma lactate and glucagon at 4 h. At this time the animals were hypotensive. There was an increased release of amino acids from muscle tissue, except for the BCAA which were rapidly oxidized [13]. The gram-negative bacteremia also impaired gluconeogenesis. The intravenous injection of E.coli in baboons gave similar results with a 100% mortality after 42 h and leukopenia, hypotension, hypoglycemia, and hypoinsulinemia [14]. The intravenous administration of Pseudomonas aeruginosa in dogs over a 5 h period induced hypothermia, leukopenia, hypotension, hypoglycemia, and low insulin levels [15]. There was a mortality rate of 70% within 24 h, whereas restoration of blood glucose levels to normal reduced the mortality to 12.5%.

The intraperitoneal administration of bacteria in rats also leads to peritonitis and septic shock with 100% mortality within 24 h [17–19]. The mortality is dose dependent, and the animals either succumb or remain healthy without any stage in between. The animals show leukopenia. Metabolic parameters have not been studied except liver mitochondrial respiration, which seemed unimpaired [18].

The parenteral administration of bacteria is advantageous in that it allows precise control over the dosage and strains of bacteria and is completely reproducible. It does not exactly mimic the human situation. The host is suddenly overwhelmed with the bacterial challenge and is unable to compile a full expression of host defense mechanisms. In the clinical situation, there usually is a septic focus, which intermittently but persistently showers the body with bacteria of one or several strains. These models are more suitable for studies of different drug effects and bacterial clearance kinetics than for metabolic and nutritional studies. If such studies are undertaken with these models, one must bear in mind that they only represent the shock phase with exhausted energy production and decreased metabolic rate.

The hemodynamic and metabolic response is different if fluid resuscitation with lactated Ringer is provided. This has been shown in a study of intraarterial infusion of E.coli in non-fasted dogs [20]. An initial dose of 10^{10} E.coli was given over 30 min to saturate the reticuloendothelial system and then an additional dose of 5×10^{9} over 30 min one hour later. This induced a temporary shock state followed by a hyperdynamic, hypermetabolic phase 6–12 h later, lasting at least 72 h. Besides great similarities to human sepsis in general and in hemodynamic response, this model also hormonally and metabolically resembled what is commonly seen in humans with sepsis (table I). The metabolic rate was increased 25%, and the energy for this increase was primarily provided by increased oxidation of free fatty acids (FFA) and triglycerides. There was an increased release of FFA and a markedly elevated triglyceride synthesis. Glucose production was maintained at the control value, and the rate of glucose oxidation was not significantly altered. Plasma insulin and glucagon concentrations were elevated.

The use of fed dogs was important for the response, and the use of two injections with an hour's interval mimicking the clinical situation is necessary for inducing the prolonged hyperdynamic and hypermetabolic situation. Although all responses observed in the model are not identical to those seen in humans with sepsis, the general alterations in metabolic profile and hormonal milieu share great similarities. Results of protein metabolic studies in this model are awaited with great interest.

When interpreting results from studies with administration of one strain of bacteria, it is important to remember that in most septic patients several organisms are involved at the same time. The simultaneous metabolic and hormonal effects on the host of several organisms and especially anaerobes are not yet clearly defined.

Implantation of Fecal Material, Bacteria, or Infected Foreign Material

In order to mimic the clinical situation with polymicrobial septicemia of intraabdominal origin, administration of feces or different strains of bacteria has been tried. Intraperitoneal implantation of pooled fecal inoculum in rats resulted in few deaths within the first 24 h but became progressively lethal with 76% of the animals dying by 5 days postinfection [21]. Most animals had positive polymicrobial cultures from blood and peritoneal fluid throughout the experiment. The animals had a hyper-dynamic circulatory state, increased colonic temperature, and an elevated metabolic rate (table I). They were anorectic and lost weight. They exhibited low glucose and alanine and increased lactate levels. In this study fluid resuscitation was not included. The septic rats showed hemodynamic and metabolic alterations which are similar to those seen in humans with peritonitis and severe sepsis. There is, however, a difference with the low glucose and alanine levels, but the reasons for this are not clear.

The disadvantage of administration of feces is the induction of an uncontrolled situation in which both the dose and the strain of bacteria are hard to quantify. The reproducibility of the model remains to be shown. In addition many animal species are resistant to their own fecal material.

This model has been refined by quantitation of the most prevalent bacteria in rat feces and, thereafter, gelatine capsules have been prepared with precisely measured amounts of E.coli, Bacteroides fragilis, and other common organisms together with barium sulphate as adjuvant agent [22]. With this model, there is initially acute peritonitis, E.coli bacteremia, and in surviving animals development of intraabdominal abscesses with anaerobes. In a further modification with the addition of sterile rats feces, we have had a predictable mortality of 55% within 72 h [23]. The animals were anorectic and lost body weight during the first 5 days. Another modification of the same model with similar strains of bacteria included nutrient broth in the gelatine capsule, which was also wrapped with cellulose [24]. Gentamicin was administered for the first 24 h and then the animals were heavily resuscitated with fluids. This resulted in a more attenuated course with a 50% mortality within a week. The rats had respiratory alkalosis, hyperglycemia, and high lactate levels.

By repeated implantation of capsules with a reduced number of bacteria for 4 weeks, intermittent periods of sepsis was induced in rats [25]. The animals were lethargic, their food and water intake was low, and body weight decreased. The total white blood cell count (WBC) increased progressively. This model permits studies of the long-term effects of episodic septicemia on metabolism and organ failure. The influence of intraabdominal operations must be considered, however.

Another approach used to create sepsis is to infect fractures or implant infected material into the hind limb of an animal. By bandaging fractured femur with cotton gauze which had previously been cultured with cecal contents, it was possible to induce sepsis in rats for 24–72 h [26]. The animals exhibited hyperglycemia, low ketone body levels, and elevated urinary nitrogen excretion. By placing umbilical tape contaminated with an animal's own enteric flora subcutaneously and intramuscularly in one hind limb, a septic state was created in dogs for 48–96 h and thereafter, complete recovery [27]. These animals showed a hyperdynamic circulation, elevated rectal temperature, and a respiratory alkalosis. There was an increased oxygen consumption and high blood lactate levels.

Injection of 5% calcium chloride with E.coli and Enterobacter aerogenes in one hind limb of dogs resulted in a hyperdynamic circulatory state for 24–96 h with elevated body temperature, respiratory alkalosis, and increased oxygen consumption [28]. The model was progressively lethal within 3–9 days.

These models of sepsis from an infected extremity seem to mimic human sepsis in several ways. They are especially useful for the study of regional metabolic differences and of the contribution from the septic focus to the host reaction. All the models of implantation in the peritoneal cavity or an extremity are well suited for metabolic studies. With adequate fluid resuscitation, a stable hyperdynamic phase is observed. Several metabolic alterations are common to human sepsis, e.g., increased metabolic rate, decreased ketogenesis, and protein catabolism. The models are probably not as easily reproducible as the models of parenteral administration of bacteria, but appear reasonably standardized.

Ischemic Organ and Bowel Perforation Models

The surgical devascularization of a segment of intestine and perforation creates strangulation and constant contamination of the abdominal cavity. This approach has been most widely used in cecal ligation models in rats, where the cecum is ligated below the ileocecal valve so that intestinal continuity is maintained [1]. The best results have been obtained if fasted animals are used and the ligated cecum is perforated once or twice to violate the integrity of the bowel. This is a simple and inexpensive technique.

During the first 10–16 h the animals appear mildly ill associated with a hyperdynamic circulation, if the animals are well hydrated. At this time blood cultures are positive. Between 16 and 24 h the animals are progressively hypodynamic. The progression of sepsis and mortality rate varies with the length of fasting prior to surgery and the number of cecal perforations. Mortality at 24 h ranges from 46 to 75%.

The metabolic alterations following this insult have been rather well characterized (table I). The rats are hyperglycemic in the early phase and have high insulin levels [29]. Comparing lipoprotein lipase levels and triglyceride levels in E.coli bacteremic rats and ligated rats, it was found that there was no hypertriglyceridemia and reduced lipoprotein lipase levels in rats after cecal ligation [10]. Perhaps trauma associated with peritonitis or the symbiotic relationship among microorganisms in these infections may partly explain the differences. It was also found that there was a decreased release of FFA from adipose tissue contrary to findings in humans [30]. This finding was, however, made in cecal ligation without perforation and without any blood culture examinations. The gluconeogenic capacity of the liver was depressed in one experiment with this model, which is not consistent with findings in humans, where gluconeogenesis often is increased [31]. This is also in contrast to findings in pigs [32]. After cecal ligation the animals exhibit protein catabolism with a significant amino acid release from muscle tissue (except BCAA) and increased hepatic uptake [33] as well as plasma amino acid changes similar to findings in humans (elevated phenylalanine and tyrosine; decreased BCAA-levels) [34].

This model shares many common metabolic features with human sepsis. It is, however, less reproducible than other models. The reaction is dependent on the length of the fasted state of the animal and bacterial content of the intestine at the time of perforation. The duration of sepsis too short. A certain mortality will also be due to the anesthesia and trauma of the operation. The contribution of the operative trauma to the metabolic changes is also not clear.

References

1 Wichterman, K. A.; Baue, A. E.; Chaudry, I. H.: Sepsis and septic shock – A review of laboratory models and a proposal. J. surg. Res. *29:* 189–201 (1980).

2 Wilmore, D. W.: Alterations in protein, carbohydrate, and fat metabolism in injured and septic patients. J. Am. Coll. Nutr. *2:* 3–13 (1983).

3 Siegel, J. H.; Cerra, F. B.; Coleman, B.; Giovanni, I.; Shetye, M.; Border, J. R.; McMenamy, R. H.: Physiological and metabolic correlations in human sepsis. Surgery *86:* 163–193 (1979).

4 Dodds, W. J.: The pig model for biomedical research. Fed. Proc. *41:* 247–255 (1982).

5 Andersson, O. K.; Lundgren, T.-I.; Revhaug, A.; Østerud, B.; Giercksky, K.-E.: Controlled endotoxinemia in pigs. A suitable model for in vivo studies of some haemodynamic, humoral and cellular reactions. Acta chir. scand. *150:* 599–606 (1984).

6 Waisbren, B. A.: Gram-negative shock and endotoxin shock. Am. J. Med. *36:* 819–824 (1964).

7 Postel, J.; Schloerb, P. R.; Furtado, D.: Pathophysiologic alterations during bacterial infusions for the study of bacteremic shock. Surgery *141:* 683–692 (1975).

8 O'Donnell, T. F.; Clowes Jr., G. H. A.; Ryan, N. T.; Blackburn, G. L.; Weisser, A.: Experimental endotoxinemia: Does it simulate metabolism in septic shock? Surg. Forum *26:* 25–26 (1975).

9 Groves, A. C.; Woolf, L. I.; Duff, J. H.; Finley, R. J.: Metabolism of branched-chain amino acids in dogs with Escherichia coli endotoxin shock. Surgery *93:* 273–278 (1983).

10 Scholl, R. A.; Lang, C. H.; Bagby, G. J.: Hypertriglyceridemia and its relation to tissue lipoprotein lipase activity in endotoxemic, Escherichia coli bacteremic, and polymicrobial septic rats. J. surg. Res. *37:* 394–401 (1984).

11 Pass, L. J.; Schloerb, P. R.; Pearce, F. J.; Drucker, W. R.: Cardiopulmonary response of the rat to gram-negative bacteremia. Am. J. Physiol. H*246:* 344–350 (1984).

12 Wolfe, R. R.; Burke, J. F.: Glucose and lactate metabolism in experimental septic shock. Am. J. Physiol. R*235:* 219–227 (1978).

13 Woolf, L. I.; Groves, A. C.; Duff, J. H.: Amino acid metabolism in dogs with E.coli bacteremic shock. Surgery *85:* 212–218 (1979).

14 Hinshaw, L. B.; Benjamin, B.; Holmes, D. D.; Beller, B.; Archer, L. T.; Coalson, J. J.; Whitsett, T.: Responses of the baboon to live Escherichia coli organisms and endotoxin. Surgery *145:* 1–11 (1977).

15 Postel, J.; Schloerb, P. R.: Metabolic effects of experimentel bacteremia. Ann. Surg. *185:* 475–480 (1977).

16 Steinberg, S. M.; Dehring, D. J.; Gower, W.-R.; Vento, J. M.; Lowery, B. D.; Cloutier, C. T.: Prostacyclin in experimental septic acute respiratory failure. J. surg. Res. *34:* 298–302 (1983).

17 Martinell, S.; Falk, A.; Haglund, U.; Myrvold, H.: Peritonitis and septic shock – An evaluation of two experimental models in the rat. Eur. surg. Res. *17:* 160–166 (1985).

18 Decker, G. A. G.; Daniel, A. M.; Blevings, S.; Maclean, L. D.: Effect of peritonitis on mitochondrial respiration. J. surg. Res. *11:* 528–532 (1971).

19 Browne, M. K.; Leslie, G. B.: Animal models of peritonitis. Surgery Gynec. Obstet. *143:* 738–740 (1976).

20 Shaw, J. H. F.; Wolfe, R. R.: A conscious septic dog model with hemodynamic and metabolic responses similar to responses of humans. Surgery *95:* 553–561 (1984).

21 Lang, C. H.; Bagby, G. J.; Bornside, G. H.; Vial, L. J.; Spitzer, J. J.: Sustained hypermetabolic sepsis in rats: Characterization of the model. J. surg. Res. *35:* 201–210 (1983).

22 Bartlett, J. G.; Onderdonk, A. B.; Louie, T.; Kasper, D. L.; Gorbach, S. L.: Lessons from an animal model of intraabdominal sepsis. Archs Surg. *113:* 853–857 (1978).

23 Hansson, L.; Alwmark, A.; Christensen, P.; Jeppsson, B.; Holst, E.; Bengmark, S.: Standardized intraabdominal abscess formation with generalized sepsis: Pathophysiology in the rat. Eur. surg. Res. *17:* 155–159 (1985).

24 Tranberg, K.-G.; Bjornson, H. S.; Fischer, J. E.: A model of sustained hyperdynamic intraabdominal sepsis in the rat (submitted for publication).

25 Kirton, O. C.; Jones, R.; Zapol, W. M.; Reid, L.: The development of a model of subacute lung injury after intraabdominal infection. Surgery *96:* 384–392 (1984).

26 Blackburn, G. L.; Moldawer, L. L.; Usui, S.; Bothe, A., Jr.; O'Keefe, S. J. D.; Bistrian, B. R.: Branched chain amino acid administration and metabolism during starvation, injury and infection. Surgery *86:* 307–315 (1979).

27 Hermreck, A. S.; Thal, A. P.: Mechanisms for the high circulatory requirements in sepsis and septic schock. Am. Surg. *170:* 677–695 (1969).

28 Yuan, X.; Wu, Z.; He, L.; Cai, Z.: Natural course of septic shock in a canine model. Cardiorespiratory and metabolic parameters. Chin. med. J. *97:* 197–204 (1984).

29 Wichterman, K. A.; Chaudry, I. H.; Baue, A. E.: Studies on peripheral glucose uptake during sepsis. Arch. Surg. *114:* 740–745 (1979).

30 Ryan, N. T.; Blackburn, G. L.; Clowes, G. H. A., Jr.: Differential tissue sensitivity to elevated endogenous insulin levels during experimental peritonitis in rats. Metabolism *23:* 1081–1089 (1974).

31 Clemens, M. G.; Chaudry, I. H.; McDermott, P. H.; Baue, A. E.: Regulation of glucose production from lactate in experimental sepsis. Am. J. Physiol. R *244:* 794–800 (1983).

32 Imamura, M.; Clowes, G. H. A., Jr.; Blackburn, G. L.: Liver metabolism and gluconeogenesis in trauma and sepsis. Surgery *77:* 868–880 (1975).

33 Lindberg, B. O.; Clowes, G. H. A., Jr.: The effects of hyperalimentation and infused leucine on the amino acid metabolism in sepsis: An experimental study in vivo. Surgery *90:* 278–290 (1981).

34 Jeppsson, B.; Freund, H. R.; Gimmon, Z.; James, J. H.; von Meyenfeldt, M. F.; Fischer, J. E.: Blood-brain barrier derangement in sepsis: Cause of septic encephalopathy? Am. J. Surg. *141:* 136–142 (1981).

Bengt Jeppsson, MD, Dept. of Surgery, University of Lund, S-221 85 Lund (Sweden)

Dietze, Grünert, Kleinberger, Wolfram (eds.), Clinical Nutrition and Metabolic Research. Proc. 7th Congr. ESPEN, Munich 1985, pp. 385–400 (Karger, Basel 1986)

Tumor-Bearing Animals as Models of Nutrition Research

M. H. Torosian, J. M. Daly

Dept. of Surgery, Memorial Sloan-Kettering Cancer Center, Cornell University Medical School, New York, USA

Animal/Tumor Models: Effects of Nutrition on Tumorigenesis and Growth

The relationship between cancer, dietary intake, and the nutritional status of the tumor-bearing host is complex. Well-controlled animal-tumor systems have been used to investigate this intricate relationship. Nutritional alterations significantly influence spontaneous tumor development, growth of previously established tumors, and biochemical, immunologic, and metabolic processes of the tumor-bearing host [1–5]. Tumor response and host toxicity to anti-neoplastic therapy are, in part, dependent on the nutritional status of the host which may be altered by changes in dietary therapy [6–10].

Tumorigenesis and Tumor Establishment

Numerous studies have shown that protein-calorie deprivation results in a reduced incidence of spontaneous tumorigenesis and a decreased rate of establishment of transplanted tumors [1, 4, 11, 12]. Tannenbaum and Silverstone in 1953 reported that protein and calorie restriction significantly inhibited spontaneous tumorigenesis in many tumor systems in the mouse and rat [1]. Refeeding significantly stimulated both spontaneous tumorigenesis and tumor development in transplantable tumor models. In 1950 Green et al. documented delayed establishment of transplanted

Walker-256 carcinosarcoma in protein-depleted rats [13]. In 1971 Ross et al. demonstrated a reduced incidence of spontaneous benign and malignant tumors with underfeeding in COBS rats [14]. In this study, a pattern of tumorigenesis was established early in life and remained stable with subsequent nutritional changes.

Carcinogen-induced tumors are also influenced by nutrient provision. White in 1961 reported that protein-calorie deprivation significantly reduced the incidence of numerous carcinogen-induced malignancies in rats and mice [15]. In 1973, Moore et al. confirmed this finding in DMBA-induced breast tumors in Sprague-Dawley rats [16]. Thus, protein-calorie deprivation in animal/tumor systems is associated with a decreased incidence of spontaneous and carcinogen-induced tumors and inhibition of tumor establishment with transplantable tumors.

Tumor Growth

Once tumor establishment occurs, subsequent tumor growth is significantly influenced by nutrition as shown in figure 6. Tumor volume, tumor weight, cellular mitotic activity, DNA, RNA and protein synthesis, and cell cycle changes have been used as parameters of tumor growth. Several investigators have documented accelerated tumor growth in rat and mouse models with ad libitum oral feeding of protein and carbohydrate diets [17, 18]. In 1978, Daly et al. demonstrated significant stimulation of the Walker-256 carcinosarcoma in Sprague-Dawley rats within 48 h of initiating oral nutritional repletion in previously malnourished animals [17]. A similar rate of increase in tumor volume was demonstrated in the Morris hepatoma of orally repleted Buffalo rats [3]. Stimulation of tumor growth was not selective, however, as evidenced by a constant tumor weight to host weight ratio in nutritionally depleted and repleted animals. Starvation, combined reduction of protein and calories, and oral feeding of protein-free diets have resulted in decreased tumor growth in several tumor systems including the Walker-256 carcinosarcoma, mammary adenocarcinoma, and rat sarcoma [12, 19, 20].

Accelerated tumor growth has been noted with provision of parenteral nutrition. In 1975, Steiger et al. demonstrated increased growth of the AC-33 mammary adenocarcinoma in Lewis/Wistar rats with total parenteral nutrition (TPN) [6]. Parenteral amino acids with or without hypertonic dextrose were responsible for tumor stimulation in this system.

Although no change in tumor weight to host body weight ratio was observed, stimulation of tumor protein synthesis and a significant increase in the percentage of tumor cells synthesizing DNA occurred with the provision of TPN [10]. In 1976, Cameron and Pavlat demonstrated increased growth and a higher index of mitotic activity in the Morris hepatoma of Buffalo rats receiving intravenous nutrition [21]. In 1981, Cameron observed increased H^3-thymidine uptake in tumor cells of animals receiving TPN [22]. In their study preferential growth of the Morris hepatoma occurred with parenteral nutrition as evidenced by a significant increase in the tumor weight to host body weight ratio. In 1983, Popp et al. reported similar results in methylcolanthene-induced sarcomas in Fischer-344 rats [23]. Tumor growth occurred to a greater extent than growth of the host lean body mass with excessive TPN administration. A direct correlation was observed between tumor weight and the rate of nutrient substrate infusion in this study.

Isolated studies have reported no significant stimulation of tumor growth with parenteral nutrition. In 1982, Kishi concluded that 7 days of TPN did not accelerate growth of the Walker-256 carcinosarcoma in Wistar rats [24]. However, a greater than two-fold increase in tumor weight occurred in animals receiving TPN compared to animals given D5W in their study. Although a level of statistical significance ($p < 0.05$) was not achieved, a small number of animals were studied and a definite trend toward increased tumor growth occurred in animals given TPN. In 1985, King et al. studied changes in tumor weight, protein content, and H^3-thymidine incorporation into DNA in Morris hepatoma transplanted into ACI-N rats [25]. It was concluded that TPN with or without fat did not increase tumor weight, protein content, or H^3-thymidine uptake in comparison to oral feeding. However, protein intake was 25% greater in animals receiving oral diets. Relative to fasting animals and groups of rats receiving oral nutrition, TPN with glucose and TPN with fat demonstrated a significant increase in tumor weight. Thus, the majority of experimental evidence demonstrates that nutritional repletion of malnourished rats and excessive nutrient administration stimulates growth of animal tumors.

In an attempt to selectively retard tumor growth, several investigators have induced specific dietary deficiencies in tumor-bearing animals. In 1959, Munro measured the RNA content in hepatoma and host liver in rats fed a 25% protein diet and compared it to animals fed an isocaloric, protein-free diet [18]. Although no change occurred in RNA content of tumor tissue, a decrease in RNA content of host liver was observed in rats ingesting the protein-free diet. In 1977, Ota et al. measured protein content and found similar results in Buffalo rats with Morris hepatomas [2]. In animals given protein-free diets, tumor protein content remained unchanged while liver protein content decreased. In 1980, Daly et al. similarly demonstrated no change in protein content of Walker-256 carcinosarcoma in Sprague-Dawley rats given protein-free diets as shown in figure 1 [19]. Apparently the tumor was able to effectively incorporate protein at the expense of host tissue during periods of dietary protein restriction. In 1977, Reilly et al. demonstrated decreased growth of MCA-induced sarcomas in rats during starvation; however, DNA-specific activity increased in the tumor and decreased in host liver [20]. These studies confirmed the concept of the tumor as a 'nitrogen trap' and documented that tumors are successful competitors with host tissues for nutrient substrates during periods of limited dietary supply.

Deficiencies of selective amino acids have resulted in continued tumor growth and host nutritional depletion [26, 27]. Studies performed in rats, mice, and hamsters with essential amino acid deprivation demonstrate minimal tumor inhibition [26–29]. In fact, accelerated tumor

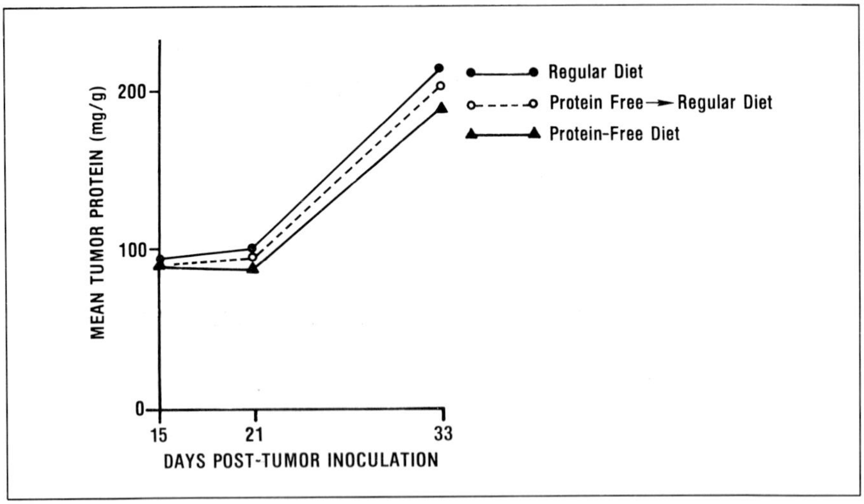

Fig. 1. In Sprague-Dawley rats bearing Walker-256 carcinosarcoma, mean tumor protein concentration (mg/g) remained similar in three groups of animals. One group received a regular diet ad lib, a second group received a protein-free diet ad lib, and a third group was switched from a protein-free diet to a regular diet 15 days after tumor implantation. This demonstrates that the tumor acts as a 'nitrogen trap'.

growth has been observed with moderate leucine restriction in adenocarcinoma-bearing mice and with exclusive administration of branched-chain amino acids in AC-33 adenocarcinoma of rats [29, 30].

Two studies have documented selective tumor inhibition with diets deficient in specific amino acids. In 1973, Jose and Good fed tumor-bearing mice casein-restricted diets to reduce plasma levels of cysteine, methionine, and tryptophan [31]. A reduction in the tumor weight to host body weight ratio occurred and was associated with a reduction in serum blocking antibody. The authors hypothesized that tumor inhibition in mice given casein-restricted diets occurred by decreasing titers of serum blocking antibody without altering cell-mediated immunity. In 1971, Theurer demonstrated preferential reduction in the growth rate of BW20232 adenocarcinoma of C57BL mice fed diets deficient in phenylalanine, valine, or isoleucine [29]. A proportional reduction in tumor and host weight occurred using oral diets deficient in tryptophan, threonine, leucine, or methionine.

Selective starvation of tumor cells with maintenance of normal host cells have been attempted by inducing specific deficiencies of micronutrients, including vitamins, trace metals, and electrolytes. In a rat model, folate deficiency impaired growth of the Walker-256 carcinosarcoma but did not alter growth of the Murphy-Strum lymphosarcoma [32]. Regardless of its effects on tumor growth, prolonged folate deprivation causes significant toxicity [32, 33]. Pantothenic acid deficiency caused fibrosarcoma growth retardation in rats; however, host growth was impaired to a similar degree [34]. Decreased riboflavin availability has been induced by administering riboflavin analogs such as lyxoflavin and galactoflavin [35]. Tumor regression occurred after administration of these riboflavin analogs; however, host effects were not documented [36]. Pyridoxine-deficient diets and pyridoxine inhibitors have independently been shown to cause tumor regression in several rat and mouse models [37–39]. Vitamin A and its derivatives are effective inhibitors of chemical carcinogenesis in multiple epithelial systems including mammary gland and urinary bladder [40–42]. Animals fed diets deficient in retinoids (vitamin A and its natural and synthetic analogs) develop an increased number of malignancies following exposure to chemical carcinogens [43, 44]. The effect of vitamin C on cancer development is controversial, but, several studies indicate that vitamin C decreases the incidence of squamous cell carcinoma in mice exposed to ultraviolet radiation [45, 46]. Vitamin K antagonists or dietary deficiency of vitamin K significantly reduced the number of spontaneous metastases in mice with Lewis lung carcinoma [47].

Trace metal deficiencies, particularly zinc and magnesium, influence tumor growth under experimental conditions. DeWys and Pories in 1972 demonstrated significant reduction of tumor establishment in zinc-deficient animals transplanted with either Walker-256 sarcoma or Lewis lung carcinoma [48]. The duration of survival of zinc-deficient animals was significantly greater than the length of survival in pair-fed, control animals. Zinc deficient animals with L1210 leukemia similarly demonstrated increased duration of survival compared to control animals [48]. The toxicity of prolonged zinc deficiency, however, precludes dietary deprivation of this trace metal for extended periods. Young and Parsons reported 40% reduction in growth of the Yoshida hepatoma and Walker sarcoma in magnesium-deficient rats [49]. Similar results were observed by Mills et al. in 1983 in transplanted mammary adenocarcinoma in rats [50].

Potassium deficiency has been shown to effectively inhibit tumor growth in tumor-bearing animals. Isolated potassium deficiency decreased growth of the Yoshida hepatoma and Walker-256 carcinosarcoma in rats by 30–60% [49]. With combined deficiencies of potassium and magnesium, tumor growth was reduced by 45–85% [49]. Ryan et al. demonstrated similar growth inhibition of ascitic tumor cells in vivo with potassium depletion [51].

Effects of Nutrient Intake and Presence of a Tumor in the Host

Nutrient intake significantly influences body weight, body composition, nitrogen balance, rates of tissue protein synthesis, visceral protein levels, and immunocompetence in the tumor-bearing host [3, 52–54]. These nutritional, metabolic, and immunologic changes have been well documented with oral and parenteral nutrition in a variety of animal tumor systems (figs. 2–5). The controversy which remains is whether nutritional support preferentially benefits the host or tumor.

Host Nutritional Status and Substrate Metabolism

In 1975, Steiger et al. analyzed body weight, liver weight, and serum albumin levels in adenocarcinoma-bearing rats after 10 days of parenteral nutrition [6]. Tumor-bearing animals given parenteral amino acids alone, hypercaloric glucose alone, or hypocaloric glucose exhibited nitrogen wasting with markedly negative nitrogen balances. In 1977, Oram-Smith et al. measured nitrogen balance in this same experimental system and demonstrated nitrogen equilibrium in animals receiving TPN [55]. In

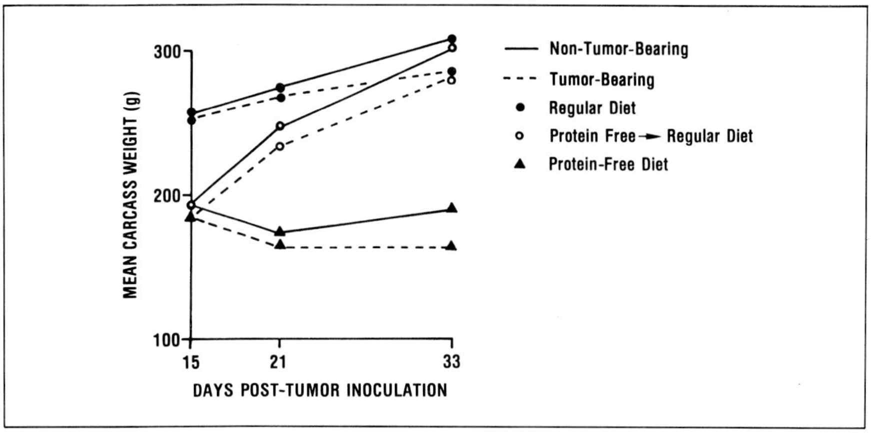

Fig. 2. Changes in mean carcass weight over time and with dietary manipulation in tumor-bearing rats paralleled those in non-tumor-bearing rats.

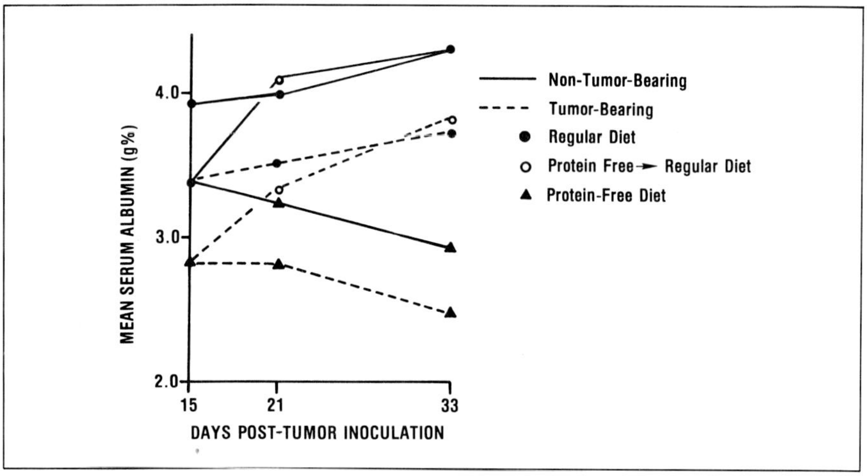

Fig. 3. Mean serum albumin levels were consistently lower in tumor-bearing rats compared with non-tumor-bearing rats in all three dietary groups.

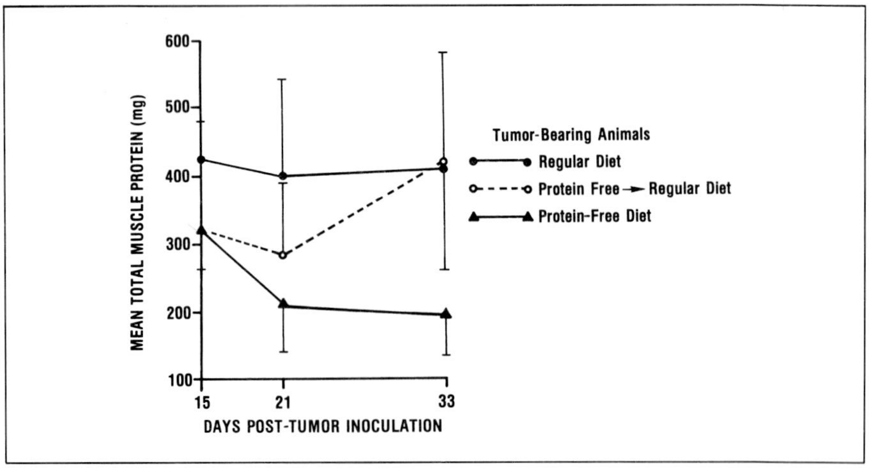

Fig. 4. Mean total muscle protein decreased significantly in tumor-bearing rats maintained on a protein-free diet compared with other dietary groups.

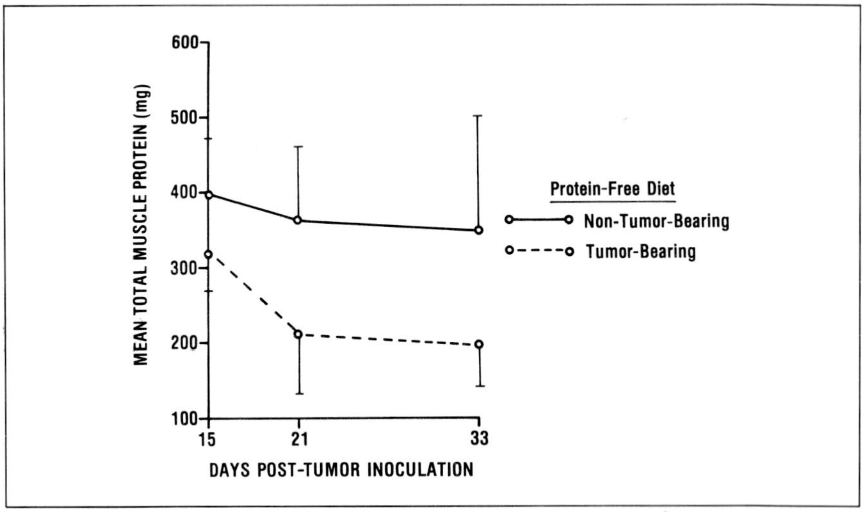

Fig. 5. Mean total muscle protein continues to decrease in tumor-bearing rats until very low levels were reached at day 21. In contrast non-tumor-bearing animals were able to adapt to a protein-free diet by maintaining their mean total muscle protein.

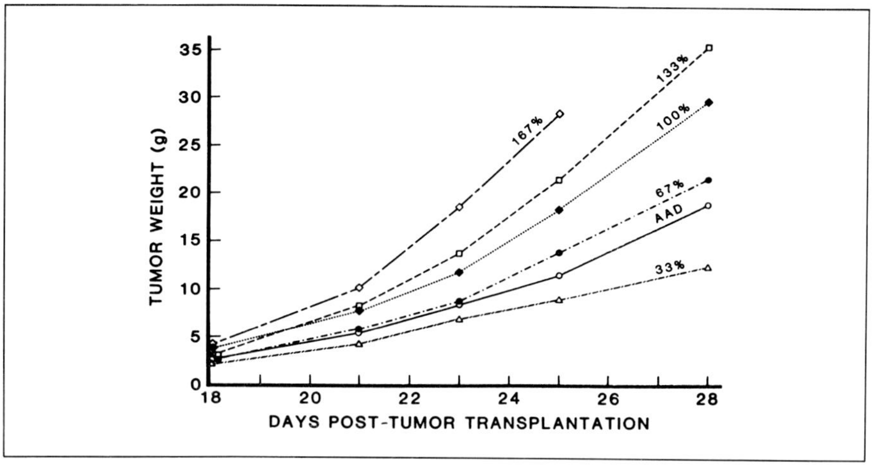

Fig. 6. Mean tumor weight increased maximally in rats who were overfed (167% and 133%), resulting in early deaths. Reduction in caloric intake (33%) retarded tumor growth [69].

1980, Buzby et al. demonstrated significant host weight gain and positive nitrogen balance over a 4-day period in animals given adequate amino acids and calories [53]. Fat-based TPN was slightly more effective that carbohydrate-base TPN in promoting weight gain in this study.

Daly et al. and Ota et al. demonstrated that increased body weight of hepatoma-bearing Buffalo rats occurred with either oral or parenteral nutrition [2, 3]. Provision of an isocaloric protein-free diet resulted in continued weight loss. Daly et al. subsequently demonstrated that oral protein repletion of malnourished Sprague-Dawley rats with Walker-256 carcinosarcoma accelerated both tumor and host growth within 48 h [17]. In animals with small tumor burdens (less than 5% carcass weight), oral nutritional repletion resulted in a return to normal of serum albumin concentration, liver and muscle protein content, and carcass weight within 6 days of initiating nutritional repletion. In malnourished animals with large tumors (greater than 25% carcass weight), serum albumin concentration returned to normal, but liver and muscle protein content and carcass weight remained significantly lower after oral repletion compared to well nourished tumor-bearing animals [3, 19].

In 1977, Cameron et al. demonstrated that TPN could prevent weight loss characteristically seen in hepatoma-bearing rats given ad libitum oral feeding [56]. However, no significant change in duration of survival was observed in animals receiving TPN and, in fact, tumor growth was stimulated out of proportion to increases in host weight gain. In 1983, Popp et al. found similar results in sarcoma-bearing Fischer 344 rats given TPN [23]. Although carcass weight increased with TPN administration, mean tumor weight increased to a greater extent than lean carcass weight with increased levels of substrate infusion.

Immunocompetence

Both humoral and cellular immunity are depressed in animals with severe protein restriction [52, 57–60]. Law et al. in 1974 demonstrated decreased titers of antibodies, decreased number of IGM-producing cells, decreased in vitro lymphocyte response to mitogens, and decreased delayed hypersensitivity in Sprague-Dawley rats after 6 weeks of protein-free nutrition [61]. Protein repletion 48 h before antigen stimulation was necessary for full expression of the immune response. Initiating protein repletion 48 h after sensitization resulted in a subnormal immunologic response.

In 1978, Daly et al. demonstrated that only 30% of Buffalo rats bearing Morris hepatoma demonstrated a positive delayed hypersensitivity response to intradermal PPD after 2 weeks on an oral protein-free diet [62]. Protein repletion with 7 days of TPN or oral ad libitum feeding restored PPD-immunocompetence to 91% and 78% of animals, respectively. Only 17% of animals remaining on protein-free diets for the 7-day period demonstrated PPD skin test reactivity. Body weight significantly increased in animals receiving protein repletion; continued loss of weight occurred in animals given the protein-free diet. Thus, restoration of immunocompetence and body weight was observed in malnourished tumor-bearing animals receiving adequate protein and calories.

Chemotherapy-Related Toxicity

Few well-controlled animal studies have been performed to objectively determine the influence of nutritional status on host toxicity from chemotherapy. In 1975, Steiger et al. administered 5-fluorouracil to Lewis-Wistar rats receiving either TPN or parenteral 5% dextrose [6]. In animals receiving TPN, positive nitrogen balance and significant weight gain occurred despite chemotherapy administration. In 5-fluorouracil-treated animals given 5% dextrose, nitrogen balance was negative and weight loss occurred. However, TPN did not prevent the myelosuppressive activity of the 5-fluorouracil as both groups of animals demonstrated an identical degree of peripheral leukopenia [6]. In 1975, Souchen et al. demonstrated a lower incidence of gastrointestinal toxicity to 5-fluorouracil and a two-fold increase in mean survival rate in animals receiving TPN compared with rats receiving an oral diet [63].

In 1982, Torosian et al. demonstrated a significant reduction in methotrexate toxicity with improved nutritional status in Lewis-Wistar rats with AC-33 adenocarcinoma [8]. Clinical signs of toxicity including hair loss, lethargy, and diarrhea, and leukopenia were reduced in well-nourished animals compared to protein-depleted animals. At high doses of methotrexate (20 mg/kg), 100% mortality occurred in malnourished animals versus no mortality in the well-nourished group. In 1984, Mihranian et al. documented decreased plasma clearance and increased serum levels of methotrexate in malnourished animals accounting for increased drug toxicity [9]. Grossi et al. suggested that increased methotrexate toxicity in malnourished rats was related to reduced liver and bone marrow levels of dihydrofolate reductase, the major enzyme inhibited by methotrexate [64].

Tumor Response to Chemotherapy

Although stimulation of tumor growth by nutrient administration has been generally regarded as detrimental to the host, recent reports have demonstrated that these changes in tumor metabolism may be exploited to therapeutic advantage. In 1981, Daly et al. reported improved tumor response to chemotherapy in rats provided with continuous parenteral or intra-jejunal feeding [7]. It was postulated that continuous substrate administration stimulated tumor cell proliferation and significantly improved tumor response to chemotherapy. Reynolds et al. demonstrated similar results with oral nutritional repletion of Sprague-Dawley rats with Walker-256 carcinosarcoma treated with methotrexate [65]. In 1983, Torosian et al. demonstrated improved tumor response to chemotherapy in AC-33-bearing Lewis-Wistar rats receiving 48 h of parenteral nutrition [10]. After only 2 h of TPN, a significant increase in the percentage of S-phase tumor cells, or DNA-synthesizing cells, was demonstrated [66]. Improved anti-neoplastic activity was observed with cycle-specific agents (methotrexate, adriamycin) but not with cycle-nonspecific chemotherapy (cytoxan) [67]. This phenomenon occurred independent of host nutritional status and was primarily due to the amino acid moiety in TPN [10]. Selective potentiation of tumor cytotoxicity appeared to occur as no increase in host toxicity was demonstrated [10, 68].

References

1 Tennenbaum, A.; Silverstone, H.: Nutrition in relation to cancer. Adv. Cancer Res. *1:* 451–501 (1953).

2 Ota, D. M.; Copeland, E. M.; Strobel, H. W.; Daly, J.; Gus, E. T.; Guinn, E.; Dudrick, S. J.: The effect of protein nutrition on host and tumor metabolism. J. surg. Res. *22:* 181–188 (1977).

3 Daly, J. M.; Copeland, E. M.; Dudrick, S. J.: Effect of intravenous nutrition on tumor growth and host immunocompetence in malnourished animals. Surgery *84:* 655–658 (1978).

4 Begg, R. W.; Dickinson, T. E.: Systemic effects of tumors in force-fed rats. Cancer Res. *11:* 409–412 (1951).

5 Ross, M. H.; Bras, G.: Influence of protein under- and overnutrition on spontaneous tumor prevalence in the rat. J. Nutr. *103:* 963–944 (1977).

6 Steiger, E.; Oram-Smith, J.; Miller, E.; Kuo, L.; Vars, H. M.: Effects of nutrition on tumor growth and tolerance to chemotherapy. J. surg. Res. *18:* 455–461 (1975).

7 Daly, J. M.; Reynolds, H. M.; Copeland, E. M.; Dudrick, S. J.: Effects of enteral and parenteral nutrition on tumor response to chemotherapy in experimental animals. J. surg. Oncol. *16:* 79–96 (1981).

8 Torosian, M. H.; Buzby, G. P.; Presti, M. E.; Stein, T. P.; Zinnsen, K.; Mullen, J. L.: Reduction of methotrexate toxicity with improved nutritional status. Surg. Forum *33:* 109–112 (1982).

9 Mihranian, M. H.; Wang, Y. M.; Daly, J. M.: Effects of nutritional depletion and repletion on plasma methotrexate pharmacokinetics. Cancer *54:* 2268–2271 (1984).

10 Torosion, M. H.; Mullen, J. L.; Miller, E. E.; Zinnsen, K. R.; Stein, T. P.; Buzby, G. P.: Enhanced tumor response to cycle-specific chemotherapy by parenteral amino acid administration. J. parent. ent. Nutr. *7:* 337–345 (1983).

11 Sugiura, K.; Benedict, S. R.: The influence of diets upon tumor recurrence and growth in rats and mice. J. Cancer Res. *10:* 309–318 (1926).

12 White, F. R.; Belkin, M.: Source of tumor proteins; Effect of a low-nitrogen diet on the establishment and growth of a transplanted tumor. J. natn. Cancer Inst. *5:* 261–263 (1944).

13 Green, J. W.; Benditt, E. O.; Humphreys, E. M.: The effect of protein depletion on the host response to transplantable rat tumor Walker 256. Cancer Res. *10:* 769–774 (1950).

14 Ross, M. H.; Bras, G.: Lasting influence of early caloric restriction on prevalence of neoplasms in the rat. J. natn. Cancer Inst. *51:* 1095–1113 (1971).

15 White, F. R.: The relationship between underfeeding and tumor formation, transplantation, and growth in rats and mice. Cancer Res. *21:* 281–290 (1961).

16 Moore, C.; Tittle, P. W.: Muscle activity, body fat, and induced rat mammary tumors. Surgery *73:* 329–332 (1973).

17 Daly, J. M.; Reynolds, H. M.; Rowlands, B. J.; Baquero, G. E.; Dudrick, S. J.; Copeland, E. M.: Nutritional manipulation of tumor-bearing animals: Effects of body weight, serum protein levels, and tumor growth. Surg. Forum *29:* 143–144 (1978).

18 Munro, H. N.; Clark, C. M.: The influence of dietary protein on the metabolism of ribonucleic acid in rat hepatoma. Br. J. Cancer *13:* 324–335 (1959).

19 Daly, J. M.; Copeland, E. M.; Dudrick, S. J.; Delaney, J. M.: Nutritional repletion of malnourished tumor-bearing and nontumor-bearing rats; Effects on body weight, liver, muscle and tumor. J. surg. Res. *28:* 507–518 (1980).

20 Reilly, J. J.; Goodgame, J. T.; Jones, D. C.; Brennan, M. F.: DNA synthesis in rat sarcoma and liver. The effect of starvation. J. surg. Res. *22:* 281–286 (1977).

21 Cameron, J. L.; Pavlat, W. A.: Stimulation of growth of a transplantable hepatoma in rats by parenteral nutrition. J. natn. Cancer Inst. *56:* 597–601 (1976).

22 Cameron, I. L.: Effect of total parenteral nutrition on tumor-host responses in rats. Can. Treat. Rep. *65* (suppl.): 93–99 (1981).

23 Popp, M. B.; Wagner, S. C.; Brito, O. J.: Host and tumor responses to increasing levels of intravenous nutritional support. Surgery *94:* 300–308 (1983).

24 Kishi, T.; Iwasawa, Y.; Hiroshi, I.; Chibata, I.: Nutritional responses of tumor-bearing rats to oral or intravenous feeding. J. parent. ent. Nutr. *6:* 295–300 (1982).

25 King, W. W. K.; Boelhouwer, R. U.; Kingsworth, A. N.; Weening, J. J.; Weber, G.; Young, V. R.; Malt, R. A.: Total parenteral nutrition with and without fat as substrate for growth of rats and transplanted hepatocarcinoma. J. parent. ent. Nutr. *9:* 422–427 (1985).

26 Demopoulous, H. B.; Gerving, M. A.; Bagdoyan, H.: Selective inhibition of growth and respiration of melanomas by tyrosinase inhibitors. J. natn. Cancer Inst. *35:* 823–827 (1965).

27 Jensen, O. A.; Edeberg, J.; Edmund, J.: The effect of a phenylalanine-tyrosine low diet on the growth and morphology of transplantable malignant melanomas of the Syrcair golden hamster. Acta pathol. microbiol. scand. *81:* 559–568 (1973).

28 Sugionura, T.; Birnbaum, S. M.; Winitz, M.; Greenstein, J. P.: Quantitative nutritional studies with water soluble, chemically defined diets. VIII. The forced feeding of diets lacking one essential amino acid. Archs Biochem. Biophys. *81:* 448–455 (1959).

29 Theurer, R. C.: Effect of essential amino-acid restriction on the growth of female C47BL mice and their implanted BW10232 adenocarcinomas. J. Nutr. *101:* 223 (1971).

30 Torosian, M. H.; Stein, T. P.; Presti, M. E.; Leonard, J. M.; Leshiw, M. J.; Steinberg, J. J.; Buzby, G. P.; Mullen, J. L.: Effect of branched-chain amino acids on the host-tumor relationship in parenterally nourished rats. Proceedings Federation of American Societies for Experimental Biology *16:* 5987 (1983).

31 Jose, D. G.; Good, R. A.: Quantitative effects of nutritional essential amino acid deficiency upon immune responses to tumors in mice. J. exp. Med. *137:* 1–9 (1973).

32 Nichol, C. A.: The manipulation of metabolism by drugs and nutrients. Cancer Res. *29:* 2422–2426 (1969).

33 Demetrakopoulos, G. E.; Brennan, M. F.: Tumoricidal potential of nutritional manipulations. Cancer Res., suppl. 42, pp. 7565–7655 (1982).

34 Montanez, G.; Murphy, A. E.; Dunn, M.: Influence of pantothenic acid deficiency on the viability and growth of rat fibrosarcoma. Cancer Res. *11:* 834–838 (1951).

35 Bertino, J. R.; Nixon, P. F.: Nutritional factors in the design of more selective antitumor agents. Cancer Res. *29:* 2417–2421 (1969).

36 Stoerk, M. C.; Emerson, C. A.: Complete regression of lymphosarcoma implants following temporary induction of riboflavin deficiency in mice. Proc. Soc. exp. Biol. Med. *70:* 703–707 (1949).

37 Mihich, E.; Nichol, C. A.: The effect of pyridonine deficiency on mouse sarcoma 180. Cancer Res. *19:* 279–284 (1950).

38 Rosen, F.; Mihich, E.; Nichol, C. A.: Selective metabolic and chemotherapeutic effects of vitamin B_6 antimetabolites. Vitams Horm. *22:* 609–641 (1964).

39 Tryfiates, G. P.; Shuler, J. K.; Hefner, M. L.; Morris, H. P.: Effect of B_6 deficiency on hepatoma 7794 A growth rate: Activities of tyrosine transaminase and serum dehydrates before and after induction of hydrocortisone. Eur. J. Cancer *10:* 147–154 (1974).

40 Moon, R. C.; McCormick, D. L.; Mehta, R. G.: Inhibition of carcinogenesis by retinoids. Cancer Res., suppl. 43, pp. 2469s–2475s (1983).

41 Bollag, W.: Prophylaxis of chemically induced benign and malignant epithelial tumors by vitamin A acid (retinoic acid). Eur. J. Cancer *8:* 689–693 (1972).

42 Moon, R. C.; Grubbs, C. J.; Sporn, M. B.; Goodman, D. G.: Retinyl acetate inhibits mammary carcinogenesis induced by N-methyl-N-nitrosourea. Nature, Lond. *267:* 620–621 (1977).

43 Cohen, S. M.; Wittenberg, J. D.; Bryan, G. T.: Effect of avitaminosis A and hypervitaminosis A on urinary bladder carcinogenicity of N-[-4-(5-nitro-2-furyl)-2-thiazolyl] formamide. Cancer Res. *36:* 2334–2339 (1976).

44 Rogers, A. E.; Herndon, B. J.; Bewberne, P. M.: Induction by dimethylhydrazine of intestinal carcinoma in normal rats and rats fed high and low levels of vitamin A. Cancer Res. *33:* 1003–1009 (1973).

45 Black, H. S.; Chan, J. T.: Suppression of ultraviolet light-induced tumor formation by dietary antioxidants. J. invest. Derm. *65:* 412–414 (1975).

46 Dunham, W. B.; Zuckenkandl, E.; Reynolds, R.; Willoughby, R.; Mareuson, R.; Barth, R.; Pauling, L.: Effects of intake of L-ascorbic acid on the incidence of dermal neoplasms induced in mice by ultraviolet light. Proc. natn. Acad. Sci., USA *79:* 7532–7536 (1982).

47 Hilgard, P.: Experimental vitamin K deficiency and spontaneous metastases. Br. J. Cancer *35:* 891–892 (1977).

48 DeWys, W.; Pories, W.: Inhibition of a spectrum of animal tumors by dietary zinc deficiency. J. natn. Cancer Inst. *48:* 375–381 (1972).

49 Young, G. A.; Parsons, F. M.: The effects of dietary deficiencies of magnesium and potassium on the growth and chemistry of transplanted tumors and host tissues in the rat. Eur. J. Cancer *13:* 103–113 (1977).

50 Mills, B. J.; Higgins, P. J.; Broghamer, W. L.; Linderman, R. D.: Magnesium depletion

inhibits growth of established tumors. Fed. Proc. *42:* 1312 (1983).
51 Ryan, M. P.; Smyth, H.; Hingerty, D.: Effect of magnesium and potassium deficiencies on composition and cell growth in ascites tumor cells in vivo. Life Sci. *8:* 485–489 (1969).
52 Copeland, E. M.; Dudrick, S. J.: Nutritional aspects of cancer; in Hickman, Current problems in cancer, pp. 1–51 (Year Book Medical Publishers, Chicago 1976).
53 Buzby, G. P.; Mullen, J. L.; Stein, T. P.; Miller, E. E.; Hobbs, C. L.; Rosato, E. F.: Host-tumor interaction and nutrient supply. Cancer *45:* 2940–2948 (1980).
54 Mider, G. B.: Some aspects of nitrogen and energy metabolism in cancerous subjects; A review. Cancer Res. *11:* 821–829 (1951).
55 Oram-Smith, J. C.; Stein, T. P.; Wallace, H. W.; Mullen, J. L.: Intravenous nutrition and tumor-host protein metabolism. J. surg. Res. *22:* 499–503 (1977).
56 Cameron, I. L.; Ackley, W. J.; Rogers, W.: Responses of hepatoma-bearing rats to total parenteral hyperalimentation and to ad libitum feeding. J. surg. Res. *23:* 189–195 (1977).
57 Hoffman-Goetz, L.; Blackburn, G. L.: Relationship of nutrition to immunology and cancer; in Newell, Ellison, Nutrition and Cancer; Etiology and Treatment (Raven Press, New York 1981).
58 Ota, D. M.; Copeland, E. M.; Corriere, J. N.; Dudrick, S. J.: The effects of nutrition and treatment of cancer on host immunocompetence. Surg. Gynecol. Obstet. *148:* 104–111 (1979).
59 Serrou, B.; Cupissol, H.: Nutritional Support and the Immune System in Cancer Management. A Critical Review. Cancer Treat. Rep. *65:* 115–120 (1981).
60 Copeland, E. M.; MacFadyen, B. V.; Rapp, M. A.; Dudrick, S. J.: Hyperalimentation and immune competence in cancer. Surg. Forum *26:* 138–140 (1975).
61 Law, D. K.; Dudrick, S. J.; Abdou, N. I.: The effect of dietary protein depletion on immunocompetence. The importance of nutritional repletion prior to immunologic induction. Ann. Surg. *179:* 168–173 (1974).
62 Daly, J. M.; Copeland, E. M.; Dudrick, S. J.: Effects of protein depletion and repletion on cell-mediated immunity in experimental animals. Ann. Surg. *188:* 791–796 (1976).
63 Souchon, E. A.; Copeland, E. M.; Watson, P.; Dudrick, S. J.: Intravenous hyperalimentation as an adjunct to cancer chemotherapy with 5-fluorouracil. J. surg. Res. *18:* 451–454 (1975).
64 Grossie, V. B.; Ho, D. H. W.; Loo, T. L.: Effect of malnutrition on methotrexate toxicity and tissue levels of dihydrofolate reductase in the rat. Cancer Treat. Rep. *66:* 85–89 (1982).
65 Reynolds, H. M.; Daly, J. M.; Rowland, B. J.; Dudrick, S. J.; Copeland, E. M.: Effects of nutritional repletion on host and tumor response to chemotherapy. Cancer *45:* 3069–3074 (1980).
66 Torosian, M. H.; Tsou, K. C.; Daly, J. M.; Mullen, J. L.; Stein, T. P.; Miller, E. E.; Buzby, G. P.: Alteration of tumor cell kinetics by total parenteral nutrition: Potential therapeutic implications. Cancer *53:* 1409–1415 (1984).
67 Torosian, M. H.; Mullen, J. L.; Miller, E. E.; Wagner, K. M.; Stein, T. P.; Buzby, G. P.: Adjuvant, pulse total parenteral nutrition and tumor response to cycle-specific and cycle-non-specific chemotherapy. Surgery *94:* 291–299 (1983).

68 Torosian, M. H.; Mullen, J. L.; Stein, T. P.; Miller, E. E.; Zinnser, K. R.; Buzby, G. P.: Enhanced tumor response to cycle-specific chemotherapy by pulse TPN. J. surg. Res. *39:* 103–113 (1985).
69 Popp, M. et al.: Host and tumor respenses to increasing levels of intravenous nutritional support. Surgery 94: 300–308 (1983).

John M. Daly, M.D., F.A.C.S., Department of Surgery, Memorial Sloan-Kettering Cancer Center, 1275 York Avenue, New York, NY 10021 (USA)